TRANSFORMING THE DEAD

TRANSFORMING THE DEAD

CULTURALLY MODIFIED BONE IN THE PREHISTORIC MIDWEST

Edited by Eve A. Hargrave, Shirley J. Schermer,
Kristin M. Hedman, and Robin M. Lillie

THE UNIVERSITY OF ALABAMA PRESS
Tuscaloosa

The University of Alabama Press
Tuscaloosa, Alabama 35487-0380
uapress.ua.edu

Typeface: Bembo

Manufactured in the United States of America
Cover illustration: Emmons mask; courtesy of Illinois State Museum Collections
Cover design: Erin Bradley Dangar / Dangar Design

∞

The paper on which this book is printed meets the minimum requirements of American National Standard for Information Sciences—Permanence of Paper for Printed Library Materials, ANSI Z39.48-1984.

Library of Congress Cataloging-in-Publication Data

Transforming the dead : culturally modified bone in the prehistoric Midwest / edited by Eve A. Hargrave, Shirley J. Schermer, Kristin M. Hedman, and Robin M. Lillie.
pages cm
Includes bibliographical references and index.
ISBN 978-0-8173-1861-1 (cloth : alkaline paper) — ISBN 978-0-8173-8809-6 (ebook)
1. Woodland culture—Middle West. 2. Bones—Social aspects—Middle West—History—History—To 1500. 3. Human remains (Archaeology)—Middle West. 4. Burial—Middle West—History—To 1500. 5. Military trophies—Middle West—History—To 1500. 6. Indians of North America—Funeral customs and rites—Middle West—History—To 1500. 7. Indians of North America—Warfare—Middle West—History—To 1500. 8. Material culture—Middle West—History—To 1500. 9. Social archaeology—Middle West. 10. Middle West—Antiquities. I. Hargrave, Eve A. II. Schermer, Shirley J., 1946– III. Hedman, Kristin. IV. Lillie, Robin M.
E99.W84T73 2015
977'.01—dc23

2014034449

Contents

Illustrations

Figures

Tables

Acknowledgments

We would like to thank our contributors, who made this volume possible—from their initial interest and enthusiastic participation in the 2008 Midwest Archaeological Conference symposium through their perseverance and patience in the final editing phases.

Our professional colleagues' conversations, insights, suggestions, and support, including the volume's reviews, were a tremendous help throughout this process and are greatly appreciated. A special thank you goes to Thomas E. Emerson at the Illinois State Archaeological Survey (ISAS), Prairie Research Institute, University of Illinois at Urbana-Champaign, and to John Doershuk at the University of Iowa Office of the State Archaeologist for the support they provided throughout this project. A special thank you also goes to Mary Hynes (ISAS) for her amazing patience and dedication during the formatting and technical editing of the final manuscript. We also thank Rose Smith (ISAS) for her skills in pulling together the volume maps.

We also extend our appreciation to the University of Alabama Press and its editors, especially Joseph Powell and Dan Waterman, for their interest in publishing this volume and their assistance in seeing it to completion, and to Merryl Sloane, our copyeditor, for the thoroughness and consistency of her work.

Last, but not least, we are grateful for the wonderful support and encouragement we received from friends and family throughout this long journey.

TRANSFORMING THE
DEAD

1

Transforming the Dead

Shirley J. Schermer, Eve A. Hargrave, Kristin M. Hedman, and Robin M. Lillie

Across the world and through time, interactions between the dead and the living have been integral parts of cultures. The beliefs that souls exist, that attributes of the dead survive physical death, and that the dead have the potential to help or hurt the living—all are among the perceptions of life and death that dictate how the dead are treated and whether the deceased is venerated or desecrated. In *The Illyrians: History and Culture*, Aleksandar Stipčević (1977:231) provides the following vivid description of mourners at tumuli: "over the grave the mourners would eat and drink, believing that contact was thus established between themselves and the departed; they maintained that the dead person never ceased to be their kin, and his relatives would continue to take care of him and help him in trouble."

Connections between the dead and the living can be maintained in any number of ways, one of which is through the removal and curation of human skeletal elements, keeping part of the dead in direct contact with the living. In *Living with the Dead: Mortuary Ritual in Mesoamerica* (2011), Fitzsimmons and Shimada note that across Mesoamerica death was almost never accompanied by the extinction of a persona. The veneration of holy relics, including human bones and objects made from human bones, has a long (and continued) tradition in Christian and Buddhist practices. Sacred artifacts may be transported from one place of worship to another, sanctifying all locations where they reside. Devotional objects allow those who lack the means or the strength to visit actual places of veneration to make an internal or spiritual journey (Manseau 2009; Phoenix Art Museum 2012).

Culturally modified human bones, like other cultural objects, are laden with meaning. The manufacture, composition, use, and discarding of these objects all provide clues to their original function and to underlying belief systems. In the prehistoric American Midwest, the cultural modification and manipulation of human bone in the construction or display of objects is more common and more varied in form and context than the existing literature would suggest. But these objects have received little attention. The material is often misidentified as animal bone, or the objects are described as anomalous artifacts, or documentation of the cultural or archaeological context is missing. Discussions of modified human bone in the midwestern archaeological literature are primarily descriptive, and if interpretations are provided, they most commonly refer to the objects as trophies of warfare or conflict, the results of mortuary processing, or evidence of ancestor veneration (see Chacon and Dye, ed. 2007). While these interpretations may be valid, we believe that the manufacture and use of culturally modified bone is a complex process; modified bone objects can have more than one meaning; and meanings can change during an object's use-life (Gosden and Marshall 1999; Meskell 2005).

Objectives

In this volume we present a regional look at culturally modified human bone from prehistoric archaeological sites in the American Midwest. The chapters originated as presentations for a symposium at the 2008 Midwest Archaeological Conference in Milwaukee, Wisconsin, entitled *Human Bone as Cultural Object: A Midwestern Perspective.*

We focus on how the deliberate alteration and/or manipulation of a deceased individual's remains can reflect shifting social ideological perspectives of the individual, the body, and death in prehistoric societies. Our understanding of this important cultural phenomenon is fundamentally based in solid, detailed descriptions of modified bone in the relevant temporal, cultural, geographical, and archaeological contexts. The chapters are meant to encourage and facilitate further research into the meaning, function, and significance of these seemingly randomly scattered artifacts and to highlight that the level of variation in past treatments goes well beyond what a synchronic viewpoint might assume. While comparative examples of the use of human bone in ritual are abundant from a global context (e.g., Bonogofsky 2006; Bonogofsky, ed. 2011; Chacon and Dye, ed. 2007; Rakita et al. 2005; Tiesler and Cucina 2007; Tung 2012), they are less well documented for the Midwest. This book is one step toward addressing that void.

Many questions arise when investigating culturally modified bone. Are the remains from group "insiders" or "outsiders"? Are they derived from known individuals? Do they serve as a memorial? What meaning does human bone as a raw material carry? Is it spiritual? Functional? Does it retain a soul or carry power? Does possession of modified bone enhance or signify power or position? Who chooses which elements to keep and how they are to be used? Is the choice based on societal perceptions of the relationship between the soul and the body? Is the item for display or is it kept hidden, for use only on specific occasions? Does its function change throughout the use-life? Once the object is no longer considered useful, what rules, if any, exist regarding disposal of the object? These are difficult questions to address for extant cultures, and it is even more challenging to interpret actions and motives in the past.

To complicate matters, multiple cultural processes can produce identical patterns in the archaeological or osteological record (e.g., Bonogofsky 2011; Duncan 2005; Martin 2000; Simon and Steffian 1994). The archaeological context, natural taphonomic processes, and the composition of the human skeletal assemblage as a whole must be taken into consideration before interpreting culturally modified bone. Lines of inquiry that are useful for determining if patterns are intentional include redundancy within an assemblage, which might suggest that changes were deliberate rather than due to taphonomic variables (e.g., soil, insects, roots); evaluation of the archaeological and cultural context in which the remains were recovered; and review of ethnographic and ethnohistoric accounts of cultural practices that might explain the presence of certain types of cultural modification (e.g., Bonogofsky 2006; Bonogofsky, ed. 2011; Buikstra 1981; O'Shea 1984; Rakita et al. 2005; Urcid 1994).

Culturally Modified Human Bone

A critical first step in the study of culturally modified human remains is to compile detailed descriptions of how they are modified. What elements are used? What are the biological characteristics of the individual of origin? What is the context of recovery? All provide important clues to function and meaning. Bone can be altered by cutting, drilling, incising, deliberate polishing, or unintentional use-wear. Purposeful postmortem rearrangement of skeletonized body parts can transform human bone from isolated anatomical elements into something different and more complex. Although some objects have recognizable forms (e.g., awls, pipes, gorgets), providing correlates for their possible function (e.g., pipestem = smoking, gorget = adornment/ornamentation), identifying symbolic significance or ideological roles can be more difficult. We often turn to the historical and archaeological context, prehistoric and historic iconography, ethnography, or historic descriptions of myths and traditions for possible ideological motives.

Trophy taking has received a great deal of attention as an explanation for understanding modified human remains (i.e., Chacon and Dye, ed. 2007). However, there are problems in recognizing human bone as a "trophy" (Seeman 2007; also see Nawrocki and Emanovsky, this volume, and Sundstrom, this volume, for discussions of varying definitions of "trophy"), and it is difficult to conclusively distinguish between modifications related to violence as opposed to other cultural processes. Further, even warfare-related trophies can take on secondary roles (Bonogofsky, ed. 2011; Sundstrom, this volume). Owsley (1994:337) noted that "remains of scalped individuals who had received mortuary rites and burial, sometimes with associated objects, at sites not associated with violence, suggested *other cultural motives* for scalp-taking and uses of scalps other than as trophies" (emphasis added). Although Owsley referred to the taking of scalps, the same could be said of the taking of other body parts—by foe or friend, aggressor or ancestor—especially if the body part is further modified into what can be termed a "cultural object."

Existing literature provides many examples of culturally modified human bone with ascribed usage outside the realm of warfare and violence (Baby 1956, 1961; Black 1967; Bonney and Clegg 2011; Bonogofsky, ed. 2011; Bonogofsky and Graham 2011; Byers 2005; Cole and Deuel 1937; Cybulski 1978; Duncan 2005; Geller 2011; Gilliland 1975; Greenman 1967; Hall 1997; Hester 1969a, 1969b; Hoyme and Bass 1962; Jacobi and Hill 2000; Jamieson 1983; Mainfort 1986; Owsley et al. 1994; Pluckhahn 2003; Rakita et al. 2005; Seeman 2007; Sharapova and Razhev 2011; Valentin and Rolland 2011; Webb and Baby 1957; Webb and DeJarnette 1942; Williams 1975; Willoughby and Hooton 1922). Such objects are described variously as gorgets, bracelets, pendants, beads, bone tubes, oval and round disks, masks, daggers, awls and other tools, rasp-like instruments, whistles, pipe mouthpieces, rattles, or skull bowls or cups. They can be incised with geometric designs (zigzags, crosshatching, tear shapes, circles), drilled, notched, ground, polished, or covered with pigment, or they display some combination of these treatments. Ascribed functions include use in mortuary or renewal ceremonialism, including mourning activities, and use as protective talismans. Modifications can be symbolic, reflecting mythological or ideological systems. They can be a means of maintaining cosmological balance and cultural/social continuity, an outward expression of ancestor veneration, or curated ancestral relics. Decorated or modified human bone may remain meaningful to an individual, a family, or an entire culture, and change hands through time (Quigley 2001); or objects may have limited value or usefulness and eventually be discarded, either by casual or ritual means (Mensforth 2007).

Theoretical Approaches

Researchers have used a number of approaches to better understand the relationships between the living and the dead, including mortuary pattern studies (Baadsgaard et al. 2012; Case and Carr 2008; Rakita et al. 2005; Sullivan and Mainfort, ed. 2010; Tiesler and Cucina 2007), the use of human remains as trophies and/or display (Bonogofsky 2006; Bonogofsky, ed. 2011; Case and Carr 2008; Chacon and Dye, ed. 2007; Rakita et al. 2005; Tung 2012), and the social/political role of sacrifice (Martin et al. 2012; Tiesler and Cucina 2007; Tung 2012). More theoretical approaches have incorporated fragmentation theory (Chapman 2000), agency theory (Gardner 2004), gender (Arnold and Wicker 2001; Geller 2009), and social use of the dead (Chacon and Dye 2007b; Fitzsimmons and Shimada 2011; Rakita et al. 2005; Sullivan and Mainfort, ed. 2010; Tiesler and Cucina 2007).

We do not advocate for any particular approach in this volume. Rather, we feel that there is more to be gained by allowing contributors the freedom to approach the topic as they see fit. Therefore, our instructions to authors were to provide detailed descriptions and contextual information for objects, then to discuss those objects' significance within the theoretical framework most appropriate to the questions of interest. Contributing authors employ experimental/replication studies, biological and forensic approaches, ethnohistoric analogies, and cross-cultural comparisons to address how these items were made, from whom the elements were taken, how they were taken, what they might symbolize, how they may have been used, and how they were disposed of (i.e., when/if their use-life ended). Interpretations are as varied as the objects described and include the use of the artifacts for ancestor veneration or memory, as symbols of power or status, the active manipulation of remains to re-create the cosmos (terrain), mortuary ritual, the objects' role in performances, and the biography of objects.

Themes

While no one methodological or theoretical framework was imposed on the contributors, several commonalities can be found throughout the chapters in this volume. All authors, to varying degrees, provide biological information about a modified human object, a summary of its manufacturing techniques and characteristics, and the archaeological, historical, and temporal context to address their research question(s). An osteological approach (i.e., consideration of the age, sex, health, and morphology of both the individual from whom the object was derived and the individual with whom it was buried) is used by several authors and allows us to consider gender and its association with social roles and power relationships. Forensic taphonomy and experimental approaches emphasize the importance of constructing a taphonomic profile for an object. These studies permit us to examine how an object may have been manufactured, whether it was worked soon after death, and whether it was worn or handled for a long period of time before burial. The final deposition of these items—whether in "sacred" space or midden—and patterns of occurrence help elucidate whether they were intentionally deposited or lost, whether they had fulfilled their use and been discarded, whether they had their power transferred from individual to corporate group, or whether they were destroyed in order to release or extinguish whatever power they may have held.

Thematically, the authors vary in how they approach their subjects. A recurring question involves the nature and meaning of modified bone. Specifically we ask whether it is the individual bone (or tooth) as the chosen material for modification that is important or whether it is the particular individual providing the material that is most significant. The overwhelming majority of modified elements are portions of the head—cranium, maxilla, mandible, tooth. Cultures worldwide have viewed the head as the body part that best displays one's identity, or as a source of power and knowledge, and/or as a place where one's soul resides (Bonogofsky 2006; Bonogofsky, ed. 2011; Duncan 2005).

A number of authors in this volume focus on identifying the possible function of these objects. Suggestions include use as a tool, trophy, ornament, mask, pipe, initiation and defloration tool, and object of symbolic or ritual power. The selection of *human* bone is often suggested or inferred to have enhanced the power or symbolic meaning of the object (McNeill 2005).

Another approach focuses on the examination of social memory, the role of ancestors in the world of the living, and the manipulation of human remains to tell stories or to create ritual drama. Suggested explanations include fertility or world renewal, mortuary ritual, viewing the manipulation of human remains as ritual drama or display, as identity, or as a representation of the cosmological and spiritual world.

The cultural biography of objects, which focuses on the interwoven transformations between objects and people, is a common theme in several of the chapters. Objects have a life history—their form, function, and significance change through time in direct relationship to the people using the object (Gosden and Marshall 1999; Holtorf 2002; Hoskins 1998; Joy 2009; Kopytoff 1986; Meskell 2005; Spector 1993). In the context of culturally modified bone, such transformations are complex and involve changing perceptions of the object through time. A single object can have many different meanings depending on the actions of its users and as determined by the particular social and cultural landscape in which it exists at any particular point in time.

Organization of the Volume

Archaeological context is a critical component of the interpretation of material culture, particularly when exploring the significance of unusual or uncommon objects, such as culturally modified human remains. How and why these particular elements were selected and utilized depended largely on the particular social and ideological contexts in which they were created and used. We have organized the chapters into four parts. The first three are temporal—Woodland, Mississippian, and late prehistoric—and each part opens with a map presenting the locations of the sites discussed by the authors. While exceptions or arguments can be made, archaeological evidence suggests that in the midwestern United States there were broad similarities in lifestyle, ideology, social organization, and material culture during each of the broad temporal categories. The fourth section, "Perspectives," focuses on more general overviews of the topics discussed in the volume.

In the Midwest, culturally modified human bone appears as early as the Archaic period (ca. 8500–800 B.C.) and continues well into the historic period (Case and Carr 2008; Chacon and Dye, ed. 2007; Milner 1995; Robbins 1974; Smith 1997; Weltfish 1965, among others). The contributions here focus on the Woodland, Mississippian, and late prehistoric periods in Illinois, Indiana, Iowa, Minnesota, Ohio, and Wisconsin. Although all of these time periods are found throughout the midwestern region, the timing and duration of these prehistoric periods vary between regions. For instance, the Oneota tradition in northern Illinois dates to A.D. 1400–1700, yet in Iowa the dates are roughly A.D. 1150–1700. As you move through the volume, please keep in mind that the sites that are referenced are from all areas of the Midwest, each with their individual local histories and temporal sequences. Some examples of bone modification show considerable time depth and continuity in form and function (for example, bone disks, awls). Others are common to only specific periods or cultures, such as Middle Woodland Hopewell modified jaws and late prehistoric incised cranial fragments.

Woodland Period

Although Woodland cultures extended from about 2000 B.C. through about A.D. 1000, the chapters in this volume focus on modified bone objects from the Middle Woodland period (ca. 200 B.C. to A.D. 500). The Middle Woodland differs significantly from the earlier and later Woodland periods in the increased complexity of the material assemblages, the widespread use of symbolic images, and elaborate mortuary programs. Exotic materials provide evidence of long-distance trade networks; similarities in material culture and the use of particular symbols on figurines, pipes, and ceramics found across the Midwest suggest a widely shared cosmology.

Stephen Nawrocki and Paul Emanovsky (chapter 2) provide a taphonomic analysis of Hopewellian modified human jaws to determine the length of time between death and modification, and they use experimental means to identify the techniques used to create these objects. They extend the definition of "trophy" to include the curation of elements beyond the narrower warfare- and conflict-related definition.

Dawn Cobb's (chapter 3) study focuses on modified human maxillae and mandibles included as grave artifacts in Middle Woodland Hopewell burial tombs in the central Illinois River valley. She notes stylistic differences in modifications and compares them with modifications at Indiana and Ohio Hopewell sites, suggesting that differences may reflect ideology and group identity. Some modified elements may have functioned as heirlooms, while the inclusion of unmodified mandibles as mortuary artifacts may indicate that there was significance placed on the object (human mandible) rather than on the modification.

Johnston (chapter 4) describes modified jaws from the Hopewell site in Ohio, which was excavated in the early twentieth century. She combines evidence of the burial location with biological information derived from both the modified elements and their associated burials to test a set of hypotheses related to the function of these elements. She also poses the question that reappears throughout the chapters—what is the significance of using *human* bone as a material?

Christopher Carr and Anna Novotny (chapter 5) consider a ritual drama framework to theorize about Ohio Hopewell mortuary behavior, looking at how the manipulation of human remains and the positioning of bodies and associated artifacts might depict the death process, the structure of the cosmos, and human and mythical beings. Using interpretations drawn largely from Native American cosmology and mythology, Carr and Novotny see ritual drama as a means to integrate dispersed households into a larger community.

The most unusual example of culturally modified bone is presented by Anne Lee and Cheryl Johnston (chapter 6). They describe two artifacts presumably made of human bone and resembling human phalli; one appears to be from a Hopewell mortuary context, the other lacks provenience information. Looking at examples of similar artifacts throughout North America and Europe, they suggest possible uses in phallicism and fertility rituals, in initiation and defloration rituals, as symbolic male substitutes, and in utilitarian roles.

In the final chapter in the Woodland section, Shirley Schermer and Robin Lillie (chapter 7) provide examples of excised, drilled, and perforated bone from sites in Iowa. They consider the archaeological/depositional context (midden vs. mortuary) and the types of modification in exploring how these items may have functioned in society. Excised disks (rondelles) that are found only in Middle Woodland mortuary contexts suggest that they are closely linked to death and rebirth and may have been powerful curated objects.

Mississippian Period

Characteristics of the Mississippian period (A.D. 1050–1700) include a reliance on maize agriculture; the development of large mound centers with dense populations; clear evidence for social stratification; evidence for craft specialists; both large villages and scattered homesteads; and the development of a unique corpus of iconography, the Southeastern Ceremonial Complex. In contrast to the Middle Woodland period, there are significantly fewer examples of culturally modified human bone. We find this intriguing in light of the many social and ideological changes that occurred during this time period.

Eve Hargrave and Della Cook (chapter 8) use a biographical approach and experimental replication to investigate modified human bone from the Submound 51 feasting feature at the site of Cahokia. They describe an awl made from a human ulna and a proximal human femur showing polish from use and discuss the possible function of the objects, the role they played in ritual events at Cahokia, and the events that led to their eventual deposition.

Katie Zejdlik's (chapter 9) discussion also emphasizes the importance of archaeological context in ascertaining the function of culturally modified bone and provides an interesting comparison to the examples in Hargrave and Cook's chapter. In describing a modified human tibia from the Aztalan site in Wisconsin, Zejdlik evaluates whether the bone served a ritual or functional purpose, and investigates why that bone in particular was selected.

Della Cook and Cheryl Munson (chapter 10) describe examples of modified human bone from the Angel site in Indiana and discuss the significance of a large modified cranial fragment with a stepped-rim decorative edge. They illustrate the widespread occurrence of the stepped-rim design on other types of prehistoric and historic artifacts and conclude that the design element combined with the deliberate use of human bone indicate that bone objects were symbolically charged. Cook and Munson also consider ties to the larger Mississippian world.

Cheryl Munson, Della Cook, and Mary Lucas Powell (chapter 11) provide a summary of modified bone from the late Mississippian Caborn-Welborn phase (A.D. 1400–1700) in Indiana and Kentucky. Applying osteological and artifact analysis standards and archaeological context, they conclude that the most likely function for the modified mandibles was ritual display. Less clear is the purpose for the modified clavicles and ulna; the authors suggest that these may be indirectly related to preparing bone for display by the removal of arms for trophies.

Late Prehistoric Period

The late prehistoric, Upper Mississippian period (ca. A.D. 1100–1700) overlaps temporally with the Middle Mississippian but represents distinct cultural groups, most of which are located in the northern Midwest. Many sites contain evidence for extraregional trade, population movement, and the threat of violence (Birch 2010; Milner et al. 1991; Owsley et al. 2007; Santure et al. 1990). Late prehistoric sites are distinguished from Mississippian cultures by a more dispersed settlement pattern and the absence of both temple mounds and large central towns.

Using an osteological approach in association with archaeological context, Kristin Hedman (chapter 12) compares modified human bone from nonmortuary and mortuary contexts at two late prehistoric sites in northern Illinois. She proposes that the material type, individual of origin, and design motifs can increase the symbolic or ritual power of both the image and the object. Further, differences in the contexts of these objects suggest that some may have had a finite functional life, while others may have belonged to particular individuals and functioned for that individual after death.

Kathleen Blue (chapter 13) investigates modified human teeth found in both mortuary and nonmortuary contexts at sites in the Red Wing locality of Minnesota and Wisconsin. She provides a global summary of the symbolic importance of teeth through time. She also presents a unique perspective on the use of teeth to symbolize group identity but, similar to other chapters in this volume, her conclusions emphasize the importance of the transformative properties of modified human bone through time.

Robin Lillie and Shirley Schermer (chapter 14) describe examples of deliberately incised, cut, and polished human bone from nonmortuary contexts at Oneota sites in Iowa. Several of the incised designs mimic Oneota iconography found on pottery, catlinite tablets, and petroglyphs elsewhere in the region, suggesting that the bone may have served a symbolic role in the transmission of the group's ideology, mythology, and identity. A cranium covered with incised motifs appears ready for division into smaller segments (for distribution?), possibly suggesting the next stage of its use-life.

Perspectives

The final two chapters in this volume draw from ethnohistoric accounts and extraregional examples of human bone modification and the taking, use, and manipulation of body parts by early Native American groups. These accounts provide invaluable insights into possible alternative meanings behind modified human remains.

Linea Sundstrom (chapter 15) discusses "trophy taking" (e.g., scalping) in a broader and more complex way than is typically found in the archaeological literature. She focuses on definitions, cultural biases, native accounts vs. nonnative interpretations, and the modification of cultural "others." In contrast to Nawrocki and Emanovsky, Sundstrom argues that the term "trophy" should be more narrowly defined and discusses the multiple functions that scalps served in Native American groups. Her discussion about the significance of hair in many Native American cultures reminds us that, although we focus here on the significance of modified bone, there are many other aspects of the body that need to be taken into account.

The final chapter by Maria Smith (chapter 16) provides an important summary of the many themes presented throughout this volume and supplements the ideas presented with supporting examples from the ethnohistoric and ethnographic literature. Importantly, she addresses the lack of a common language in discussions of the role of culturally modified bone, one example being the myriad ways that the term "trophy" has been defined. Smith's insightful chapter also addresses the importance of recognizing and acknowledging the differences between the western and nonwestern concepts of the self, the soul, and sacred vs. secular while investigating the past. She reiterates that archaeological context is critical to evaluating pre- and postdepositional life and to understanding the life history of culturally modified bone.

Future Directions

Both improvements in methodological approaches derived from forensic and osteological studies and the application of new theoretical approaches allow researchers to interpret the significance of human bone as a cultural material in more nuanced ways than in the past. No one theoretical approach, however, is adequate for explaining the variability evident among these artifacts. Attempts to determine the function of objects recovered from archaeological contexts also provide ample opportunity for cultural appropriation and bias. We have used the term "object" throughout this volume but are conflicted as to whether that is the most appropriate term. "Object" can be interpreted as inanimate; however, these bones are generally interpreted as maintaining their sense of humanness. From some perspectives, these modified "objects" are more appropriately seen as "individuals." A number of the modified bones described here were identified during inventories conducted for the Native American Graves Protection and Repatriation Act (NAGPRA), and consultation with Native American scholars during the course of this project have helped us to understand these items as living entities. Sundstrom (chapter 15) reminds us that the interpretation of the past is often complex and that archaeologists need to incorporate Native American perspectives in their efforts. We hope that the perspectives and insights from Native American scholars and community members will enter more visibly into future discussions.

We have opened a conversation and an avenue to interpret culturally modified human remains that appreciates and acknowledges the complexity of past peoples and cultures. Intentionally selected and modified human remains appear to have served complex sociocultural roles, including spiritual or ritual use; symbolic representation of group identity, ideology, and cosmology; and remembrance of and assistance for and from the deceased. Larsen (2011) noted that postmortem modifications to human remains were necessarily "performed *by* the living *to* the dead" (emphasis added). If these modified remains (cultural objects) take on a "life after death," we need to consider the complex interactions between these two realms—the living and the transformed dead—throughout an object's life history. We need to view these remains not as representative of a single object with one purpose only. They originated from individual people with unique histories and social roles. Upon their death, specific elements were selected for modification for a myriad of reasons, as indicated throughout this volume, but the meaning and significance of the modified element changed through time in response to changing social situations and relationships with the living. The final depositional context represents the completion of its use by the living, although not necessarily by the dead.

I

WOODLAND PERIOD

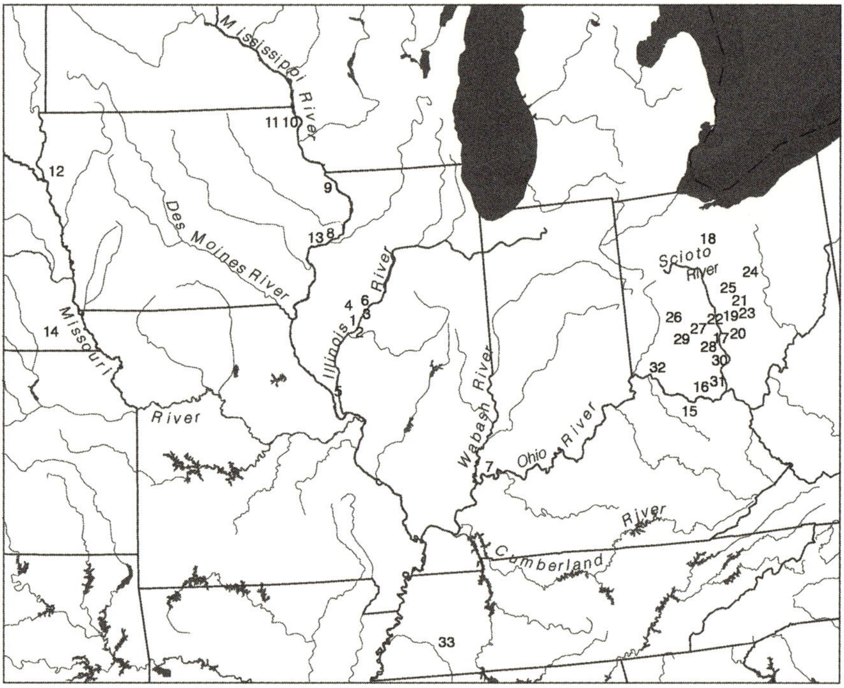

Woodland sites. *Illinois*: (1) Eveland/Ogden-Fettie (chapter 3); (2) Havana (chapter 3); (3) Liverpool (chapter 3); (4) Sister Creeks (chapter 3); (5) Snyders Mound C (chapter 4); (6) Weaver (chapter 3). *Indiana*: (7) Mount Vernon (GE) Mound (chapters 2, 4). *Iowa*: (8) Cook Farm Mound group (chapter 7); (9) Deppe Mound group (chapter 7); (10) Lane Farm Mound group (chapter 7); (11) Quandahl rockshelter (chapter 7); (12) Larson site (chapter 7); (13) Lowry Farm Mound group (chapter 7). *Nebraska*: (14) Gage County (chapter 6). *Kentucky*: (15) Mason County (chapter 6). *Ohio*: (16) Adams County (chapter 6); (17) Bournevile Mound (chapter 4); (18) Crawford County (chapter 6); (19) Florence Mound (chapter 4); (20) Harness Mound (chapter 4); (21) Hocking County (chapter 6); (22) Hopewell Mound group (chapters 4, 5); (23) Mound City (chapters 4, 5); (24) Newark earthwork (chapter 4); (25) Old Town (Frankfort site) (chapter 5); (26) Purdom Mound (chapter 4); (27) Raymond Ater Mound (chapter 4); (28) Rockhold Mound group (chapters 4, 5); (29) Ross County (chapter 6); (30) Seip Mound (chapters 4, 5); (31) Tremper Mound (chapters 2, 4); (32) Turner (chapter 4). *Tennessee*: (33) Madison County (chapter 6). (Courtesy of Illinois State Archaeological Survey, University of Illinois)

2

A Taphonomic Analysis of Hopewellian Modified Trophy Jaws

Stephen P. Nawrocki and Paul D. Emanovsky

Anthropologists have been speculating on the meaning of human "trophy" artifacts for over a century. These items, found in both prehistoric and recent contexts, often conjure up images of forbidden acts, heinous crimes, secret rituals, and deviant behavior. Just as the American public at large has at times become fascinated with tales of cannibalism, torture, and serial killing in modern society, anthropologists have sometimes spent a disproportionate amount of effort projecting these same phenomena into the distant past. Franz Weidenreich (1951:238–239) was convinced that many specimens in the Ngandong (Solo) *Homo erectus* cranial assemblage had had their foramina magnums enlarged "to obtain access to the brain to eat." In the same monograph, Gustav von Koenigswald (Weidenreich 1951:216–217) cited modern ethnographic evidence from Indonesia to suggest that those same crania were curated and used as bowls. Raymond Baby (1956) hypothesized that remnants of a more recent Hopewellian artifact, composed of worked human facial and cranial bones, were once part of an elaborate headdress, and to illustrate his point he fashioned a version of his vision from leather and recent human bones. His creative handiwork is still stored at the Ohio Historical Society in Columbus.

Unfortunately, by their very nature, the archaeological and osteological records are giant Rorschach tests onto which we sometimes project our biases, fears, and obsessions. The bones and stones that form the bases of our interpretations are often the accidental byproducts of imperfect site-formation and sampling processes, the simple physical remnants of far more complex behavioral and cultural phenomena that refuse to be fossilized. Even after a thorough analysis of all available evidence, the resulting picture is still so incomplete that we are often free to insert our own biases. Baby's reconstructed Hopewellian headdress is an excellent example of this phenomenon; it is a work of (almost) pure fancy, telling us more about its modern maker than about people who lived almost two millennia ago.

Of course, despite our tabloid-like obsession with the dark side of human nature, it is academically valid to ask what genuine trophy specimens mean and how they originated. Were our human ancestors truly violent, engaging in warfare and systematic trophy taking to assert their superiority (Seeman 1988)? Did they take away parts of their victims to somehow absorb their enemies' strength, out of a sense of awe and respect? Or did some societies invent elaborate arrays of funerary rituals for handling their revered ancestors and departed loved ones (Johnston 2002)? Can we even tell the difference in the archaeological record? The artifacts beg for description and explanation, and anthropologists have not been shy to rise to the challenge.

By "trophies" we refer specifically to objects that were intentionally acquired for use and retention as possessions or trade items, not to human bone that was incidentally or accidentally modified as a result of other processing or cultural activities. Trophies may or may not have been taken by force or violence, but it is clear that they eventually acquired complex postmortem histories. By this definition, bones that display defleshing or disarticulation marks or perimortem trauma would not be classified as trophies per se unless some other evidence of curation (such as use-polish or inclusion as special grave goods) can be identified. For example, a cranium and mandible with cut marks created during scalping and tongue removal would not be "trophies" if the bones were left behind on the field of battle, although the scalp and tongue themselves would be if the intent were to retain or modify them, even if temporarily. Bones processed solely for their nutritive value (cannibalism) would also fail the trophy test, regardless of the amount or complexity of modification they experienced (White 1992).

We understand that our focus on curation may differ somewhat from previous definitions of "trophy," a term that seems to imply warfare and conflict. In most circumstances, it is difficult if not impossible to distinguish between war trophies and items with other origins. For example, a head may have been removed from the body in exactly the same fashion regardless of whether the intent was to kill the individual, release the person's spirit, capture the warrior's strength, speed up the decomposition process, honor the individual in a postmortem ceremony, or acquire raw material (jaws) for producing an ornamental pendant with trade value. The resulting processing marks are unlikely to be specific or unique enough to allow the investigator to differentiate between these varied purposes. In other words, it is not necessarily the initial modification of a specimen that defines its significance; it is its use and distribution after acquisition that determines its meaning. Evidence of curation, then, while not a perfect litmus test, can show at least that the item had a purpose beyond the incidental.

In this chapter we examine a rare subgroup of trophy specimens: jaws that have been very heavily modified to the point where they begin to lose many of their distinguishing anatomical features. Our hypothesis is that heavily modified artifacts, because they have been extensively handled, may reveal more about the origins and postmortem histories of trophies in general than do the far more common examples that display only incidental (or even no) physical modifications. We do not specifically attempt to answer *why* these artifacts were made, nor do we systematically assess the various theories that have been offered to explain their cultural relevance or meaning. Instead, we attempt to clarify patterns in their manufacture and usage as an essential first step toward reconstructing their ultimate significance. Furthermore, our primary training as forensic scientists affords us the opportunity to approach the problem from a slightly different perspective than has been offered in the past. If indeed bone trophy artifacts have their origin in warfare and violence, then an analytical approach that is overtly geared toward identifying and interpreting the results of interhuman aggression in the *present* could prove useful.

Forensic Taphonomy

Forensic taphonomy focuses on the alterations made to human tissues and personal belongings at and after death (that is, during the perimortem and postmortem intervals) (Haglund and Sorg 1997, 2002; Nawrocki 2009). The methods used are not necessarily new or unique; rather, it is the context in which these analytical tools are applied and the specific subjects to which they are applied that define the field. Forensic taphonomists use methods originally developed in paleoecology and paleontology in the context of recent death investigations in an attempt to clarify the factual and legal circumstances of those deaths.

Forensic taphonomic analysis is typically used to (1) estimate the time since death of the decedent, (2) determine the location of death or locations with which the remains subsequently came into contact, (3) extrapolate victim and assailant behaviors related to the death event, and (4) help elucidate the cause and manner of death. This information is then used by the medicolegal system (coroners, medical examiners, prosecutors) to determine how, or if, the court should proceed in a given case.

The forensic taphonomist's approach differs from that applied by taphonomists in archaeological or geological settings. First, rather than focusing primarily on bone modification, the forensic specialist typically is able to examine the totality of the remains, including soft tissue, cartilage, skin, and hair. An in-depth understanding of the decomposition processes that affect those tissues in specific environments is therefore essential. Second, the forensic specialist looks carefully at the interaction between the remains and the deposition site itself, whether that is the ground surface, a carnivore's stomach, a shallow clandestine grave, a deeply buried coffin, or a car trunk. The approach is therefore inherently ecological, with the remains being seen as only one component of a complex microecosystem that includes other animals, plants, the soil, and climatic variables. Third, the forensic specialist must regularly identify and describe modifications made to hard and soft tissues that result from human conflict, distinguishing them from changes that arise from more mundane sources, such as rodents or roots. In this capacity, the analyst has the opportunity to examine numerous specimens whose histories are known and verified, and therefore hypotheses about causal processes can be tested more rigorously than is typically possible in (nonexperimental) archaeological contexts.

These foci tend to distinguish forensic taphonomy from human taphonomy as applied in more traditional bioarchaeological contexts (Nawrocki 1995). Although previous bioarchaeological analyses of prehistoric trophy specimens have at times incorporated some of these perspectives, few have specifically approached the issue in a comprehensive fashion with the intent of elucidating the rather narrowly defined perimortem interval and its distinguishing events from the factors that affected the remains in the postmortem interval. This forensic approach could be valuable if indeed the phenomenon of curation is an inherent component of trophy artifacts that is somehow distinct or meaningful apart from the process of simply *acquiring* the bones (as exemplified by the lack of specificity of simple dismemberment marks).

The topic of trophy specimens—either recent or ancient—is inherently taphonomic in nature. For example, consider the case of missing or displaced bones in a recent clandestine burial. It would be an essential job of the forensic taphonomist to explain the events that led to the observed anomalies. To demonstrate that a deliberate "taking" had been conducted by the assailant at death or even after initial burial, one must first exclude other depositional and postdepositional phenomena, both natural and cultural, that could explain the anomaly. Carnivore scavenging, rodent burrowing, and accidental human intrusion into preexisting burials are frequently more parsimonious explanations of skeletal disturbance than deliberate human trophy taking. Soft tissue decomposition combined with soil movement can produce odd skeletal configurations that can be misinterpreted as human intervention. The grave shaft changes dynamically as the soft tissues slowly decompose, and body parts will begin to slump as the muscles, ligaments, and tendons disappear. The bones can shift as voids open in the surrounding matrix, which has already been disturbed and is thus unstable. Gravity and percolating ground water then can move even large skeletal elements into unusual positions within the grave. As more time passes, the weight of the accumulating overburden can compress the grave shaft and its contents into a simplified, largely two-dimensional representation of its original, more complex three-dimensional arrangement, effectively erasing evidence of its once-dynamic nature.

Unfortunately, we have encountered many examples in both criminal and archaeological settings where postmortem taphonomic processes in the grave (a subspecialty called "geotaphonomy" by Hochrein [2002]) were incorrectly interpreted as a result of relying too heavily on the two-dimensional picture and interpreting the final configuration as evidence of deliberate trophy taking or intrusion. A cranium lying between the knees is not necessarily evidence that it does not belong to the rest of the skeleton nor that it had been removed at death and placed there deliberately as part of a ritual. A complicating factor in the interpretation of prehistoric trophies is that many early archaeological projects did not record the exact contexts from which those trophies were excavated, and crucial details that might have helped us to understand their perimortem and postmortem histories are no longer available (Johnston 2002).

A second intersection of forensic taphonomy with the trophy issue involves the interpretation of bone and soft tissue modifications. In a modern criminal case that could involve perimortem trauma or dismemberment, the taphonomist would immediately ask whether any abnormal marks on the skeleton were created by the assailant. If so, what types of activities and tools created those marks? Were the remains altered as fresh specimens that still possessed soft tissues, or were they modified as dry elements that had long since decomposed? Can the marks be distinguished from, or were they altered by, later autopsy procedures? How were soft tissues removed, and were these tissues curated as well? How did the characteristics of the raw materials restrict or shape the modification process? Can the marks be replicated, and how long does it take to create them? Is there physical evidence that the bones had been curated or handled after being modified? All of these questions are clearly relevant to the interpretation of prehistoric trophies, but few analyses address these issues in a systematic fashion.

Hopewellian Trophy Jaws

The Hopewell peoples of the Middle Woodland period (ca. 200 B.C.–A.D. 500) had a penchant for human bone "trophies." Although they may have inherited this tendency from Adena predecessors of the Early Woodland, during the Middle Woodland we see a proliferation and diversification of trophies that has not been seen before or since (see Nawrocki 1997 and Seeman 1988 for thorough reviews). Modified jaws (mandibles and maxillae) and isolated crania are particularly common, although a few modified postcranial elements are also known (for example, see Baby 1961).

While trophy skulls as grave goods have been found in Illinois and elsewhere (see Cobb, this volume; Johnston, this volume), it would appear that the Middle Woodland trophy skull "cult" was centered in Ohio (Johnston 2002; Seeman 1988:569). More widely distributed and (perhaps) more numerous in Middle Woodland sites throughout the Midwest are jaws of both humans and nonhuman animals. The majority of these jaws occur in isolation or, less commonly, in small clusters of two to four specimens (Nawrocki 1997:17). Some were found at the wrists or heads of interred individuals, suggesting that they were worn as pendants or charms. Most display only minimal modifications, such as simple perforations (presumably for suspension) or cut marks. Modified human maxillae are less common than human mandibles, probably because the former are difficult to separate intact from the cranium and contain less of the dense cortical bone that would help to hold them together during extensive processing. However, some careful craftspeople were able to produce maxilla artifacts, as shown by their presence at the Hopewell and Harness mounds in Ohio and at the Liverpool and Neteler sites in Illinois (Cobb, this volume; Johnston, this volume). A few jaws are incised with designs, but most do not display such modifications.

Modified nonhuman jaws are common in Hopewell contexts (Parmalee 1959). Species represented include bear, wolf, fox, cougar, lynx, bobcat, raccoon, badger, wolverine, otter, mink, weasel, beaver, porcupine, muskrat, woodchuck, deer, barracuda, and woodpecker. Some are heavily modified or ornately carved, but most display rather simple alterations, such as perforations.

This chapter focuses on two known caches of the most heavily modified Hopewellian mandibles. A third large cache was found at Snyders Mound C°103 in Calhoun County, Illinois (Braun et al. 1982), and while we have examined these human specimens as well, they are not detailed here. These assemblages are particularly interesting for a number of reasons. First, unlike the mostly isolated or paired jaws found at other Hopewell sites, each of these caches contains the artifactual remains of many individuals, creating the best opportunity to clarify the biological characteristics of the decedents. Second, the jaws display the greatest degree of modification among trophies found anywhere in the Middle Woodland or, perhaps, from any prehistoric time period in the Americas, and thus they may reveal more about their origin than unmodified specimens. Third, the pattern of modifications is very similar in all three caches, suggesting a high degree of craft specialization and continuity despite the great physical distance between their recovery locations. In particular, we were interested in how the modified remains had been manufactured, what tools produced them, whether they were processed in a fresh or dry state, and whether they had been curated. We examined and photographed all of the specimens firsthand and were also able to compare them directly to specimens from other Hopewell sites.

Mount Vernon (General Electric) Mound Cache

The first cache came from the Mount Vernon Mound (12PO885) in Posey County, Indiana, adjacent to the confluence of the Ohio and Wabash rivers (Tomak 1994). This Woodland site was heavily looted by collectors in 1988 and became the focal point for federal prosecution under archaeological protection laws (Munson et al. 1995). Many of the stolen artifacts were recovered by law enforcement agents and brought back to the General Electric Company, on whose land the mound sits. Other artifacts were gathered during a limited archaeological recovery effort (Tomak 1994). Plugged bear canines, dozens of copper celts, thousands of chert bifaces, copper earspools, copper pan pipes, cannel coal ceremonial blades, and exquisitely crafted quartz blades underscore the uniqueness and importance of the site in Hopewell society. General Electric reburied all of the artifacts and human remains, including the modified human bones, in the surviving portion of the mound in May 1994, at the request of Native American groups.

A detailed study of the human remains was conducted in 1994 before the reburial, and the results were published in a monograph released by General Electric (Nawrocki 1997). Included in the assemblage were 42 fragments of at least 22 human hemimandibles (9 left and 13 right). A minimum of 13 different decedents are represented in this cache, although the extensive modifications and a great many missing teeth made it difficult, if not impossible, to securely link left and right sides. Therefore, it is possible that more than 13 individuals are present. A total of 44 mandibular teeth are associated with these jaws, 37 of which articulate directly. There is no evidence to suggest that modified maxillae or entire trophy skulls were present at Mount Vernon. However, the assemblage did include a single perforated human metacarpal, a trophy type that is not known from any other Middle Woodland site (although a single, perforated left first proximal manual phalanx is known from Hopewell Mound 25).

Unfortunately, we do not know the original context of the cache within the mound or whether the specimens were placed as grave goods in a single burial. Fragments of unmodified cranial and postcranial bones of a very large, middle-aged adult male were present in the assemblage, suggesting that at least one individual had been interred in the mound. Two lightly worn maxillary teeth of a second (probably teenaged) individual were also present, as were many tiny cremated (calcined) bone fragments, at least some of which were probably human.

Analysis of the decedents from whom the jaws were taken reveals that all were likely young or middle-aged adults, with no evidence of any subadults or adults of advanced age (Nawrocki 1997). Based on dental measurements, both males and females are present in the assemblage, consistent with the results of Johnston's (2002) analysis of Ohio Hopewell trophy specimens. Frequencies of carious lesions and enamel hypoplasias are very low, and there is no evidence of antemortem tooth loss. Therefore, dental health can be characterized as fairly good. Analysis of the dental microwear suggests a typical Middle Woodland diet with a heavy reliance on nuts or similar hard foods (Schmidt and Helmkamp 1997).

Four main types of modification are present in the Mount Vernon mandible assemblage: grinding, superficial scratching (abrasion striations), perforation, and polishing. The most significant process was grinding, which resulted in the removal of the majority of bone material required for shaping the specimens. The reduction process occurred as follows. The mandibular symphysis has been snapped or cut in the midline, and the resulting surfaces have been ground flat, producing two separate hemimandibles with no remaining connection between them. The inferior portion of the body (corpus) and ramus of each hemimandible has been ground away, exposing the tooth roots and removing many root apices. Grinding marks on the inferior surfaces are generally transversely (mediolaterally) oriented with respect to the long axis of the corpus. The coronoid process and mandibular condyle have been removed, and the superior portion of the ramus has been ground flat. At least two perforations are present on each hemimandible, one in the approximate center of the ramus and a second on the body just below the premolars. The perforations display circular channel marks within, indicating that they were drilled from both sides by a narrow object, probably a stone awl.

Figure 2.1 presents one of the right hemimandibles. It is incomplete, and a postmortem fracture separates the posterior (ramus) portion from the anterior (body) portion. Note the additional perforation at the top of the ramus (indicated by arrow), which has been nearly removed during processing. It seems unusual to go to the trouble of perforating the specimen and then to destroy

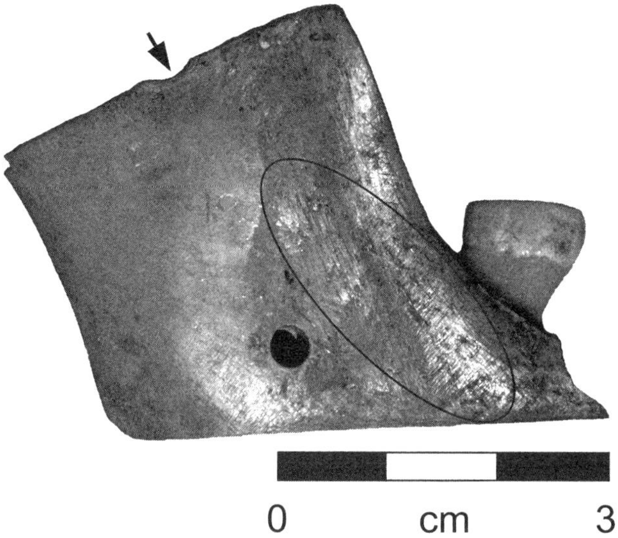

2.1. Mount Vernon Mound, human right hemimandible 19, external view. The ramus has been ground superiorly and inferiorly, and both scratches and grinding marks are visible on the external surface (*circled area*). The arrow points to a partially obliterated perforation. A postmortem fracture separated the corpus from the ramus just anterior to the third molar. (Photo by Stephen Nawrocki)

the perforation through further modification. We have noted this same phenomenon at other Hopewell sites and suggest that these specimens may have had two different postmortem "lives"—one as a more complete specimen similar to the modestly modified (mostly intact) mandibles found at various Ohio sites (Seip Mound 1, Hopewell Mound 25, and Harness Mound) (Nawrocki 1997; Seeman 1988), and then a second life as a more highly modified artifact. It is also possible that the upper perforation, which occurs at one of the thinnest spots of the mandible, was added early in the process to allow suspension on a drying rack or in a charnel house or boiling pot so that soft tissues could be removed prior to further (final) processing.

Scratch marks (Figure 2.1) are prominent on the nonground surfaces of the Mount Vernon jaws and can also be observed on many Hopewellian trophy specimens. These scratches are sometimes aligned in clustered sets; in other areas, they are more randomized. They display rounded or U-shaped channels, indicating that they were created by dull objects, such as grains of sand or siliceous rushes, rubbed repeatedly on the surface. True cut marks made by bladed instruments, such as chert flakes, typically display V-shaped channels. While stray cut marks can be found on these and other Hopewellian trophies, they are nearly always greatly outnumbered by scratch marks. The extensive scratching did not remove a significant amount of bone and thus was not part of the shaping process. Rather, these marks may reflect the freshness of the human remains at the time of processing; perhaps the jaws were processed fairly shortly after death, before all soft tissues could decompose naturally. Using abrasives would remove traces of periosteum, ligament, tendon, and muscle and may have helped to remove irregularities of color. In forensic cases, decomposing soft tissues and other environmental factors often create irregular color patterns on the surfaces of bones. For example, iron in the blood stains the bone red or purple around perimortem wounds or in areas that are gravity dependent (i.e., on surfaces facing or in direct contact with the ground, which are also likely to be more shielded from the bleaching effects of the sun). Contact with leaves and decaying plant material produces brownish tannin stains, and algae, mold, and fungus can produce other colors ranging from green to pink to black. Some of these color changes occur quite soon (hours or days) after death; extended surface exposure or subsurface burial tends to ameliorate these color irregularities, reducing contrast and homogenizing the bone's appearance. The depth of staining varies, but at least some can be removed by thorough cleaning or light abrasives.

Tremper Mound Cache

Tremper Mound in southern Ohio was excavated in the early 1900s and described in a monograph by William Mills (1916a). Among the many artifacts and cremated human burials found in this Woodland mound was a large cache of modified human and nonhuman jaws. The collection consists of burned hemimandibles, hemimaxillae, and teeth that have been drilled, incised, and flattened on one or more surfaces. Housed at the Ohio Historical Society in Columbus, the collection was not thoroughly described until the early twenty-first century (Emanovsky 2002). The Tremper cache is the only known cache that is dominated by nonhuman jaws, although it includes at least two fragments of worked human mandible (Johnston et al. 1997; also see Johnston, this volume).

Four animals are present in the Tremper assemblage: cougar (16 fragments of 7 animals), bobcat (4 fragments of 2 animals), canid (9 fragments of 5 animals), and bear (32 fragments of 13 animals). The canid category could include coyote, dog, or wolf, as the degree of modification makes it difficult to distinguish between these closely related species. Similarly, bear could include both grizzly and black bears. The cougar and bobcat specimens are represented entirely by mandibles, while the canids and bears are represented by both mandibles and maxillae, although maxillae dominate. It is likely that the shortened faces of the felids (cats) made it impossible to construct a viable maxillary trophy artifact, while the elongated faces of dogs and bears made maxillary trophies feasible.

The overall pattern of modification of the Tremper specimens is very similar to that observed at Mount Vernon, including the patterns of grinding, scratching, perforation, and polishing. However, the Tremper assemblage does show some unique features. For example, all have been burned or smoked, some reaching the point of calcination. Many of the specimens had red ochre applied. The presence of ochre in the scratches and grinding channels suggests that the coloration was applied as a last step. Some specimens (particularly felids) display decorative incising on the anterior edges of the ramus and coronoid processes.

The Tremper mandibles have been ground along the inferior border to the point where the sockets are exposed; tooth root apices have been removed. Grinding striations are primarily oblique or parallel with the long direction of the bone. The mandibular condyles have been removed; the coronoid process is frequently left intact in the felid specimens, but has been removed in the canid and bear specimens. The symphyseal surfaces have been ground flat, and so opposite sides were not designed to articulate together. Perforations are present at both ends of many specimens, as at Mount Vernon. The Tremper maxillae are also split in the midline and have had their palates removed by grinding. The root tips are exposed similar to the mandibles. The hemimaxillae are perforated at either end and generally look like the mandibular fragments. Both upper and lower jaws retain teeth, including incisors, canines, premolars, and molars. However, many of the canid and bear artifacts are shorter than the human specimens from Mount Vernon, having had the rami completely removed (similar to the Snyders Mound specimens). Surface scratches are present on only 26 percent of the Tremper jaws, although these marks may be more difficult to discern due to the burning. There are few identifiable cut marks.

Figure 2.2 illustrates an important feature of many specimens from both Tremper and Mount Vernon. The ground apices of the tooth roots sometimes project below the inferior ground surface of the mandibular body. The best explanation for this phenomenon is that the specimen was still fresh enough to preserve the periodontal ligaments and other soft tissues surrounding the tooth roots while it was being ground. Over time (specifically, after burial), the ligaments decayed, allowing the teeth to drop farther down into the sockets. In forensic casework, periodontal ligaments are known to decay rapidly,

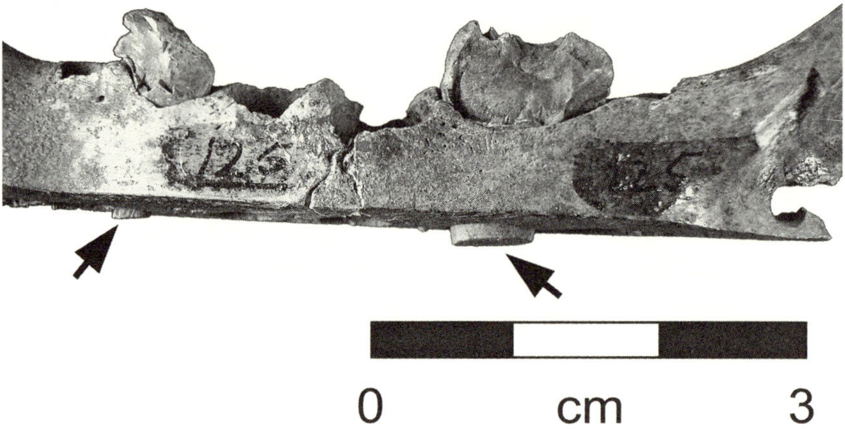

2.2. Tremper Mound, cougar left hemimandible FC-6, external view. Note how the ground tips of the tooth roots (*arrows*) project below the inferior margin of the corpus. (Photo by Stephen Nawrocki)

and the single-rooted anterior teeth frequently fall from the alveoli long before the skin, tendons, major joint ligaments, and cartilage are destroyed. The presence of endogenous bacteria and mucous membranes in the mouth, nose, and throat, which naturally attract necrophagous insects, helps to accelerate the decay of soft tissues in the facial region. If the jaws were removed from the decedents fairly quickly after death and processed manually to remove surface tissues, the periodontal ligaments could have dried (mummified), allowing the teeth to be held securely in the artifacts during later use and curation. Then, when they were eventually buried, the combination of ground water and bacteria would be sufficient to completely destroy the ligaments. Alternatively, if the jaws were boiled early in processing, as remains are commonly prepared in modern forensic cases, the periodontal ligament would quickly dissolve as the proteins in its collagen fibers denature. The single-rooted teeth would therefore fall out during curation and be lost prior to burial unless an adhesive was used to affix them in their sockets.

Therefore, the presence of single-rooted teeth in modified trophy jaws may be an important clue to the timing and extent of processing. Unfortunately, the Tremper assemblage is hard to assess because of damage caused by burning and postmortem fracturing. However, many of the jaw fragments include sockets for the anterior teeth, and a number of anterior tooth roots are present but now dissociated from the jaws. Of the 44 human teeth present in the Mount Vernon assemblage that are known or suspected to belong to the

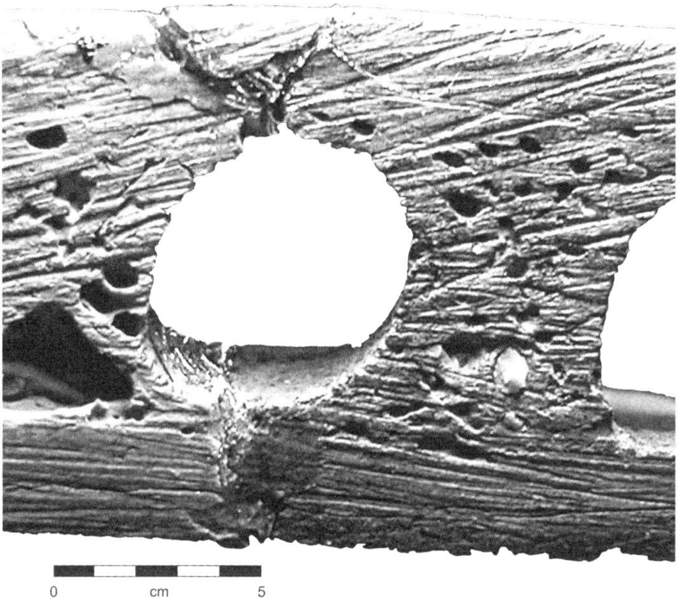

2.3. Tremper Mound, cougar left hemimandible FC-6, inferior view. The visible grinding striations cluster in multiple directions. (Photo by Stephen Nawrocki)

modified jaws, 1 is an incisor, 5 are canines, and 9 are premolars; furthermore, 11 incisor alveoli, 3 canine alveoli, and 13 premolar alveoli are preserved in an open (empty) and undamaged state. The careful and deliberate preparation of the anterior sections of the jaws strongly suggests that the craftspeople were attempting to preserve the anterior teeth in position as part of the final artifact, a premise supported by the fact that a number of other Hopewell trophy jaws still include anterior teeth. It is likely that the uncontrolled looting of the Mount Vernon jaws resulted in postmortem loss of single-rooted teeth. Therefore, in the absence of evidence of an adhesive used in the sockets (which, if organic, may also have decayed, leaving no trace), the presence of single-rooted teeth at Mount Vernon would seem to suggest that the jaws were processed (a) soon after death and (b) without boiling, resulting in mummified periodontal ligaments that held the teeth in place during their lives as curated possessions.

Figure 2.3 is a high-contrast image illustrating the grinding marks on the inferior surface of the corpus of the same cougar specimen shown in Figure 2.2. Note that adjacent marks are parallel, but clusters of marks in different areas of the object run in slightly different directions. This variety in grinding striation direction occurs as the specimen is rubbed in slightly different directions by the grinding medium, much the same as a woodworker moves the sandpaper when smoothing a piece of wood.

How do we know that grinding was the method of choice in producing these specimens? Many authors have referred to these as "cut jaws," implying the use of stone flakes or blades and sawing or scraping as the primary shaping technique. Cutting might seem more feasible as a means of producing such straight lines. However, the linear striations on the flattened surfaces are U-shaped in cross section, and there is no evidence of V-shaped cut marks along the edges of the modified surfaces.

Emanovsky (2002) tried to replicate the Mount Vernon and Tremper trophy jaws using fresh and dry human and animal hemimandibles. The specimens were drawn repeatedly along a fine-grained sandstone base, applying pressure to the inferior border of the body with each stroke. More than a centimeter of bone was removed in just under 90 minutes, producing an artifact that duplicated the same basic pattern seen in the prehistoric specimens. The inferior edge of the body is straight and square, and continued grinding would have exposed the tooth roots. It is clear that with practice and a more careful selection of raw materials (such as a coarser grindstone), the specimen could have been shaped fairly quickly into nearly any desired configuration.

The inferior edge of the experimental mandible displays grinding striations that are slightly narrower but very similar to those seen in the prehistoric caches. Toward the end of the grinding session, the direction of movement was deliberately altered in order to observe the effects on the striations. The last few draws across the sandstone block were made transversely, producing transversely oriented striations overlapping all the others. However, the easiest way to handle the specimen was to draw it lengthwise or slightly obliquely along the long length of the mandibular body, in which case the striations were oriented exactly as depicted for the Tremper jaw in Figure 2.3.

A Taphonomic Profile for the Mount Vernon and Tremper Caches

Of central importance to any taphonomic analysis is the construction of a taphonomic profile for the specimen or assemblage (Nawrocki 2009; Nawrocki et al. 1997; Schultz et al. 2003). The profile is composed of two parts. First, a description is made of any modifications to the remains, cataloging all insults that were not present during the normal lifetime of the individual. Second, the analyst extrapolates the general or specific causes of those modifications, in the process referring to previous studies or observations that tie those modifications to real-world causal agents, such as rodent gnawing or gunshots. A taphonomic profile is therefore both a description and a series of hypotheses that can be tested once the remains are identified (in forensic contexts) or when other specimens come to light or can be replicated (in archaeological contexts) (Nawrocki 2009).

The human and nonhuman animal jaws in the Mount Vernon and Tremper caches were all modified in a similar fashion using the same general reduction sequence. They therefore display a constellation of specific features that can serve as a profile against which specimens from other sites can be compared. Analysts may also refer to this profile when reviewing existing collections for previously unidentified trophy specimens, or when examining eroded fragments of jaws and teeth that do not seem to belong in a particular burial.

The inferior border of the mandibular corpus has been removed by grinding, leaving well-defined, U-shaped striations that may be transversely, obliquely, or longitudinally oriented with respect to the long axis of the jaw, depending on the direction that the specimens were drawn during the final stages of production. The tooth sockets are usually exposed and the root apices are ground away, especially in the anterior teeth (which sit lower in the jaw than the posterior molars in humans). The resulting inferior margins of the jaw are square, contrasting with the curving lower edge of an unworked mandible. The mandibular condyle and coronoid process are removed, and the superior border of the ramus is ground flat, usually sloping downward toward the posterior border in humans. The anterior and posterior borders of the ramus may or may not be ground, depending on the degree of shaping desired by the artisan. In some nonhuman specimens (particularly felids), the majority of the coronoid process may be retained and incised along its leading and trailing edges. In bears and canids, the ramus is completely removed by grinding, leaving only the corpus, and in this respect these specimens are similar to the heavily ground human mandible sections from Snyders Mound C°103 (Braun et al. 1982).

The human mandibular symphysis is snapped or cut in the midline and then ground flat, producing striations on the medial (lingual) surfaces of the symphysis and the corpus that are similar to those found on the inferior corpus. The mandibles of adult carnivorous mammals are generally unfused, and so less grinding is necessary to produce a flat medial surface. The lower central incisors may be removed or damaged during this phase of processing, especially in humans. In addition, telltale grinding facets may be created on the lingual surfaces of the (especially third) molar tooth crowns as the symphysis is being worked. Grinding facets are less frequently seen on the buccal surfaces of the tooth crowns. Lingual and buccal facets display clear grinding striations and are important because they may be the only indicators of trophy specimen status for loose teeth. Perforations were drilled near the front and back of each specimen, presumably for suspension as jewelry or for mounting on clothing. Partial obliteration of some perforations suggests that the specimens may have been suspended prior to or during the formal reduction sequence. Nonhuman animal maxillae have been processed in a fashion that is similar to how the mandibles were treated. Opposing sides are split along the midline, and the hard palate is removed completely. Tooth roots are exposed by grinding along the superior border.

Multiple lines of evidence suggest that the jaws were processed initially in a fresh state, while they still retained at least some soft tissue. First, most bone surfaces that are not ground display fine, U-shaped, superficial scratching marks that may be clustered or randomly oriented. These scratches did not serve to shape the specimens but appear to have been produced with loose sand or a similar abrasive that was applied to remove connective tissues or to even out irregular surface staining that occurred during decomposition. Second, the ground tips of the tooth root apices frequently fall below the ground inferior surface of the jaw, indicating that the periodontal ligaments were in place in the alveoli while the specimens were being ground. These ligaments were allowed to mummify and thus held the single-rooted teeth in place during the curational life of the artifacts, as evidenced by the presence of incisors and canines in the caches despite the fact that their tips had been removed by grinding, which would have loosened them even further in the absence of soft tissues. Together, these findings indicate that the jaws were not removed from subsurface burials or surface depositions that were more than a few days or weeks old, depending on the season and geographic location of the death. Instead, we must consider scenarios where the remains of the recently deceased were being accessed and harvested.

The high degree of modification of the Tremper and Mount Vernon jaws has erased most evidence of defleshing cut marks, so it remains unknown how much soft tissue had to be removed in order to acquire the specimens. The thin, easily accessible soft tissues of the face, jaws, and throat tend to decompose more quickly than tissues located in other areas of the body, particularly the limbs. In modern forensic casework, the bones of the face and jaws are frequently exposed after only a few days of warm weather. It is therefore possible that the jaws at least could have been harvested fairly shortly after death, with little defleshing or disarticulation being needed. The acquisition of complete trophy skulls, on the other hand, would require additional processing. The scalp and major muscle masses on the sides and back of the head usually decay more slowly than the facial tissues, and they can mummify if conditions are right, producing a tough protective coating that can retain an intact hair mat. Tissues of the neck tend to follow the decay trajectory of the face, and we have encountered numerous cases where the cervical vertebrae, mandible, and hyoid are free but the dried upper scalp is present.

Further detailed analysis of the more complete and less thoroughly modified trophy skulls from Ohio should help to clarify their processing history. Particularly relevant is the presence and proportion of scratching marks to cut marks and the distribution pattern of the cut marks relative to major muscle masses and ligaments. For example, the trophy skull included in Burial 5 of Hopewell Mound 2 displays numerous cut marks to the temporal bone and upper mandible, suggesting that the intact temporalis muscles were removed; the specimen also shows numerous scratches over most surfaces. Other specimens from the Hopewell Mound group display similar modifications (Johnston 2002; Seeman 1988). Our preliminary observations lead us to believe that at least some of the Ohio trophy skulls were sufficiently covered with soft tissues when initially processed to require both manual defleshing with stone knives and considerable detailed cleaning with abrasives.

Both of the assemblages that we examined display evidence that trophy jaws were curated or used after the processing was completed. Polishing and smoothing of edges and projections are particularly evident on the medial and lateral surfaces of the jaws, perhaps the result of long-term suspension on clothing or of handling. The burning of the Tremper specimens makes it difficult to see polishing, but they do not display any signs of the warping and twisting that would be found on bones burned in a fresh state (Baby 1954; Emanovsky 2002). This evidence suggests that the specimens were curated for some years after manufacture, allowing them to dry completely and lose their contained fat and collagen through bacterial action. Only then were they burned, perhaps when their owner died.

The complex sequence of modification and reduction of the Mount Vernon and Tremper jaws stands in contrast to the less complex modifications of many other skull and jaw trophy specimens at other Middle Woodland sites. While the basic grinding procedure is straightforward, replication studies demonstrate that it takes time and care to produce these artifacts. It is possible that we are seeing evidence of a small number of craftspeople who made these objects for very specialized purposes. It may be beneficial to reexamine curated bones from other Hopewell sites to determine whether additional specimens have been missed. The taphonomic profile of these artifacts is unique and may be recognized even on degraded specimens.

Discussion

This chapter offers two broad suggestions regarding human bone trophy specimens. The first is that a careful analysis of the production methods of highly modified and curated trophy jaws as represented by the Mount Vernon and Tremper Mound caches can give us different, perhaps unique, insights that may not be as forthcoming from the numerous isolated, less extensively modified specimens (including complete skulls) that have been found at various sites dating to the Middle Woodland period. Although small in size and limited in the number of anatomical features they present for analysis, the jaws in these caches nonetheless provide a more substantive sample for determining the biological characteristics of the decedents, who were more likely to have lived and died in the same general time frame and geographic region when compared to samples drawn from multiple mounds or sites. Furthermore, because the artifacts were extensively handled both during production and afterward, the details of the reduction and manufacturing process are more discernible and their status as curated items is more securely demonstrable.

Second, a forensic perspective that is overtly focused on the process of soft tissue decomposition, on the complex interplay between human remains and the surrounding depositional environment, on signatures of perimortem violence, and on distinguishing between the closely linked perimortem and postmortem intervals can help to ferret out additional clues regarding the history of these items. Before we can assess whether the artifacts are likely to be war trophies, revered ancestors, and/or ritual pieces, it could be helpful to determine, for example, whether the jaws were harvested from recently deceased, fully decomposed but unburied, or previously interred individuals. Clearly, the problem of trophy specimens is in no small part a taphonomic one, and thorough taphonomic profiling is an essential first step in the attempt to discern the cultural meaning of these artifacts. While the forensic perspective employed here does not produce radically different interpretations of these specimens than might have been offered by an analyst using traditional taphonomic and osteological methods, it does help to reframe the discussion and apply a body of experimental and observational data that may not be completely familiar to bioarchaeologists. In particular, a thorough understanding of the patterns of human soft tissue decomposition is important.

Another perspective brought by the forensic approach is a focus on determining the circumstances of death. In this respect, Hopewellian trophy specimens present at least one dramatic anomaly: few, if any, of them display any clear evidence of perimortem trauma that can be traced back to the death event and that might be indicators of a violent end for the decedent. None of the Mount Vernon, Tremper Mound, or Snyders Mound jaws display perimortem fractures of the remaining portions of their rami, corpi, alveoli, or teeth. Excluding dismemberment or other cut marks that *could* have occurred after death rather than having caused it, our examination of Early and Middle Woodland trophy specimens produced no clear and irrefutable evidence of death-related violent trauma. Johnston (2002:84), who is forensically trained also, came to a similar conclusion in her examination of many of the same specimens. In our experience with nonballistic interpersonal violence in modern forensic casework, perimortem fractures to the facial skeleton and teeth, while not ubiquitous, are certainly common enough that we would expect at least a few clear examples of facial trauma in the Hopewellian material if they were being acquired predominately through warfare. We must caution, however, that even in forensic cases, the interpretation of perimortem trauma is rarely straightforward. The bioarchaeological literature contains many erroneous assessments of postmortem fractures as death-related perimortem trauma, interpretations that were based on misunderstandings of fracture biomechanics and that would not survive scrutiny in a court of law. Helping to clarify the presence and extent of perimortem trauma in the bioarchaeological record may be the most significant contribution that the forensic perspective can make to this discussion.

Conclusion

Imagine a scenario in which anthropologists of the distant future locate, excavate, and analyze a serial homicide site from the ruins of a major American city. The victims' remains were altered in a fashion that was atypical of most other burials from that time period. Some bones display dismemberment marks, ritual modifications, and signs of selective curation and preferential treatment. Some of the unused portions of the victims are commingled, others have been scattered and discarded. While taphonomic analysis might be able to describe in great detail how the bones were modified and deposited, and osteological analysis could describe or even identify the victims, anthropologists of the future would be hard-pressed to understand the cultural significance and "meaning" of the modified remains without comprehending the highly unusual and stochastic phenomenon of a serial killer. The tendency would be to explain these artifacts in terms of "normal" cultural phenomena, such as warfare, ancestor worship, or religious acts—none of which would adequately explain the complex origin of the remains.

Hopewellian trophy jaws present a similar problem. Even with a solid understanding of how they were manufactured, an appreciation of the characteristics of the individuals from whom they were taken, and clear evidence of their long-term curation, do we understand their cultural significance any better? Unfortunately, it is difficult to construct testable hypotheses that can eliminate alternative theories explaining the artifacts' meaning. What do war victims look like compared to revered relatives? How do enslaved captives compare to voluntary sacrificial lambs? How would the pattern of cut marks, grinding, and polishing differ among these alternative sources? Without knowing the broader cultural context in which these artifacts were once embedded, our theories may reflect more about our own biases regarding the past than about the ancient world as it actually existed. Even the presumably straightforward hypothesis that war trophies are more likely to be composed of young adult males (Seeman 1988) is built on numerous untested assumptions about the practice and significance of warfare in prehistoric America. Furthermore, even if we find that the jaws were indeed derived from young adult males, we cannot reject the nonwar theories outright because other cultural patterns could, conceivably, produce the same demographic pattern (for example, systemic reverence for males who died of disease or accidents before marrying off their children). Johnston (2002; also see Johnston, this volume), in her attempt to test three alternative theories of the significance of trophy specimens from the Hopewell Mound group, rejected two and failed to find strong support for the third, leaving us with no real alternative—despite analysis of one of the largest and best-documented samples of culturally modified remains available.

Similarly, does knowing that all of the species represented by the Tremper jaws are predatory carnivores help us to understand their meaning? After hunters acquired the animals, they may have sold the jaws to specialized craftspeople, who produced and then sold the amulets to wealthy or important chiefs as signs of courage and prestige, to shamans or midwives as magical charms, to priests as religious icons, or, for all we know, to children as toys. Each time the jaws changed hands through this chain of production and consumption, their meaning and symbolism became more complex and more difficult for us to decipher. Therefore, solving the riddle of trophy jaws and skulls is dependent not only on completing detailed taphonomic and osteological analyses of the specimens themselves but also on our ability to construct a comprehensive picture of the cultural and behavioral context of a society from the broader archaeological record.

Acknowledgments

We would like to thank Tom Beard, Martha Otto, Cheryl Johnston, and the Ohio Historical Society for access to the specimens described here, and Christopher Schmidt and Matthew Williamson for their critical assistance during the data collection phase of the study. Comments provided by an anonymous external reviewer were extremely helpful in helping us to clarify and frame our ideas.

3
Objectifying Middle Woodland Mortuary Practices through the Inclusion of Modified Human Jaws

A Central Illinois River Valley Case Study

Dawn E. Cobb

The Native American Graves Protection and Repatriation Act's federally mandated inventory of human skeletal remains provided researchers with the opportunity to examine the Illinois State Museum's anthropology collections in their entirety. Included in these collections is a sample of intentionally modified human maxillae and mandibles. A review of the archaeological literature demonstrated that modified human jaws were present in several Middle Woodland mound sites in the central Illinois River valley (Baker et al. 1941; Cole and Deuel 1937; McGregor 1952; Meinkoth et al. 1995; Schoenbeck 1946, 1947; Shields 1978; Taylor 1929; Walker 1952; Wray and MacNeish 1961). Similarly worked human jaws were documented in the lower Illinois River valley, the central Mississippi valley, the Ohio valley, southwestern Indiana, and northwestern Georgia (Braun et al. 1982; Farnsworth and Atwell 2015; Jeffries 1976; Mills 1907, 1909b, 1916b; Nawrocki 1997; Perino 1968; Seeman 1988). These modified human jaws were found in Middle Woodland burial tombs as grave artifacts. They were either placed on an individual or were placed with the body much like a pottery vessel is included in the grave.

Why were modified human jaws incorporated into Middle Woodland mortuary practices? This chapter seeks to identify temporal and regional patterns through an analysis of the variation in cultural modification and their archaeological context. The significance of these objects in the Middle Woodland mortuary program is also explored by examining the cultural and temporal context of these items, where they were found on the landscape, and their placement in individual graves. Once we know how they are made and can identify variations in style and context, we are able to talk about human behavior and how social identity is reflected through mortuary behavior.

Review of Woodland Period Mortuary Practices

Mortuary practices of the Middle Woodland period are distinct from those of the Early Woodland and Late Woodland periods in the central Illinois River valley (Table 3.1). Esarey (1986:242) summarized this notion succinctly: "the interface of the Early and Middle Woodland periods marks a time of striking technological, ideological, and probably social, transformation. Changes in subsistence practices, ceramic technology, and mortuary ceremonialism in the period subsequent to Red Ochre and the Marion phase (Early Woodland) are radical and impressive." "Red Ochre" is best described as a set of burial practices that bridges Late Archaic *and* Early Woodland phases across the Midwest (Duane Esarey, personal communication 2013). In contrast to the Early and Late Woodland periods, the Middle Woodland mortuary program is characterized by the construction of larger complex mounds with ramps, elaborate log crypts, and subfloor tombs often containing the remains of one or more individuals, isolated crania, secondary burials, and an abundance and variety of local and exotic associated grave artifacts (Brown 1979; Cole and Deuel 1937; Moorehead et al. 1928). The mound constructed over log crypts and subfloor tombs was clearly intended for a specific segment of the local Middle Woodland societies (Baker et al. 1941; Cole and Deuel 1937; McGregor 1952; Meinkoth et al. 1995; Schoenbeck 1946, 1947; Shields 1978; Taylor 1929; Walker 1952). Fire was a component of Middle Woodland mortuary traditions and is evidenced by hearths in tombs and on tomb ramps. These hearth features were originally interpreted as cremation pits (Cole and Deuel 1937; Walker 1952; Wray and MacNeish 1961), but subsequent research by Asch (1976) and Buikstra (1976) demonstrated that human cremations were rare during the Middle Woodland, unlike during the Early Woodland period. Cremation, reported for some Early Woodland mounds, is not associated with Middle or Late Woodland mortuary treatments (Baker et al. 1941; Brown 1979; Cole and Deuel 1937; Eggan 1930; Ritzenthaler and Quimby 1962).

In stark contrast, Early and Late Woodland mounds lack the elaborate subfloor tombs and crypts seen during the Middle Woodland period, typically include a larger cross section of the population, and contain less variety of exotic artifacts; further, the burial positioning of the deceased is primarily flexed, semiflexed, or bundled. The Late Woodland mortuary program differs from both the Early and Middle Woodland periods in the introduction of deliberate postmortem processing of the dead. On a Late Woodland habitation site located on the bank of the Illinois River, human bone fragments are present in refuse pits and scattered across the site surface (Esarey et al. 1998). Cuts made on these scattered and discarded human bone fragments clearly show that dismemberment and defleshing occurred (Harn 1998). This indicates that, for the first time in the central Illinois River valley, retrieval of the dead for secondary burial sometimes occurred prior to full decomposition. Secondary burials from the Early and Middle Woodland periods do not

Table 3.1. Woodland Period Mortuary Traits in the Central Illinois River Valley

	Mound Location	Mound Structure	Burial Location in Mound	Burial Type	Diagnostic Artifact Types
Late Archaic/ Early Woodland transition 800–250 B.C.	absent or low mounds over natural ridges adjacent to river bottomlands, in habitation areas, bluff crests	absent or prepared surfaces of natural ridges or low mounds over natural ridges	absent or burials placed on ground surface and in pits below ridge surface	flexed, semiflexed, bundled, cremation	red ochre in graves, ovate cache blades, turkey-tail blades, copper awl, beads and plaque, shell beads and gorgets, Havana and Neteler Stamped pottery
Middle Woodland 250 B.C.– A.D. 250	floodplain, bluff base terrace, bluff top	dome- and conical-shaped, prepared mound floor, central subfloor tombs, log crypts, ramps, single or multiple tombs, crematory basin, intrusive burial pits in mound fill	subfloor tomb, above tomb, ramp, mound fill	extended, flexed, semiflexed, bundled, cremation, isolated skulls	modified human and animal jaws, shell and pearl beads, platform pipes, worked copper, worked animal bones, exotic raw materials (mica, galena, hematite), marine shells, projectile points, Hopewell pottery
Late Woodland A.D. 300–900	floodplain, bluff top ridges, habitation areas, stream-edge mortuary facility, isolated graves at margin of habitation area	low, dome-shaped	ground surface, accretional burial pits in mound	flexed, semiflexed, bundled	notched and stemmed points, boatstone, limestone discoidal, snail and shell beads, mussel shell spoons, Maples Mills pottery

have cut marks, which suggests that remains were gathered and reburied long after the individual's death.

Evidence for long-distance trade is present throughout the Woodland period. What distinguishes Middle Woodland from earlier and later periods is the variety of artifacts and materials present (e.g., marine shell ornaments, copper beads and adzes, drilled bear canines, effigy and platform pipes, elaborately decorated ceramics, obsidian tools and flakes, mica, and galena), which is indicative of a much-expanded trade network (Braun 1986; Brose and Greber 1979; Struever and Houart 1972) (Table 3.1). As an example, Illinois pipestone platform pipes are found in a variety of village and mortuary contexts in Illinois, but they are only found in mortuary sites in Ohio (Emerson et al. 2013). In contrast, certain rare classes of artifacts, in this case modified and decorated human jaws, are only found in Middle Woodland mounds. While their presence in graves is uncommon, their infrequent placement in tombs and with particular individuals implies that the recipients played a specific role in the local community. Such objects served to emphasize differences in social position—much more clearly than associated mortuary objects from the Early or Late Woodland periods.

The significance of modified human jaws in mortuary contexts is emphasized by their frequent association with a limited subset of artifacts, as noted by Farnsworth and Atwell (2015). The most common items include pearl, shell, and copper beads; split and drilled bear canines; copper axes and adzes; celts and blades; and platform pipes. Middle Woodland mortuary items not found in association with modified human jaws include pottery vessels, flint blades and points, worked animal jaws, worked and unworked animal teeth (excluding bear), and mica. The specific and restricted nature of the associated suite of artifacts found with modified human jaws suggests that the combination of particular items and the exclusion of others are intentional and important to the spiritual well-being of the deceased.

Modified Animal Jaws

Modified animal jaws occur in mortuary contexts throughout Illinois's prehistory, but during the Middle Woodland there was a significant increase in the manufacture and use of these bone ornaments, both human and animal (Parmalee 1959). Modified objects include cut and worked maxillae and mandibles, some with polishing or perforations. Thirteen animal species represented by modified skulls, jaws, and teeth include both predator and nonpredator species at 10 Middle Woodland sites in Illinois (Parmalee 1959). Parmalee identifies the predator species as black bear, gray wolf, bobcat, and mountain lion and the nonpredator species as fox, raccoon, squirrel, wolverine, otter, badger, coyote, domestic dog, and whitetail deer. Teeth of raccoons, foxes, and squirrels were also perforated and worn as necklaces or used as headdress decorations on human burials (Parmalee 1959:87, Figure 1). Parmalee observed that while most bones of birds and mammals worked into various tools and ornaments are found in prehistoric habitation sites, those of predators, like the black bear and gray wolf, are found primarily in association with Middle Woodland burials. The intentional choice was to hunt these predators for their valued skulls and teeth rather than for meat, hence the absence of postcranial remains of predators in midden and trash pits at prehistoric archaeological sites in Illinois. Parmalee (1959) believed that modified human and animal jaws were for personal ornamentation but that they also signified or had meaning as symbols of religion or bravery. Deuel (1952) offered two alternative meanings of these modified jaws. He believed that the predator jaws were chosen because of the powerful animals they represented. By extension, modified human jaws were important because they represented brave enemies. In both instances, the purpose behind the modified elements was trophy taking. The alternative hypothesis presented by Deuel was that the human jaws had religious significance and may have represented a relative or friend (ancestor worship).

Another interpretation of the modified jaws is the belief that there exists a metaphorical link between humans and predators when one considers the possible meaning of the mouth. This is where the animal holds its power, and in humans this can be seen as the power of the voice. As humans, our expression of ourselves through our voices can be viewed as a social tool or "weapon." In animals, the teeth are seen by humans as something to avoid because of their use in defense or hunting. If you harness or capture the source of the "weapon," the source of the power is captured.

As modern researchers, we will not truly know the reasons for modifying human and animal jaws. Multiple interpretations have been offered, and each is plausible in the context of Middle Woodland mortuary practices. One is the predator-prey theory offered by Deuel (1952) and Parmalee (1959). Predator animals are chosen for the specific elements that represent their power. When their jaws or teeth are worn or carried, you have conquered them. Deuel (1952) offered two explanations for the modified human jaws. One is similar to the predator theory: you have captured or conquered a human enemy. The other is ancestor worship. Parmalee (1959) agreed with Deuel in that the human jaws could be symbolic of religion or bravery.

Another explanation is that the modified animal and human jaws represent a form of honoring the perceived role of the animal spirit, which may be important to society beyond being predatory in nature. This relationship could be interpreted as totemic, mythic, or symbolic. I propose that the intent was to honor the animal rather than the more confrontational meaning of man vs. beast. Humans are included in my interpretation because they belong to the animal kingdom. Supporting evidence for this is the presence of human, predator, and nonpredator modified jaws at Middle Woodland sites in Illinois.

Archaeological Context of Middle Woodland Modified Human Jaws

This section describes the archaeological context of modified human jaws in terms of their physical location on the landscape, their placement in grave features, where they occur relative to the body, and the presence of other associated artifact types. The central valley is a 135 km stretch of the Illinois River with Chillicothe as the northern boundary and the Sangamon River near Beardstown as the southern boundary (Woermann 1902–1904). The study area encompasses the floodplain, terrace slopes, and both bluff edges. Over the past hundred years, professional and amateur archaeologists have investigated 9 Middle Woodland mound sites in this region. These sites are listed in Table 3.2, from north to south as they occur in the valley. Fewer than half of the 117 Middle Woodland mounds in this region have been excavated. The majority of the excavated mounds are located on the floodplain and terrace. Farnsworth and Atwell (2015) noted that floodplain mounds (e.g., Liverpool, Ogden-Fettie, Neteler, Sister Creeks, and Weaver) are early Middle Woodland constructions in the central Illinois valley. Internal construction and datable artifacts from these floodplain mounds support this assessment (Cole and Deuel 1937; Farnsworth 2004; McGregor 1952; Moorehead et al. 1928; Taylor 1929). A modern radiocarbon date from a preserved log tomb in Liverpool F°77[1] produced an uncalibrated date of 60 B.C. +/- 70 (ISGS-1853) (Farnsworth and Atwell 2015). Toward the latter part of the Middle Woodland period, there is a shift in the placement of mounds from the floodplain to the nearby terraces (Dickison) and bluff tops (e.g., Hannah, Weaver, Clear Lake, and Frederick) in this region (Farnsworth and Atwell 2015). The Weaver site is unusual in that it has both floodplain and bluff crest Middle Woodland mounds. The later shift in locality may reflect a desire to avoid seasonal flooding. Relocating habitation and mortuary sites to higher ground would also facilitate burial and access to the mounds during periods of high water.

Of the excavated mounds, only 25 percent contain modified human jaws (see Table 3.2). Ninety-four percent of the modified human jaws occur as grave offerings in floodplain and terrace mounds, specifically at Weaver, Liver-

Table 3.2. Geographical Locations of Central Illinois River Valley Middle Woodland Mounds

	Floodplain Mounds	Terrace Mounds	Bluff Crest Mounds	Number of Modified Human Jaws*
Hannah (11P77)	0	0	2	0
Dickison (11P5)	0	12	0	2
Weaver (11F61)	14	0	36	1
Liverpool (11F24)	4	0	0	10
Sister Creeks (11F15)	0	23	0	8
Ogden-Fettie (11F58)	0	26	0	3
Clear Lake (11MN1, 11T1)	0	0	3	0
Neteler (11MN2)	5	0	0	7
Frederick (11SC11)	0	0	4	0
Total	23	61	45	31

Note: *Paired hemimandibles are counted as a single item.

pool, Sister Creeks,[2] Ogden-Fettie, and Neteler. Middle Woodland mounds located away from the river on the bluff crests contain only 6 percent of the modified human jaws. It is significant that floodplain mound sites have a higher count of modified human jaws.

A total of 281 individuals are reported from the excavated mounds[3] (Table 3.3). Most individuals (62 percent) were interred in tombs while 38 percent were interred in intrusive pits. Only 5 percent of all individuals buried in the mounds have modified human jaws directly associated with them (Baker et al. 1941; Cole and Deuel 1937; McGregor 1952; Meinkoth et al. 1995; Moorehead et al. 1928; Morse and Morse 1965; Perkins 1965; Ribick 2004; Schoenbeck 1946, 1947; Shields 1978; Taylor 1929; Walker 1952; Wray and MacNeish 1961). Although additional modified human jaws are reported in the archaeological literature, only those with reliable contextual documentation are included in this chapter.

Thirty-one modified maxillae and mandibles are reported in the literature. They occur primarily in tombs and secondarily in nontombs, or intrusive pits (Table 3.4). One modified mandible is present from Liverpool, but its specific mound and burial provenience are not known. Nearly all (73 percent) modified jaws are found in association with single primary interments, but a few are included with multiple (13 percent) primary individuals and bundled (13 percent) remains. The majority of the modified human jaws are placed directly on or beside the body. Typically, maxillae are placed on the individual's

Table 3.3. Mound Context of Modified Human Jaws

	Mounds Present	Mounds Excavated	Mounds with Modified Jaws	Skeletons in Tombs	Skeletons in Intrusive Pits	Modified Jaws Reported*	Modified Jaws Reanalyzed
Hannah (11P77)	2	1	0	18	1	0	0
Dickison (11P5)	12	2	1	34	24	2	0
Weaver (11F61)	38	17	1	61	25	1	0
Liverpool (11F24)	7	3	3	11	1	10	7
Sister Creeks (11F15)	23	2	2	9	3	8	7
Ogden-Fettie (11F58)	26	13	3	13	0	3	1
Clear Lake (11MN1, 11T1)	3	1	0	7	5	0	0
Neteler (11MN2)	5	2	2	0	30	7	1
Frederick (11SC11)	4	4	0	21	18	0	0
Total	120	45	12	174	107	31	16

Note: *Paired hemimandibles are counted as a single item.

Table 3.4. Burial Associations of Modified Human Jaws

	Tomb	Nontomb	By Skeleton	On Skeleton	No Skeleton Association
Maxillae	3	1	2	1	1
Mandibles*	12	2	1	12	1
Total	15	3	3	13	2

Note: *Paired hemimandibles count as a single item.

chest and mandibles are placed on or around the forearms and wrists. In Liverpool F°79, a maxilla was found on an individual's chest and a pair of hemimandibles was found around a wrist of the same skeleton (Dickson ca. 1945).

Two maxillae were found next to skeletons at Liverpool F°77, one between two skeletons in a tomb and the other below the feet of an individual in an intrusive pit (Cole and Deuel 1937). At Sister Creeks F°61-2, eight mandible fragments (six left and two right) were found on the lower arm of an adult skeleton (Schoenbeck 1946, 1947). The same placement of paired hemimandibles is found at Sister Creeks F°61-4, Ogden-Fettie F°166 and F°192, and Neteler MN°6 (Schoenbeck 1946, 1947; Shields 1978). A single bundle burial in Ogden-Fettie F°36 and Neteler MN°9 each have an associated hemimandible with them, but the notes do not clearly state whether the mandibles were on or beside the bundles (Cole and Deuel 1937). Two isolated crania at Neteler MN°9 had two modified maxillae with them but, like the bundle burials, the maxillae are noted as present only and no placement is given (McGregor 1952). In two mound contexts, Cole and Deuel (1937) reported instances where a modified jaw was found some distance from the body. One is a maxilla from Liverpool F°77 that was found in a fire basin in the corner of the tomb. The other is a paired hemimandible from Sister Creeks F°54 that was found about a foot away from a skeleton. Its location is interpreted as being in a medicine bundle with a projectile point, three hawk claws, and 85 small beads (Cole and Deuel 1937).

The inclusion of modified human maxillae and mandibles is potentially one of the most informative categories of mortuary artifact due to the relatively rare occurrence in Middle Woodland tombs and due to the varied styles of production. The presence of this object seems to signify that the recipient held an important social position in the community. But to whom did the donor jaws belong? Some researchers (Deuel 1952; Moorehead 1922; Webb and Snow 1945) believed that the curation of modified jaws represented either ancestor worship or war trophies. Seeman (1988, 2007) studied modified jaws and crania from Middle Woodland sites in Ohio. Citing examples of trophy taking in Mississippian art and from ethnographic examples from Native American Plains groups, Seeman suggested that modified jaws represent conflict-related trophies derived from adult males since males were most commonly involved in warfare. Seeman (2007) also proposed the idea of a metaphorical link between animal predators and humans. The Ohio data have shown that human jaws were the most frequently modified species followed by wolf, bear, mountain lion, and bobcat (Seeman 2007). In Ohio Middle Woodland sites, animal jaws were interpreted to have meaning as predator jaws. If you display evidence of having conquered an animal predator, you are displaying your success over that animal and its power. Therefore, displaying both predator and human jaws could be connected to warfare and trophy taking (Seeman 2007).

Demographic Attributes of Modified Jaws

Examination of the available modified human jaws followed standard osteological methods (e.g., dental eruption and attrition) to determine age at death (Buikstra and Ubelaker 1994; Smith 1991; Ubelaker 1978; White and Folkens 2005). Most donor jaws are from young adults. The Liverpool sample includes three young adults, two middle-aged adults, and two adults (>20 years). The Sister Creeks hemimandibles are from three young adults, two middle-aged adults, and four adults (>20 years). The hemimandibles from Ogden-Fettie and Neteler are each from a young adult. Sex estimates for modified jaws are limited since modification tends to remove or alter areas of the mandible used to estimate sex (e.g., gonial angle, symphysis, and ramus).

Age and sex data for those individuals buried with modified jaws are limited to an adult male from Sister Creeks Mound F°54, from Ogden-Fettie Mounds F°166 and F°192, and from Neteler MN°9 (Cole and Deuel 1937; McGregor 1952; Shields 1978). Neither age nor sex data are available for the individuals from Liverpool, Sister Creeks Mound F°61, or Neteler MN°6, although the available reports for each site seem to indicate that most were adults.

Cultural Modifications of Human Jaws

Of the 31 modified human jaws recorded in the archaeological literature of the central Illinois River valley, only 16 were available for reexamination by the author (Table 3.3). The missing modified jaws are 2 mandibles from Dickison (Walker 1952), 1 mandible from Weaver (Wray and MacNeish

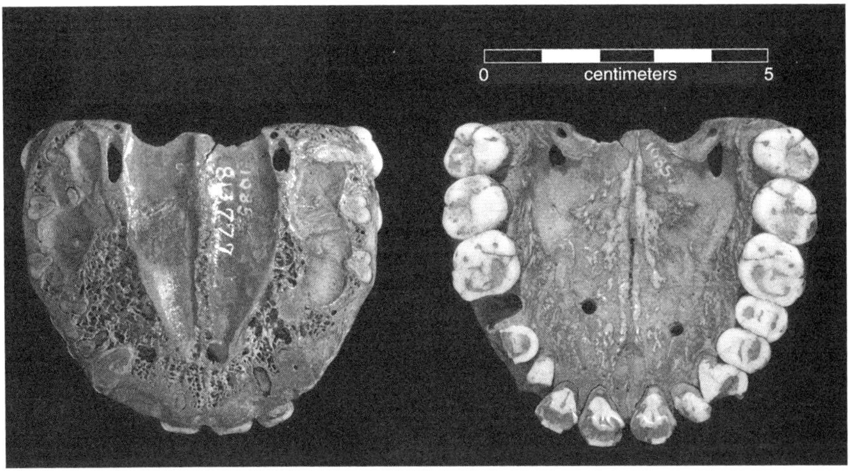

3.1. Superior and inferior surfaces of a modified human maxilla, Liverpool F°77. (Courtesy of Illinois State Museum Achives)

1961), 3 maxillae from Liverpool (Cole and Deuel 1937), 1 mandible fragment from Sister Creeks (Schoenbeck 1946, 1947), 2 mandibles from Ogden-Fettie (Cole and Deuel 1937; Shields 1978), and 4 to 5 maxillae and 1 mandible from Neteler (McGregor 1952). Information included in the following regarding these missing examples is derived from the limited descriptions in the literature and field records.

Maxillae

The maxillae have been modified by separating the inferior portion from the nasal bones and both zygomatics. The bones of the maxillary sinus and nasal aperture are reduced and ground smooth to follow the natural curvature of the palate. Exposed tooth roots are also ground to this level, leaving only the dental arcade, alveolar bone, and palate (Figure 3.1). Two perforations made in the palate, one on either side of the anterior incisive suture, are most likely for suspension. The holes are beveled but not polished.

Four maxillae are present from Liverpool F°77 and F°79, and each is covered with red ochre and/or green mineral staining. These decorative alterations were made subsequent to their reduction (Table 3.5). All features (cancellous and cortical bone, sinus cavities, and tooth dentine and roots) of the Liverpool F°77, Tomb 4, maxilla are stained (Figure 3.2). The superior surfaces are thickly covered with red ochre. Green mineral staining is evident beneath the red ochre on the cancellous bone and tooth roots. The natural bone color of the superior maxilla is completely obscured by the green and red staining. On the inferior surfaces, red ochre staining covers the majority

Table 3.5. Intersite Modification Styles

	Dickison	Weaver	Liverpool	Sister Creeks	Ogden-Fettie	Neteler
Maxillae	0	0	7	0	0	4–5
modified[a]	–	–	7	–	–	4–5
stained/painted	–	–	4	–	–	–
unknown[c]	–	–	3	–	–	4–5
Mandibles[b]	2	1	3	9	3	2
modified[a]	2	1	3	7	3	2
stained/painted	–	–	3	2	1	0
squared posterior	–	–	–	6	1	1
rounded posterior	–	–	1	0	–	0
notched posterior	–	–	–	3	–	1
unknown[c]	2	1	2	3	2	1

Notes: [a]Modified = cut, ground, perforated, polished.
[b]Hemimandible pairs count as a single item.
[c]Unknown = no reported modification (e.g., reduction, grinding, or staining).

of the palate and the alveolar bone, but patches of natural bone coloration are present. The occlusal surfaces of the teeth, including the exposed dentine, have patchy red ochre staining. Green staining is also present on the inferior maxilla, primarily on the left posterior palate, the exposed dentine, and within the alveolar sockets of three missing teeth (M^3, I^2, and I^1). On the right inferior surface, the exposed dentine of the three right molars is also lightly stained green. The maxilla from Liverpool F°77, Tomb 5, is lightly stained with red ochre on the superior and inferior surfaces, but the exposed dentine is not stained. The staining is darker on the superior surfaces, especially over the anterior portion of the alveolar bone. There is no green staining on this maxilla. Two commingled human teeth have been placed in each of the above maxillae to complete the dental arcades, either prehistorically during the modification process or historically by the original collector.

Two modified maxillae from Liverpool F°79 have red ochre and green mineral staining. One has moderate red ochre staining that covers most of the bone, including the superior and inferior surfaces, dental calculus, and exposed dentine. Green mineral staining is present on the center of the superior and anterior surfaces and covers exposed tooth roots and most of the exposed nasal cavity. In addition, some of the enamel on the anterior teeth is missing postmortem, and the exposed dentine is stained green. The other maxilla from F°79 has both prehistoric modifications and modern repairs. The pre-

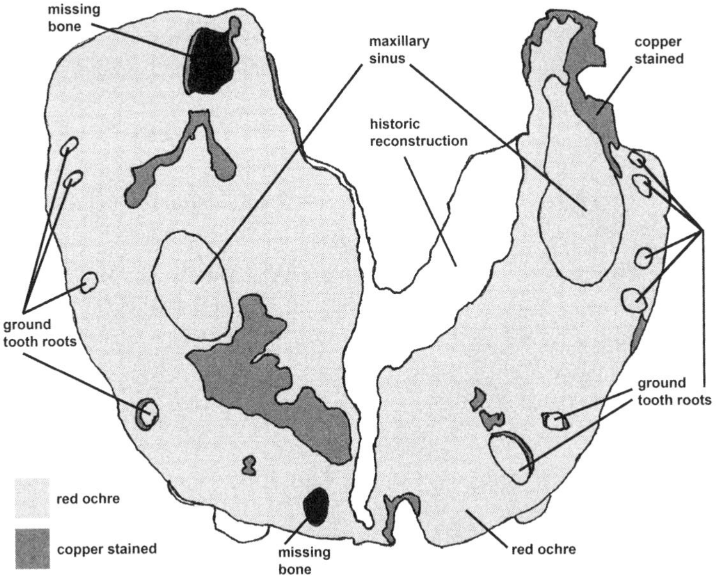

3.2. Sketch of a maxilla (superior view), showing red ochre paint covering copper staining, Liverpool F°77, Tomb 4. (Courtesy of Illinois State Museum Archives)

historic modification includes red and green staining of the superior surfaces with the red ochre covering the green mineral staining. The green discoloration is evident on the exposed cancellous bone and around a tooth root on the right superior maxilla. The inferior bone surfaces and exposed dentine are not stained. The modern repair is a partial reconstruction with plaster that covers approximately 60 percent of the palate. Features of the normal bone and the original modifications are replicated, and these include the palatine, the alveolar sockets for two right molars (M^2 and M^3), and light red staining over the plaster. The plaster was colored red to mimic red ochre.

Although the maxillae from Neteler MN°9 are not available for analysis, McGregor (1952:65) reported that they were each ground and perforated. He did not provide any details regarding additional decoration.

Mandibles

All hemimandibles have been worked and ground to reduce the height of the body and the width of the ramus (Figure 3.3). The coronoid processes and mandibular condyles of the ramus are removed, and the bone is separated into halves at the chin along the symphysis. The inferior body of the man-

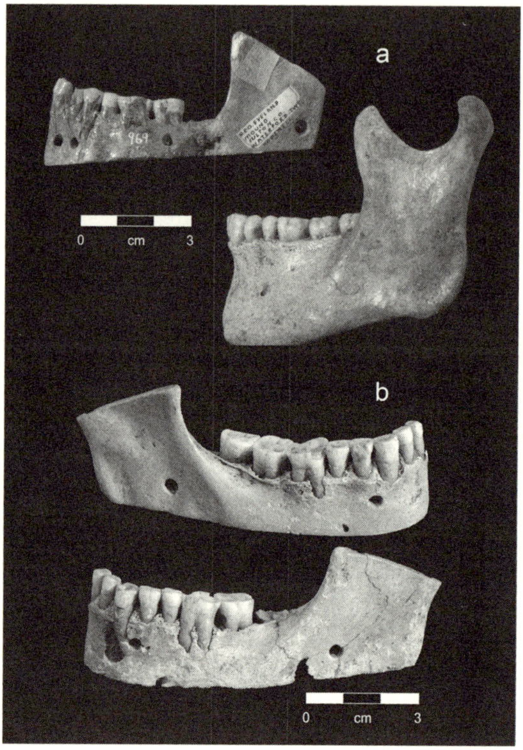

3.3. (a) Final modification of a human mandible (*top*) compared with an unmodified human mandible (*bottom*); (b) modified human hemimandibles, Sister Creeks F°54. (Courtesy of Illinois State Museum Archives)

dible, including the tooth roots, is reduced to the level of the mental foramen. These modified surfaces are ground flat, smoothing all natural contours of the bone. Cancellous bone is exposed on all ground surfaces, and striations are clearly visible (Figure 3.4). The lingual surfaces of the hemimandibles are also ground, typically from the second molar to the posterior ramus and often on the lingual crown and root surfaces of the third molars. All hemimandibles are perforated through the width of the anterior body and the ramus, at the level of the mental foramen. The holes are typically placed near the canine and the center of the ramus. Most of the holes are beveled; one mandible has polish along the edges of the perforation. In addition to the reduction of the ramus, this area of the mandible has been further modified by angling the superior margin posteriorly, rounding the superior margin, or notching the posterior margin.

The mandibles are lightly stained red and/or green. Three hemimandibles are present at Liverpool F°77, F°78, and F°79. The F°77 hemimandible is a left body fragment with two teeth (M_1 and M_2). A single perforation is drilled through the width of the body immediately anterior and posterior to

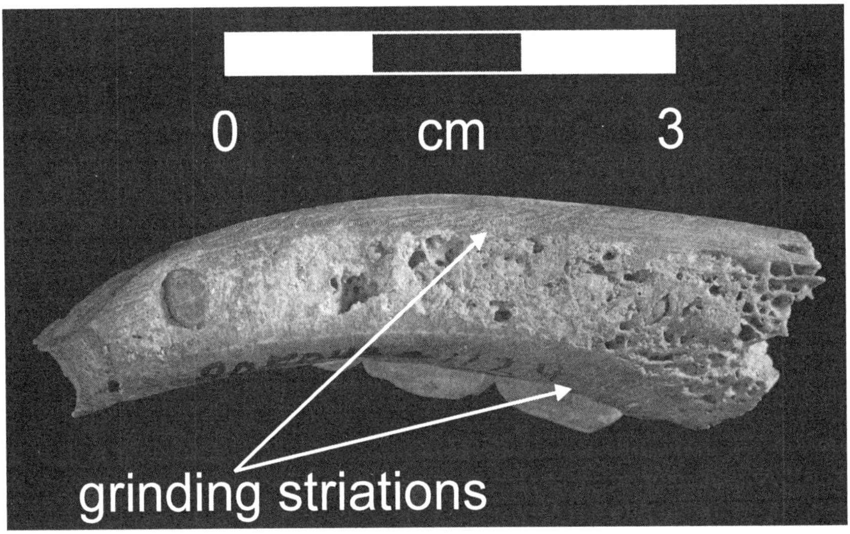

3.4. Grinding striations on an inferior mandible, Liverpool F°78. (Courtesy of Illinois State Museum Archives)

these teeth for a total of two perforations. The fragment is broken through both of the perforations, and it is not known if additional perforations were present elsewhere on the bone. The buccal surface of the body and the molar roots are decorated with red ochre. Green staining is evident on the inferior surface, on the lingual roots of the second molar, and in the alveolar socket for the third molar. A left hemimandible body fragment from Liverpool F°78 has five teeth (M_2 to C). A single perforation is located between the premolars and another is posterior to the second molar. The latter perforation is broken in half, and the rest of the posterior mandible is missing. Red staining is evident on the buccal and inferior surfaces, and green staining is evident on the inferior and lingual surfaces at the second and third molars. Complete and paired hemimandibles from F°79 are each double perforated: on the anterior body and on the ramus. The superior margins of each ramus are rounded, incised in a scallop pattern, and polished. These surfaces are also lightly stained with red ochre (Figure 3.5).

The mandible bodies from the Sister Creeks site (F°54 and F°61) are each reduced and perforated similarly to those from Liverpool. The hemimandibles from F°54 are complete, and the superior rami are cut square and angled posteriorly (see Figure 3.3). The posterior margin of the left ramus is ground until flat. The posterior right ramus retains its natural curvilinear shape. Both hemimandibles are polished, especially on the ground surfaces

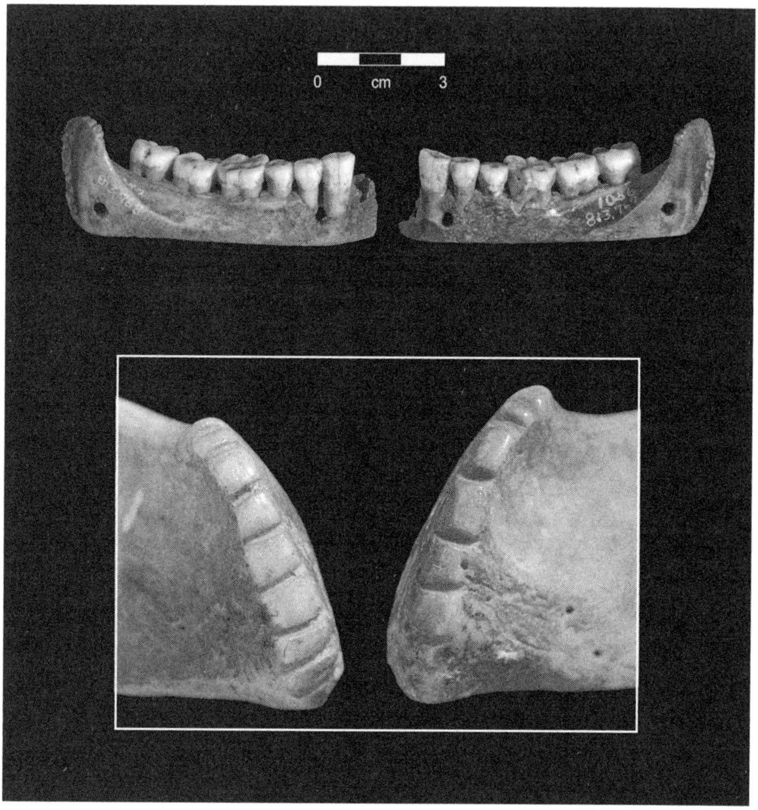

3.5. Modified human hemimandibles, Liverpool F°79 (*top*); detail of rounded and incised mandibular rami, Liverpool F°79 (*bottom*). (Courtesy of Illinois State Museum)

and the perforation margins. Unlike the Liverpool examples, neither bone is stained. Nine (six left and three right) modified mandible fragments from F°61 were combined in the original private collection and could not be differentiated by specific burial provenience. Each of these fragments is modified and ground as previously described, with several exceptions. None have green staining and only two left fragments have light red ochre staining on the buccal surfaces. Three left mandible fragments have square-cut superior rami and notched posterior rami (Figure 3.6). The superior rami of six other fragments (three right and three left) in the sample are broken, and this modification cannot be confirmed. A right mandible fragment has 11 cut marks on the posterior ramus margin just superior to the gonial angle. These are likely disarticulation cuts from separating the mandible from the cranium. This sug-

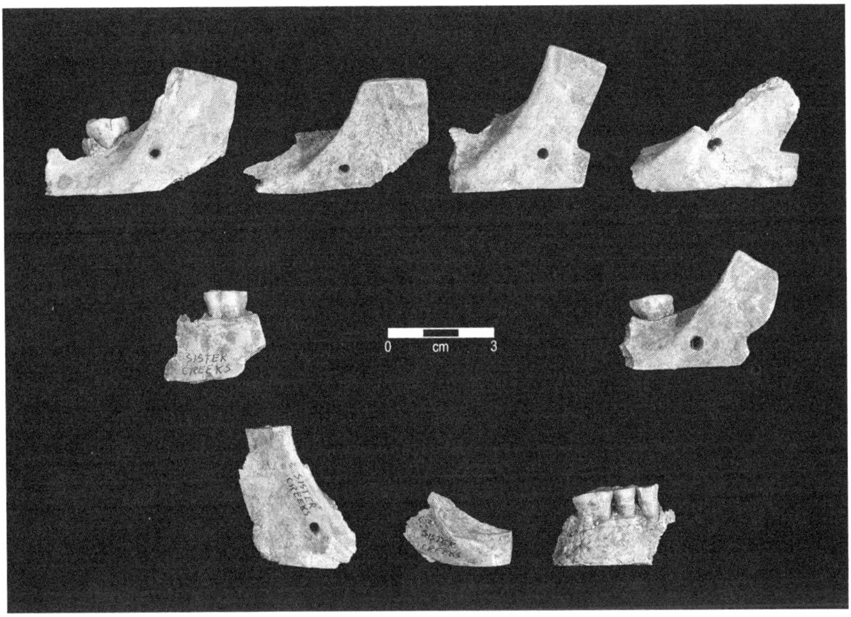

3.6. Modification styles of posterior mandibular rami, Sister Creeks F°61. (Courtesy of Illinois State Museum)

gests that the mandible was removed for modification fairly soon after death and before the complete decomposition and disarticulation of the donor.

The superior rami of the complete Ogden-Fettie F°166 hemimandibles are squared and angled posteriorly (see Figure 3.3a). The margin of the left posterior ramus is worked until flat, but the right is not. Multiple holes are drilled into each hemimandible, but not all of the holes perforate the width of the body. Both halves have two complete perforations on the anterior body and one on the posterior ramus. The right mandibular portion has three additional perforations on the body inferior to the second and third molars, but only two of these holes are completely drilled. The third hole does not penetrate through the body. The left half has four additional perforations inferior to the second and third molars. Three of these are incomplete, and only one perforates through to the lingual surface. Both hemimandibles have broken at one of the holes drilled through the body near the third molar. The multiple holes drilled in these bones may represent either a mistake during manufacture or, more likely, an attempt to repair the broken items. These hemimandibles reportedly had an additional modification of the ramus not noted in previous studies. A ramus was separated from the mandibular body and perforated for ornamentation (Dickson ca. 1945; Shields 1978). This modification could not be confirmed because the ramus is not included with the hemimandibles. Dickson (ca. 1945) reported that the ramus was found lying near the arm and may have been worn as a bracelet, like the paired mandible halves. Farnsworth and Atwell (2015) believed that the placement of the mandibles on the forearms could be attributed to their being used as decoration on clothing or to their being strung on cordage or a leather thong that was then placed with the deceased. Neither of these bones is stained.

One entire hemimandible pair from Neteler MN°6 was available for documentation. The superior ramus of the right hemimandible is angled posteriorly, squared, and notched. It has three complete perforations, one on the anterior body and two on the posterior ramus. The left hemimandible has the two anterior perforations, but the ramus is missing, and additional stylistic modifications, if once present, are not observable. Neither of these bones has red or green staining.

It is important to note that none of the green-stained maxillae or hemimandibles was found in direct contact with a copper artifact. Green mineral staining on bone occurs when it is in direct and prolonged contact with copper or copper alloy items (Buikstra and Ubelaker 1994; Schindelholz and Storch 2001). The green staining in this sample, however, is more than a surface expression on the maxillae and mandibles. It extends into the cancellous bone. There are two possible explanations for the green staining. One is that the green mineral staining existed on the bones prior to their being selected for modification. Perhaps the donor individual was buried with one or more copper objects, which stained the bone. The intentional selection of these discolored bones implies that specific individuals were chosen, perhaps for their status in life and perhaps for their stained jaws. The inclusion of copper items on the remains of the deceased and the subsequent selection of green-stained jawbones suggest that the donor was a person of significant status in the community. Could the donor have been an ancestor worthy of veneration, as was suggested by Deuel (1952)? The alternative explanation is that the staining occurred after the reduction of the jaws. Three of the four modified maxillae from Liverpool have green staining on the superior surfaces, and one is stained on the inferior surface as well. Although the green staining is mostly covered by red ochre, it appears to cover much of the superior surfaces and is a darker, more intense coloration. The maxillae may have been covered in copper and curated until they were needed for inclusion with the deceased. Green staining on mandibles is only present at Liverpool. The discolored surfaces are the lingual and inferior. Logically, these surfaces must have lain on a copper object (i.e., been curated) after being modified. Unlike the maxillae, the green staining on the mandibles is light and patchy, which likely reflects less contact time with copper.

The presence of red ochre staining on both modified maxillae and mandibles becomes important when we consider the sequence of events leading up to their deposition in a tomb. When green staining is present on the maxilla, it has been covered with red ochre. In the Liverpool examples, red ochre was heavily applied to one of the maxillae and lightly to moderately applied to the other three. Clearly, the green mineral staining was present on these maxillae before they were covered with red ochre. The action of applying red ochre over the green-stained bone shows an intentional choice in the object to be decorated. What is important about the three maxillae with light to moderate red ochre staining is that the staining occurs over all the bone surfaces. If the maxillae were chosen to be placed on the remains as ornamentation, only the superior or the inferior surface would be visible, depending on how the bone was oriented on the body. Red ochre would then be sprinkled over the remains as part of the burial process and would only affect the exposed surface of the maxilla. This is not the case with the other three maxillae from Liverpool. The fact that all surfaces of these maxillae have red ochre staining demonstrates that these bones were not modified for a single burial event; the decoration represents a deliberate application of pigment. They were reused multiple times, as evidenced by the multiple colored surfaces. The heavy application of red ochre on one maxilla can be interpreted as a reapplication of the pigment. The light to moderate red ochre on the other three maxillae can be interpreted as their being curated and reused for different people or for different ritual events.

On each of the hemimandibles, the green staining is primarily located on the lingual and inferior surfaces, and the red ochre staining is located on the buccal and occlusal surfaces. This differential staining could occur if the donor mandible were from an individual who had been buried with a copper object on the chest or around the neck. The light red staining likely occurred during the burial process as red ochre was scattered over the remains. Therefore, both the green mineral staining and the red ochre staining of the hemimandibles are unintentional decorations.

The maxillae occur in early Middle Woodland contexts where red ochre predominates in the mortuary program. Hemimandibles also occur during the early Middle Woodland, but they are retained as part of the mortuary program throughout the Middle Woodland whereas the maxillae are not. The green discoloration on both the maxillae and the mandibles occurred as an unintentional decoration of these elements. The bones became stained from direct and prolonged contact with a copper item during the original burial process or after the initial reduction of these elements. The red ochre staining occurred by either a direct or an indirect application of the pigment. The direct staining occurred when the red ochre pigment was applied to the maxilla. An example of this is from Liverpool F°77, Tomb 4. In contrast, indirect red ochre staining occurred on the modified maxillae and mandibles when the pigment was sprinkled over the remains during the burial process. The modified jawbones would have been placed on the body and then subsequently became stained after the application of the red ochre. This would account for only certain surfaces being stained. Alternatively, the red ochre staining of all surfaces of the Liverpool maxillae could have been the result of the items having been stored and only brought out for infrequent use in rituals and/or for additional modification, such as adding more pigmentation.

The absence of polish along the edges of the perforations on the modified maxillae and hemimandibles suggests that these objects were not regularly worn as ornaments. One explanation is that the ornaments were temporarily interred with a deceased individual and retrieved from the individual for specific rituals at a later time. Simply put, modified human jaws were created for the dead and not the living.

Comparison of the Central Illinois River Valley Samples

A comparison of the six central Illinois River valley sites with modified human jaws shows clear differences among them in the elements modified and in the style of modification. The primary difference is that both maxillae and mandibles are found at Liverpool and Neteler, while only mandibles are found at Dickison, Weaver, Sister Creeks, and Ogden-Fettie (Figure 3.7). Two unmodified human mandibles are also reported from Sister Creeks (central pit of F°54 and the log tomb of F°61). These items may represent intentional offerings, but they may also be elements that were left behind when cleaning out the tomb. Because their exact purpose and association are unknown, they have been removed from the data set.

The modification techniques of reducing, grinding, and perforating are similar among the six sites, but the decorative styles vary. Rounded and incised rami are found at Liverpool, while squared and notched rami are characteristic of Sister Creeks, Ogden-Fettie, and Neteler. The decorative use of red ochre pigment also differs between sites. At Liverpool red ochre was used on each modified jaw. The application of red ochre varied from light to heavy with the maxillae receiving the heaviest application of the pigment and the mandibles having the lightest application. Two of the nine hemi-

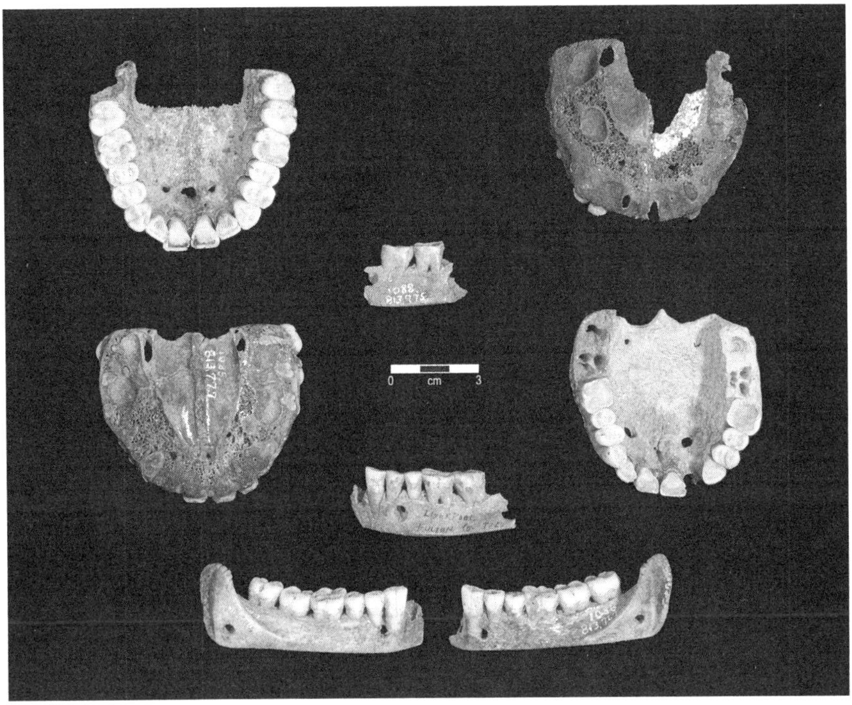

3.7. Modified maxillae and mandibles, Liverpool F°77, F°78, and F°79. (Courtesy of Illinois State Museum)

mandible fragments from Sister Creeks F°61 have light red ochre on them. Green mineral staining is found in association with red ochre staining only at Liverpool, where three maxillae and two hemimandibles have both colors on them; on two maxillae, the red ochre clearly covers the green staining. In contrast, the mandibles from Sister Creeks F°54, Ogden-Fettie, and Neteler have no red or green staining.

Comparison of Indiana and Ohio Data with Central Illinois Data

Modified human crania and mandibles are also known from Middle Woodland sites in Ohio and Indiana (Mills 1907, 1909b, 1916b; Nawrocki 1997; Seeman 1988, 2007; Webb and Snow 1945). Table 3.6 compares the traits of Ohio and Indiana modified human bone with the central Illinois River valley examples. In Ohio and Illinois, modified jaws are found primarily in burial contexts and, less frequently, in nonmortuary contexts (e.g., secondary deposits in caches, disturbed contexts). Modified human jaws from Indiana

Table 3.6. Comparison of Modification Styles from Ohio and Illinois

Ohio Trait	Element Modified	Central Illinois River Valley Trait	Element Modified
burial artifacts	cranium	burial artifacts	mandible
nonburial deposits	mandible	nonburial deposits	maxilla
cleaning/disarticulation	maxilla	disarticulation	adult canine
cutting		cutting	
grinding		grinding	
painting		perforation	
polishing		painting	
perforation		polishing	
young to middle adults ($n = 39^a$)		young to middle adults ($n = 17^b$)	
predominately males		sex undetermined	

Notes: [a]There are references in the literature to 14 additional specimens in Ohio. [b]There are references in the literature to 19 additional specimens in Illinois.

were recovered from Mount Vernon Mound, which had been significantly disturbed by looting activities. Therefore, none of those examples have primary contextual information. Similar manufacturing techniques and decorations occur in all regions.

In Ohio, cleaning striations and disarticulating cuts are the most common form of modification; the cranium is the most frequently modified element, followed by the mandible and maxilla. Ohio researchers have interpreted these cuts and scrape marks as the end result of defleshing and dismemberment and not as the result of decapitation and mutilation (Seeman 1988, 2007; Webb and Snow 1945). In contrast, no evidence for modified crania is present in central Illinois during the Middle Woodland period. The mandible is the most frequently modified bone followed by the maxilla in the central Illinois River valley. Striations are clearly visible on all specimens, but disarticulation cuts are absent or have been deliberately obliterated. One exception is a mandible fragment from Sister Creeks F°61, which has cut marks on the margin of the posterior ramus. At Mount Vernon Mound (12PO885) in southern Indiana, Nawrocki (1997) identified 39 modified hemimandible fragments representing 21 individuals. No maxillae are reported from the site. The modifications include reduction by grinding, perforation, and polishing, and the rami are squared. At the Tremper and Snyders sites in Ohio, the rami are also squared (Stephen Nawrocki, personal communication 2008). Similar modification techniques were used in Ohio and Indiana, but the central Illinois River valley shows the greatest regional variation in decorative styles. In Ohio and Indiana, the modified jaws are young to middle-aged adults, with mostly males represented. Females are also reported from Indiana (Nawrocki 1997). Sex was not determined for any of the modified examples in the central Illinois sample.

Conclusions

This chapter summarizes the archaeological context of modified human jaws in the central Illinois River valley and identifies patterns in manufacture, decoration, placement, and association that shed light on their broader significance in Middle Woodland mortuary behavior. Modified human jaws are found exclusively in Middle Woodland mounds. Although these mounds are located on all landform types in the valley, almost all modified human jaws are located in floodplain and bottomland settings. In these locations, the jaws are found primarily in log tombs and placed on adult skeletons. The low occurrence of the modified jaws in Middle Woodland mounds when compared to other artifact classes clearly demonstrates that the items were restricted to a select subset of the population.

Modified human mandibles are more common than maxillae in the central Illinois River valley. Both element categories are included in the mortuary program during the early Middle Woodland period (Liverpool, Ogden-Fettie, and Neteler), but by the latter part of the Middle Woodland only mandibles are present in the graves at Weaver and Sister Creeks. Perhaps the mandible became the preferred bone for modification because of its ease of manufacture. Another distinction between the maxillae and the mandibles is the amount of decoration. Two maxillac from Liverpool are painted or heavily coated with red ochre, and in these instances the red ochre covers green-stained bone. The use of a heavy red ochre pigment on these items makes sense given the early Middle Woodland context. Red ochre is an important component of Late Archaic/Early Woodland mortuary practices, and the tradition of heavy red ochre use continued into the early Middle Woodland period. However, the emphasis on red ochre as a primary mortuary trait became less important toward the latter part of the Middle Woodland period. The staining of the hemimandibles illustrates this point. Red- and/or green-stained hemimandibles are present at Liverpool and Sister Creeks F°61, where the staining is light, while hemimandibles from Sister Creeks F°54, Ogden-Fettie, and Neteler have no staining. The light staining appears to be unintentional. Green staining likely resulted from the donor individual being buried with a copper object in contact with the maxilla or mandible. Red staining is attributed to the sprinkling of red ochre over the body as part of the burial ritual.

Both maxillae and mandibles are perforated, likely for suspension, but the internal surfaces and edges of the perforations are not typically polished. In the central Illinois River valley sample, there is only one pair of modified hemimandibles (from Sister Creeks F°54) with polish on the perforations. The remaining modified mandibles exhibit polish only on the outer surfaces of the bone, indicating that they were handled or carried often, perhaps in a bag or similar container. The convex curvature of the external mandibles contributes to their being polished more than the concave inner surface. An alternative theory is that the bone became polished from repeated handling as it was passed from generation to generation. The absence of polish within the perforations indicates that, if these elements were suspended on clothing or used as ornaments at one time, they were worn infrequently. What we are seeing archaeologically is the end product of their use through their inclusion in a tomb.

The presence of modified human and animal jaws in Middle Woodland mortuary contexts is significant when we consider their meanings. It is worth noting that modified human and animal jaws do not co-occur with the same individual. However, the fact that these objects are only found in Middle Woodland mortuary contexts indicates that they carried great significance in the Middle Woodland world view or religion.

There is a 500- to 600-year span of Middle Woodland occupation in this region, and thousands of people have lived and died there. If modified human jaws were a common mortuary item in the Middle Woodland, like shell beads, there would be more than the 31 examples known from the archaeological record. It is much more likely that these objects were prepared and handed down from generation to generation specifically for the death of an individual with an important role in the community. If a tomb is cleaned out and the primary individual's skeleton is reorganized into a bundle and moved in preparation for the tomb's reuse, then the modified human jaws placed with that individual could be passed to his or her successor. Modified human jaws are almost exclusively found with primary interments, in tomb contexts, and only with a restricted subset of Middle Woodland mortuary artifacts, thereby signifying their particular status. When one religious or political leader in a society dies, another will assume the leadership responsibilities. The items of status are placed in the tomb until the new leader's death, when they will be transferred to him or her. An alternative theory is that the modified human jaws are kept with the body until the remains are reorganized into a bundle. The jaws are then curated until they are needed for another leader's death. If their limited use is due to curation, then it is not surprising that modified human jaws became rare and valued objects.

A further distinction must be noted about the choice of mound location and what it could represent in the central Illinois River valley. As previously stated, Middle Woodland mounds occur at floodplain, terrace, and bluff crest localities, and modified human jaws occur in all of these locations. By far, the greatest number and variety of jaws occur in the early to middle Middle Woodland floodplain mounds. While the small sample size makes it difficult to assign definitive meaning to these mortuary objects, we can infer some social meaning. Individuals having a specific social role are given modified human jaws in death along with a subset of Middle Woodland mortuary objects, such as pearl, shell, and copper beads; split and drilled bear canines; copper axes and adzes; celts and blades; and platform pipes (Farnsworth and Atwell 2015). Early in the Middle Woodland period, these individuals are placed in tombs that occur in floodplain and terrace mounds. Toward the late Middle Woodland period, the location of similar mounds shifts to the bluff crest. The floodplain setting of the earliest Middle Woodland mounds, with their complicated tombs holding presumably important people, helped to create a ritual landscape specific to the floodplain, with stronger and older ties to the Middle Woodland people's history and ideology. Through time, these early floodplain mounds became valuable links to the ancestors and the spirit world and assumed a higher status, symbolic meaning, or cultural importance distinct from later bluff top mounds and burials.

Suggestions for Future Research

Research projects should always ask new questions of the data and should strive to take the research in new directions. Many scholars have done just that by reexamining the wealth of data available in existing archaeological collections. This chapter has focused on modified human jaws as objects of significant social status in Middle Woodland mortuary contexts in Illinois. While decorative styles, red ochre application and copper staining, and Woodland mortuary practices provide clues to the source or origin of the modified jaws, lead or strontium isotope analysis might determine if these jaws were items of long-distance trade or if they were derived from the local population.

Another unresolved issue involves the significant decrease in the frequency of modified human jaws in later Middle Woodland mounds. Modified human jaws appear to be restricted to the Middle Woodland period in Illinois. What cultural/social changes were occurring at the end of the Middle Woodland that might explain the changes in mortuary behavior and the disappearance of modified jaws? Did the later people replace the modified human jaws with another object to signify the same status, or was status reflected in another manner? Did status itself change meaning and form? If people had a significant social status in the later Middle Woodland, was it expressed in another way?

Acknowledgments

The following institutions granted access to their collections and graciously allowed the documentation of the modified human jaws: the Illinois State Museum, the Dickson Mounds Museum, the Illinois State Archaeological Survey at the University of Illinois, and the Upper Mississippi Valley Archaeological Research Foundation. Doug Carr at the Illinois State Museum photographed the remains and provided the digitized sketch. His efforts are greatly appreciated. I am grateful for the constructive criticisms provided by Hal Hassen, Julie Bukowski, Duane Esarey, Alan Harn, Ken Farnsworth, and each of the volume editors. Last, I want to acknowledge the anonymous reviewers who helped to turn my paper into this chapter. My thanks to all of you.

Notes

1. The site nomenclature used is from the University of Chicago system established in the early to mid-twentieth century. The inclusion of ° in a site number indicates a mound (e.g., F°77). The inclusion of ^{v} indicates a village site (e.g., F^{v}1284).

2. The Schoenbecks identified mound F°60 based on the 1937 University of Chicago map of the Sister Creeks mounds. Meinkoth and colleagues' (1995) reanalysis of the same data identified the mound as F°61. Mound F°61 is used in this chapter.

3. Detailed information from these sites is limited due to incomplete excavations, a lack of systematic documentation, poor curation records, and an absence of skeletal analysis by physical anthropologists. There have been 281 individuals documented in nine mound sites in the central Illinois River valley. Reliable skeleton counts are reported in the archaeological literature for the excavated mounds at Hannah, Dickison, Weaver, Liverpool F°77, Sister Creeks, Ogden-Fettie, Clear Lake, Neteler, and Frederick. Only estimated skeleton counts exist for Liverpool F°78 and F°79, and they are excluded from the total count of individuals.

4
More than Skulls and Mandibles

Culturally Modified Human Remains from Woodland Contexts in Ohio

Cheryl A. Johnston

Culturally modified human remains have been recovered from a number of mortuary sites in midwestern North America and express a wide range of formal, depositional, and contextual variation. In Ohio, sites that have yielded culturally modified human remains are, for the most part, attributable to the Middle Woodland cultural phenomenon known as Hopewell. Between approximately 200 B.C. and A.D. 400 (Greber and Ruhl 1989), Hopewell thrived in parts of what is now the eastern half of the United States. Hopewell is known for an elaborate material culture and the construction of numerous mounds and earthworks. It is strongly and richly expressed in south-central Ohio and is named for the typesite (33RO27) located in Ross County, Ohio, on land that once belonged to Mordecai Cloud Hopewell.

It is not clear whether the people responsible for the material remains associated with Hopewell were all part of a single culture (Greber 1991). However, the archaeological record establishes that the material culture of contemporaneous people living during this time period in parts of the eastern portion of the United States shared aspects of symbolism and ideology, stylistic elements and raw materials, and mortuary behavior.

Unique among the varied and often exotic Hopewell grave inclusions were culturally modified human remains. These provide evidence of biological variation as anatomical elements, and these "objects" also express stylistic variation as artifacts. Their manufacture and intentional deposition were unusual and presumably culturally meaningful actions in the context of Hopewell traditions.

Defined broadly, "culturally modified human remains" include any human skeletal material that has been deliberately changed by humans from the state the material was in at the time of death, the time of interment, or the time of final disposition. These include cremated remains, bundle burials, and reinterments, as well as carved long bone shafts, drilled crania, and cut and ground mandibles and maxillae. Excluded are modifications caused by events that occurred during the life of the decedent, such as cranial shape alteration caused by a cradleboard or bindings (Johnston 2002). A more narrow definition of "modified bone," which is used in this chapter, includes only human remains that have been incised, drilled, ground, cut (i.e., worked), or intentionally arranged and deposited in the same manner as other cultural objects, such as worked copper or lithic artifacts.

The types and distribution of modified cranial bone from Middle Woodland contexts varies across the Midwest (Seeman 1988; also see Cobb, this volume). An examination of culturally modified human remains from Illinois (Snyders Mound C), Indiana (Mount Vernon Mound), and Ohio (Turner Mound, Hopewell Mound group, Seip Mound, Harness Mound, Purdom Mound, Tremper Mound, Mound City, and Raymond Ater Mound) reveals some patterns in the distribution of human vs. nonhuman culturally modified remains and the types of modification applied to each. Examples of modified cranial elements from Indiana and Illinois resemble the Ohio material from Tremper in degree and type of modification. The Illinois, Indiana, and Tremper examples have been modified in ways similar to many of the Ohio culturally modified nonhuman mandibles, which are often split at the symphysis and heavily reduced by grinding to the extent that only small sections of alveolar bone and associated teeth remain (Johnston et al. 1997). In contrast, modified crania from the majority of Middle Woodland Hopewell sites in Ohio (Johnston et al. 1997) have undergone only minimal modification that includes drilling and striations. They do not exhibit heavy grinding resulting in the removal of relatively large portions of bone nor the splitting of mandibles at the symphysis.

Ultimately, the goal of a bioarchaeological study such as this one is to discover something about the breadth and nature of past human variation with the hope that we will learn something about ourselves. First, however, we must try to tease out variables that can be used in the reconstruction of past human behavior. From such reconstruction we may glean knowledge of the organizing principles that governed social behavior. The theoretical program of mortuary analysis set forth by Binford (1971) and Saxe (1970) predicts that this can be accomplished. The Saxe-Binford program holds that the manner in which people treat and dispose of their dead is conditioned by social, political, and personal relationships. Hence, logical arguments can be constructed that relate mortuary behavior to sociological variables.

In order to address questions about social organization, cultural practices, and ideology using mortuary evidence, the archaeological record must be used to identify the characteristics of the deceased individuals and the treatment accorded the deceased by the living (Saxe 1970). Mortuary practices during the Ohio Hopewell period are characterized by considerable variation in grave construction, in the placement and material of associated burial objects, and in the treatment of the corpse. The age, sex, and genetic or social relationship of individuals interred in Hopewell contexts also vary and are often poorly understood. Before we can identify potential patterns, relationships, and meanings, the relevant variables must be identified and examined. Specifically, in this chapter, the focus is on one aspect of mortuary behavior: the cultural modification of human remains and their placement in a mortuary context. The demographic composition of both the modified human elements and the individuals associated with the modified elements from the Hopewell Mound group (33RO27) are examined in order to evaluate the significance of these particular objects in the social and ritual sphere of Hopewell.

Culturally Modified Cranial Remains from Ohio Woodland Contexts

Culturally modified human cranial remains from Woodland contexts in Ohio have historically been referred to as "trophy skulls." Included are skulls, crania, and jaws that have been drilled, ground, incised, or shaped in a variety of ways and often, but not always, deposited with interred skeletons or cremations, seemingly as funerary objects. Most examples have come from Middle Woodland Hopewell contexts, but Early Woodland and even Archaic examples exist. It seems a worthy goal to reexamine the use of the term "trophy skull" in recognition of the variability present in the modified elements and their association with individual burials.

These objects have been recovered from varied contexts: single interments, multiple interments, post molds, and caches containing nonhuman bone and other material. For example, Burial 41 from Mound 25 at the Hopewell Mound group is a triple burial that includes three extended adult females, a set of modified jaws (Figures 4.1, 4.2), and a modified male skull (Figure 4.3). The modified jaws are drilled and notched. Other examples of culturally modified cranial remains from Ohio Middle Woodland sites include a drilled and notched mandible from the Edwin Harness Mound and heavily modified maxillae from Burial 34, Mound 25, of the Hopewell Mound group (Figure 4.4). The variability in culturally modified human remains from Hopewell contexts points to a bigger picture in which it becomes clear that more than one cultural phenomenon led to their production and deposition.

To understand the cultural significance and possible role of these elements, we need to consider several lines of evidence: the nature of modification, the

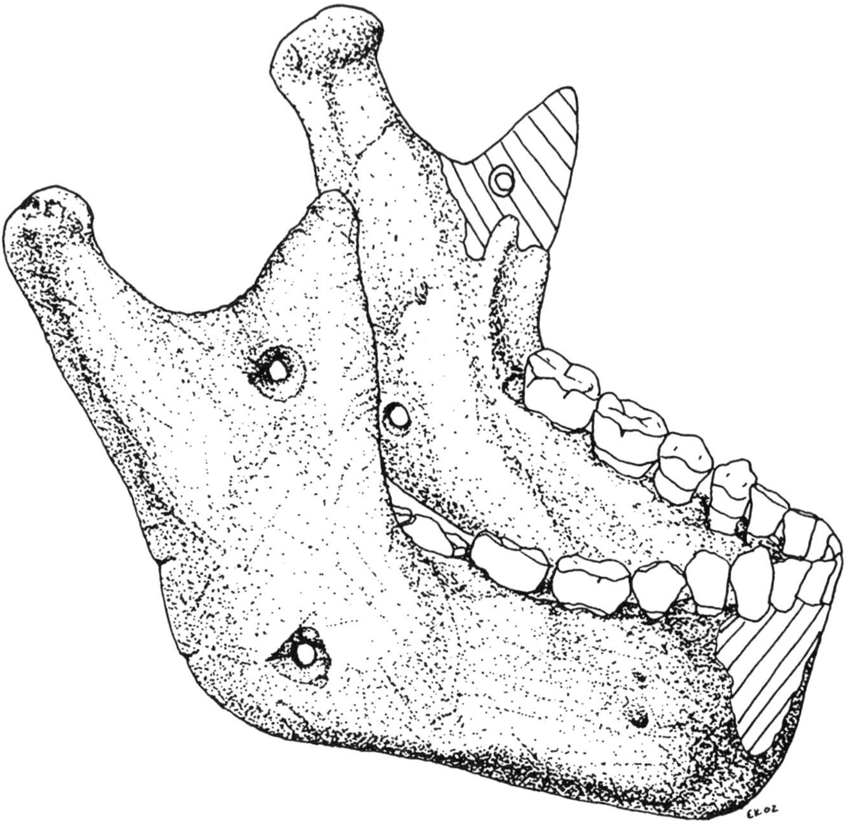

4.1. Culturally modified mandible from Burial 41, Mound 25, Hopewell Mound group. (Drawing by Erica Keener)

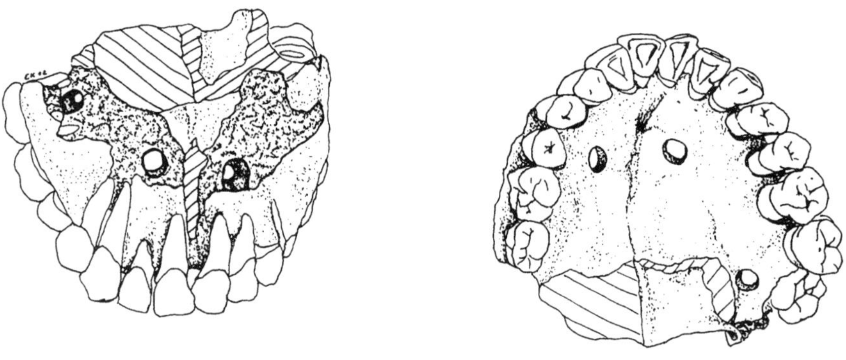

4.2. Culturally modified maxillae from Burial 41, Mound 25, Hopewell Mound group. (Drawing by Erica Keener)

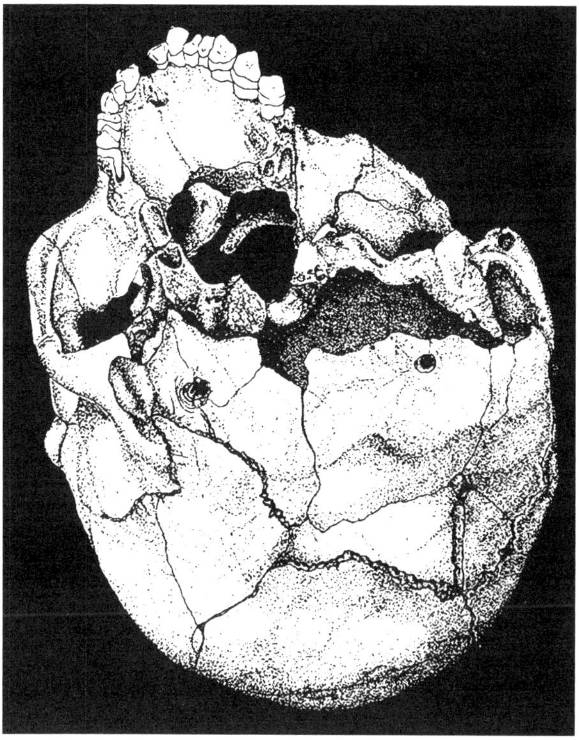

4.3. Culturally modified cranium from Burial 41, Mound 25, Hopewell Mound group. (Drawing by Erica Keener)

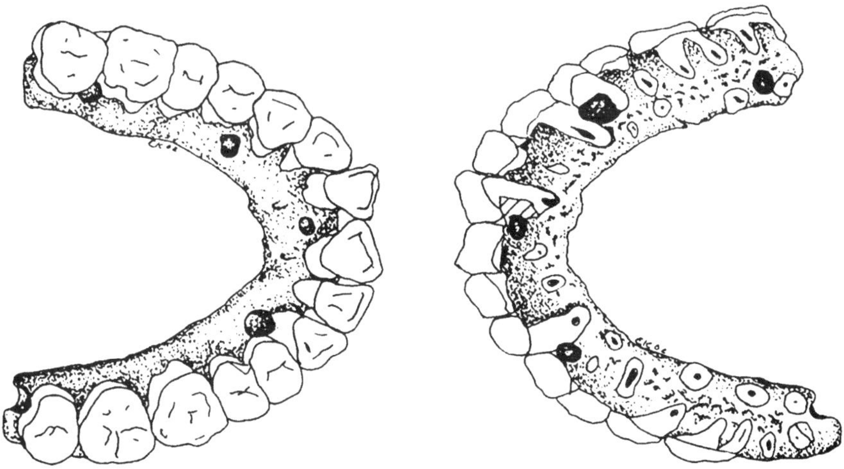

4.4. Culturally modified maxillae from Burial 34, Mound 25, Hopewell Mound group. (Drawing by Erica Keener)

biological attributes of modified bones, the biological attributes of the individuals with whom they are associated, and the archaeological contexts in which they are found. Presented here are tests of several hypothesized cultural roles (i.e., trophy, revered ancestor, memento mori, ritual object) of culturally modified human remains based on age and sex estimates of skeletonized human remains from the Hopewell Mound group (33RO27). Specifically, I consider the following:

- the ages and sexes of the individuals represented by culturally modified human cranial remains,
- the ages and sexes of the individuals interred with culturally modified human cranial remains,
- a comparison of the age and sex distribution of culturally modified human cranial remains vs. the age and sex distribution of the population at large.

History

Previous interpretations of culturally modified human remains focused on the role in life of the person from whom the remains were derived (Mills 1909a; Moorehead 1968; Seeman 1988; Shetrone 1926; Webb and Snow 1945). Until relatively recently, only two interpretations of their significance were entertained in the literature—trophies of war and revered ancestors (Mills 1909a; Moorehead 1968; Shetrone 1926). The trophy explanation assumed that the modified human remains were initially gathered from enemies by the victors during episodes of warfare. In contrast, the revered ancestor interpretation holds that the person represented by the modified bone was important in some way to his or her own living relatives, to the person with whom the modified bone was interred, or to the living relatives of the decedent.

The most complete published survey to date of Hopewell "trophy skulls" is provided by Seeman (1988; see also Nawrocki 1997; Owsley et al. 1994). Prior to Seeman's study, the consensus had been that culturally modified human remains fit the revered ancestors interpretation better than they fit the trophy interpretation (Seeman 1988; Webb and Snow 1945). This was largely based on an assessment of a cache of drilled skulls from Turner (Willoughby and Hooton 1922) in which Hooton incorrectly identified the individuals as old adults. The idea that these remains were revered ancestors seemed better supported by the evidence at the time and was thus the accepted explanation for culturally modified human remains until Seeman (1988) challenged this idea. Stimulated by the introduction of new age and sex estimation techniques in the 1980s, Seeman reevaluated the revered ancestor and trophy interpretations. It seems reasonable that if the key to understanding the significance of these remains was the age and sex of the "donor" individual, then perhaps a more complete and accurate assessment of age and sex could lend strength to one interpretation over the other.

Seeman favored a trophy interpretation based largely on ethnographic examples of human trophy taking and display from Plains groups of Native Americans, archaeological representations of trophy taking on Mississippian art objects, and a reassessment of the age and sex of the modified elements. Examples of representations of severed human heads in Ohio Middle Woodland art also exist and are even more relevant to interpretations of Hopewell culturally modified human remains than is Mississippian art. However, they are not very informative. For example, the Wray figurine from the Newark Earthworks (a Middle Woodland site with geometric earthen enclosures in Licking County, Ohio) depicts a human dressed in a bearskin (complete with bear head and claws) wearing earspools and holding what appears to be a severed human head (also wearing earspools) in his/her lap. While the depiction of a severed head stimulates thoughts of a potential connection to culturally modified human remains, the ritualistic nature of the Wray figurine does not help us choose between the trophy and revered ancestor interpretations. Another depiction of a severed human head noted in Ohio Hopewell art is on a pipe from Seip (a Middle Woodland site in Ross County, Ohio) in which a dog holds a human head in its mouth. Similarly, it is hard to make an argument that this depiction supports one interpretation over the other.

Seeman compiled a list of Middle Woodland culturally modified human remains, including their present location, presence or absence of several modification variables (including drilling, polishing, cutting, and application of "red paint"), age, and sex. Of the 40 or so examples he documented, Seeman reported age and sex estimates for fewer than half. According to Seeman, young males outnumber old males and females; hence the conclusion that the trophy interpretation is supported. Three aspects of this conclusion are noteworthy. First, there are a lot of missing data, which gives rise to the question of whether Seeman's use of age and sex is helpful. Second, Seeman does not clearly indicate who produced the age and sex estimates nor the methods used. Third, hypotheses were not formulated and objectively tested. The conclusions amount to an opinion, yet the use of the term "trophy" to describe these modified human elements has stuck even though the variability in the modified bones and their contexts suggests otherwise.

Although Seeman's study seems to lend support to the trophy interpretation, his conclusion that males predominate has been questioned. Konigsberg and Frankenberg (1993) used missing data theory and Ohio Hopewell craniometric data collected by Charles Snow, Georg Neumann, and Earnest Hooton to demonstrate that there is no statistical evidence for a biased sex ratio in a sample of Ohio Hopewell "trophy skulls." In addition, a reexamination of many of the culturally modified human remains included in Seeman's report, plus additional examples from the Mount Vernon Mound (Johnston et al. 1997; Nawrocki 1997), shows that it cannot be statistically determined whether males outnumber females. This conclusion holds for the sexes reported in Seeman's paper and in the more recent works. These results, and the fact that sex had not been assigned to many of the Hopewell culturally modified human remains, has rendered the trophy and revered ancestor interpretations equally well supported (or unsupported) by the age and sex evidence.

It was thought that the age and sex of the individuals from whom these objects were made held the key to their interpretation. If the preponderance of the "donors" were young males, it was assumed that they fit the profile of individuals likely to be involved in conflicts with other groups, though the presence of young female donors would not cause the trophy idea to be summarily rejected. Advanced age and maleness were attributes that supported the revered ancestor interpretation, but old females could be revered ancestors as well. Although the idea that age and sex are key to interpreting culturally modified human remains was stated in the literature, no one had framed testable hypotheses in order to scientifically support or reject the idea. In other words, there was no scientific basis upon which to accept or reject one interpretation—trophy or revered ancestor—over the other.

In 1993, Konigsberg and Frankenberg proposed the memento mori ("tokens of remembrance") and ritual object ("heads collected for a particular ritual") interpretations. They suggested that to understand the significance of culturally modified human remains, we must also examine all the unmodified human remains from the same contexts (i.e., in a mound). To do this is to take a step backward from the previous strategies, where researchers sought to understand the role of culturally modified human remains in Hopewell ideology by focusing on the age and sex of those individuals from whom the modified bones were derived.

To objectively evaluate the robustness of the primary explanations regarding Hopewell culturally modified human remains, this chapter examines these interpretations by testing several hypotheses. A trophy taking, or victory token, hypothesis is based on the assumption that older individuals and females would be less likely than young males to become trophies, since they would be less likely to be involved in a conflict between groups. A revered ancestor hypothesis predicts that the individuals represented by culturally modified human remains were chosen for modification because they were honored ancestors and could include adults of either sex. A memento mori hypothesis is based on the idea that culturally modified human remains are simply tokens of remembrance of someone who has died, while the ritual object hypothesis proposes that the significance comes more from the fact that the culturally modified remains are *human* bone than that they come from a specific individual.

Hopewell Mound Group

The implicit assumption made by Seeman (1988)—that all culturally modified human remains from Hopewell contexts were created and deposited for the same reason—seems simplistic. Paradoxically, Seeman also reported that there is sufficient variability in attributes among the specimens he examined to render the formation of a typology of culturally modified human remains uninformative. The project summarized in this chapter was designed to determine if enough demographic data could be recovered from collections of human remains from the Hopewell Mound group to test hypotheses put forth regarding their cultural significance. In order to better understand the significance of modified human cranial elements, I set out to identify and describe the biological and stylistic variations present among these modified cranial elements and, for the first time, the age, sex, and mortuary treatment of the individuals with whom they were deposited at the Hopewell Mound group (Johnston 2002).

The skeletal collections from the Hopewell Mound group were chosen for this study because they contain numerous examples of culturally modified human remains and a large burial population of at least 230 individuals described and/or excavated by Moorehead (1891, 1897, 1968) and Shetrone (1922–1925, 1926). I have examined and described all available skeletons recovered from the Hopewell Mound group (Johnston 2002). Of the 230 individuals, only 74 were identifiable with regard to mound and burial number in museum collections. Eleven age estimation methods (including dental, auricular surface, and pubic symphysis seriations) and principal components analysis were employed to estimate age at death. Sex was assigned based on one or more of 14 indicators, including seriation of cranial robusticity. Skeletal elements identifiable only as having been recovered from the Hopewell Mound group are also present in the collections of the Ohio Historical Society and the Field Museum of Natural History, but because they lack documentation, their use was limited to inclusion in seriations.

Of the 74 individuals that are identifiable with regard to mound and burial number, 37 could be assigned to a sex category, and age could be estimated for 70. However, of the 70 that could be aged, 30 were assigned the general category of "adult" due to the absence of more specific age markers. Shetrone and Moorehead each reported encountering 9 examples of modified human remains for a total count of 18 individual modified elements. Of the 18 sets of culturally modified human remains reported, age ranges were established for 12 and sex was assigned to 8 (see Table 4.1). Of the 11 individuals associated with the modified remains, age ranges were established for 8 individuals and sex assigned to 8 (see Table 4.2). Clearly, detailed demographic information for many of the individuals is missing. In light of this, hypotheses were still tested, but only tentative conclusions could be reached.

Age and sex were used to test three hypotheses regarding the role of culturally modified human remains in Hopewell culture (Johnston 2002): trophy taking/victory token, revered ancestor, and memento mori/ritual object. Trophies are expected to be young adult males, and revered ancestors are expected to be older and of either sex. Both the memento mori ("tokens of remembrance") and ritual object ("heads collected for a particular ritual") interpretations would be expected to have an age and sex distribution that parallels the mortality profile of the related burial population.

Trophy Taking or Victory Token

In most human groups the participants in conflicts are predominately young and male. In other words, the assumption is made that older individuals and females would be less likely than young males to be chosen for trophies since they would be less likely to be involved in a conflict between groups. This is supported by the work of Mensforth (2001), who looked for evidence of warfare and trophy taking in Late Archaic skeletons from Kentucky and Ohio sites. Mensforth noted that adult males predominate as victims of conflicts that lead to death. Although Milner (1995) cautioned against extrapolating a sex ratio for participants in prehistoric warfare from human skeletal samples, the tendency for there to be a greater number of the skeletons of males exhibiting evidence of antemortem and perimortem trauma associated with conflict was noted in his summary of osteological evidence of prehistoric warfare. It is a reasonable assumption that if females did participate in conflicts, they would not have been present in the same numbers as males. Therefore, the smaller the sample of culturally modified human remains, the less likely it is that a female will be represented even if conflicts were not an exclusively male endeavor.

If males were the main participants in conflicts, then it is reasonable to assume that they were the ones taking trophies and thus would more likely be

Table 4.1. Age and Sex Estimates of Culturally Modified Human Remains from Hopewell Mound Group

ID	Mound	Burial	Skeletal Age at Death (years)	Sex Assignment from Skeleton	Available for Analysis?	Investigator
150215	2	5	35–45	male	yes	Shetrone
	3				no	Moorehead
150138	7		20–30	male	yes	Shetrone
56033	18	181	20–25		yes	Moorehead
56034-1	18	181	adult		yes	Moorehead
56034-2	18	181	20–25		yes	Moorehead
56034-3	18	181	20–25		yes	Moorehead
56034-4	18	181	20–25	male	yes	Moorehead
56064	23	213	20–25	female	yes	Moorehead
	23	238			no	Moorehead
56068	24	192	15–20	female	yes	Moorehead
150173	25		adult		yes	Shetrone
150120	25	34	21–25	male	yes	Shetrone
150118	25	34	35–45	male	yes	Shetrone
	25	35			no	Shetrone
150056	25	41	25–35	male	yes	Shetrone
150172	25	41	15–20		yes	Shetrone
	26	6			no	Shetrone

Table 4.2. Age and Sex Estimates of Individuals Interred with Culturally Modified Human Remains from Hopewell Mound Group

ID	Mound	Burial	Skeletal Age at Death (years)	Sex Assignment from Skeleton	Available for Analysis?	Investigator
150214	2	5	24–49	female	yes	Shetrone
	3				no	Moorehead
41618	18	181	40–50	male	yes	Moorehead
	23	213			no	Moorehead
40173	24	191	adult		yes	Moorehead
150117	25	34	45–55	male	yes	Shetrone
150212	25	35	35–45	male	yes	Shetrone
150058	25	41-1	41–45	female	yes	Shetrone
150053	25	41-2	30–40	female	yes	Shetrone
150057	25	41-3	40–50	female	yes	Shetrone
150164	26	6	35–45	male	yes	Shetrone

interred with trophies than would females. One would then predict that the individuals with whom culturally modified human remains were interred would be adult males, though not necessarily of any particular age category.

The Hopewell Mound group individuals from whom elements were taken for modification were all 15 years of age or older, most were younger than 25 years old at death, and only three were older than 25 (see Table 4.1). Six individuals, or a third of the sample, could not be placed in a specific age range.

Females are present among both the culturally modified elements and the individuals interred with modified elements. Only two females were identified among those culturally modified, and the sex of one of these is questionable (see Table 4.1). However, more than half (55 percent) of the sample could not be sexed. Perhaps more significant, individuals buried with modified bone included equal numbers of males and females; 3 out of 11 individuals (27 percent) could not be assigned to a sex category (Table 4.2). As noted earlier in this chapter, Burial 41, Mound 25, is an interesting example of the inclusion of culturally modified human remains with female interments.

Age and sex estimates of culturally modified human remains from the Hopewell Mound group do not support an explanation of trophy taking or victory token. The presence of older individuals among the culturally modified bone and the presence of females among both the modified elements and those interred with them suggest that the modified remains had an alternative role.

Revered Ancestor

The revered ancestor hypothesis predicts that the individuals who are represented by culturally modified human remains were chosen for modification because they were honored ancestors—of the individual with whom they were buried, of the individuals who buried them, or of the living population represented by the burials at Hopewell Mound group. They are expected to be adults, but either sex might be included. However, one sex may have predominated depending on how descent was perceived.

The expectation that ancestors should be adults is based on the biological fact that in order to be someone's biological ancestor you must have left descendants. Children are incapable of reproducing, would therefore not have left descendants, and thus could not be anyone's ancestor in the biological sense of the term (Parker Pearson 1999). It is possible for a person to be considered an ancestor for cultural reasons even if the person did not leave biological descendants. However, ancestor worship often involves not only a belief in the immortality of ancestors but also a belief in their power and wisdom and represents continuity across generations (Parker Pearson 1999).

Even if a particular group's definition of ancestor does not require a biological connection by descent, it is not uncommon for there to be some requirement that the person was a well-respected elder in life. The assumption that revered ancestors are adults is sound in either case.

The revered ancestor hypothesis similarly predicts that the age and sex distributions of individuals with whom culturally modified human remains were interred will reflect the age and sex distributions of the burial population since no one is prevented, based on their age or sex, from having a revered or worshiped ancestor.

The data support the revered ancestor hypothesis to the extent that none of the culturally modified human remains associated with the Hopewell Mound group appear to have derived from individuals younger than 15 years old at death (see Table 4.1). Also consistent with the predictions of the hypothesis is that both sexes are represented among the modified remains.

Difficulty is encountered in evaluating whether or not the prediction regarding the individuals interred with culturally modified human remains is met. The hypothesis predicts that the age and sex distributions of those interred with culturally modified human remains mirror the age and sex distributions of those buried without culturally modified human remains. In other words, whatever selection process was used to decide who was buried at the site in general was used to decide who was buried with culturally modified human remains.

Missing data render the determination of the age and sex distributions of those buried at Hopewell Mound group unknowable and thus prevent an evaluation of this prediction. However, if only age is considered, an argument can be made that the age distribution of those interred with culturally modified human remains is patterned after the age distribution of the burial population, at least in terms of the proportion of subadults present. Moorehead and Shetrone shared a tendency to note if a set of remains they encountered was a subadult. The assumption that the excavators noted all of the subadults they encountered is reasonable. Using this information, it makes sense to interpret the absence of subadults in the sample of individuals interred with culturally modified human remains as the result of sampling bias. Only about 5 percent (11 of 230) of individuals interred at the Hopewell Mound group were identified as subadults by Moorehead (1891, 1897, 1968) and Shetrone (1922–1925, 1926). If it is assumed that 5 percent of the individuals interred with culturally modified human remains should be subadults (n = 11; .05 x 11 = .55), then it is reasonable to conclude that even if there was no selection process that excluded subadults, a subadult would not be expected to be present among those interred with culturally modified human remains unless this group was approximately twice as large.

This reasoning can be applied to the culturally modified human remains as well. If 5 percent of them are expected to be subadults based on the proportion of subadults in the burial population, then approximately one subadult would be expected to be present among those culturally modified elements (n = 18; .05 x 18 = .9). Based on the available evidence, no subadults are represented among the culturally modified individuals, and thus the expectation of the revered ancestor hypothesis that all of those modified are adults is tentatively met.

In summary, the revered ancestor hypothesis is tentatively not rejected because its expectations are met in terms of the absence of subadult individuals among the culturally modified. Sampling bias cannot be ruled out as a cause of the absence of subadults among those interred with culturally modified human remains. The sample is so small that definitive conclusions based on the expected absence of subadults are not appropriate.

Memento Mori and Ritual Object

The memento mori and ritual object hypotheses are considered together since they both predict that the age and sex distributions of culturally modified individuals and those with whom they were interred are patterned after the age and sex distributions of the burial population. The memento mori hypothesis is based on the idea that culturally modified human remains are simply tokens of remembrance of someone who has died (Konigsberg and Frankenberg 1993). The ritual object hypothesis holds that the significance of culturally modified human remains may lie more in the fact of their being *human* bone, rather than originating from a specific identified individual. The time and place of death as well as the availability of a particular element for a specific ritual may determine which individual's remains are modified (Konigsberg and Frankenberg 1993).

The logical arguments used for the revered ancestor hypothesis can also be used for the memento mori/ritual object hypothesis. The assumption is that the age and sex distributions of both the modified bone and the burials with modified bone should be the same as those of burials without modified bone. However, as noted above, missing data prevent an accurate assessment of the age and sex distributions of those buried at Hopewell Mound group. Based on Moorehead's (1891, 1897, 1968) and Shetrone's (1922–1925, 1926) identifications, the proportion of subadults in the group can be estimated to be 5 percent. No subadults are identified among the culturally modified individuals, and no modified bones are found in association with subadult burials; therefore, the expectation of the memento mori and ritual object hypotheses that the age distribution of culturally modified individuals is patterned after the age distribution of the burial population is tentatively not met. The lack of subadults represented among the culturally modified individuals does not support a memento mori or ritual object role. Given the small sample size, we cannot rule out recovery bias in the absence of subadults, and definitive conclusions based on the expected absence of subadults are not appropriate.

Discussion

It seems clear from this and previous studies (Johnston et al. 1997; Konigsberg and Frankenberg 1993; Nawrocki 1997) that the interpretation that modified human remains from Hopewell contexts are trophies of war, based on the expectation that they were made from skeletal elements of young adult males, cannot be robustly tested using morphological age and sex data derived from Hopewell human skeletal remains in museum collections. The collections do not provide enough intact sets of remains from which indicators of age and sex can be observed to render anything other than tentative conclusions. Other lines of inquiry that may be applied to the trophy hypothesis include studies of prehistoric warfare and trophy taking that reveal a pattern that includes the interment of multiple individuals in a grave, osteological evidence of antemortem and perimortem injuries received in conflicts, and evidence of scalping, decapitation, and removal of other body parts (Mensforth 2001; Milner 1995). Although some of the graves at Hopewell Mound group contain multiple individuals, of the 201 grave features reported by Moorehead (1891, 1897, 1968) and Shetrone (1922–1925, 1926), only 20 are double burials and only 2 are triple burials. There is also one burial feature that Shetrone called a "bundle burial," which includes skeletal elements minimally representing three adults and one subadult. There is no evidence among any of the individuals examined from Hopewell Mound group, whether interred individually or in multiples, of scavenger damage, which is sometimes seen on the remains of victims of conflict who were not buried immediately after death (Milner 1995). Evidence of antemortem or perimortem injury that might have been the result of warfare is virtually absent, as are individuals who are missing body parts from whom trophies might have been taken. No evidence of scalping was observed.

The ancestor worship hypothesis, though not rejected outright, is somewhat tenuous due to the small sample sizes of culturally modified individuals and individuals interred with them. Conversely, the memento mori and ritual object hypotheses were tentatively rejected. A larger sample might reveal a better fit (or lack thereof) between the age and sex distributions of those who were modified or who were buried with modified elements, and the rest of the burial population. However, it may be the case that subadults are not missing from the Hopewell Mound group samples because of sampling bias. Observations of culturally modified human remains from numerous other midwestern Hopewell contexts reveal an absence of subadults in general among those chosen for modification.

Why were human remains culturally modified? Most probably, there were numerous reasons. Just as the magnitude of the variation among Hopewellian earthworks has been reevaluated (Mainfort and Sullivan 1998), so should be the variation represented among Hopewell mortuary attributes, including the production, use, and deposition of culturally modified human remains. It is not necessarily the case that they were all made, used, and deposited for the same reasons, to serve the same purposes, or by the same people. Possible functions include trophies, ancestors, shamanistic equipment, parts of death bundles (see Hall 1997), and clan or group symbols, and some may have been made for reasons we will never know. It is clear that the contexts in which they are found, the people they were made from and deposited with, and the way they were made are varied, which suggests diverse meanings or significances.

How were culturally modified human remains made and used? Most were probably made from fleshed remains that had to be cleaned or from fairly fresh bone (Johnston 2002:113; also see Nawrocki and Emanovsky, this volume). There would have been no cultural prohibition against handling human remains, or there was a way to suspend it, at least for certain people participating in the Hopewell rituals (Johnston 2002:113). Given the different modification techniques used, perhaps it is the case that they were made by more than one person. Some exhibit polish, suggesting they were handled or carried in a bag, while others do not. Some were drilled, perhaps for suspension, although the lack of evidence of abrasion in and around the drilled holes suggests that, if they were suspended, it was for a short period of time or that they were not subjected to repeated movements (Johnston 2002:114; also see Cobb, this volume).

Why were culturally modified human remains deposited with certain individuals at the Hopewell Mound group? The answer to this question depends on the cultural significance of each example and the cultural significance of being buried at the Hopewell Mound group in general.

Unfortunately, there are no satisfying answers to many of our questions about Hopewell. It is worthwhile to explore what can be known based on the evidence gleaned from the archaeological record, but it is essential to recognize the limitations of the data. There are two supportable conclusions in this chapter. One is that, regardless of the function of culturally modified human remains in Hopewellian mortuary behavior, either sex could participate as donors of raw material or as posthumous recipients of culturally modified human remains as long as biological maturity had been reached. The other conclusion is that multiple stimuli existed that led to the production, use, and deposition of culturally modified human remains.

Acknowledgments

I would like to thank Paul Sciulli for his intellectual contributions to this work, Martha Potter Otto for her encouragement and advice as well as her facilitation of numerous aspects of my work with Hopewell materials, Erica Keener for the drawings of culturally modified human remains that illustrate this work, Holly Williamson for last-minute proofreading, the Ohio Archaeological Council for providing financial support for this research, and the staffs of the Ohio Historical Society, the Field Museum of Natural History, the Cleveland Museum of Natural History, and the Milwaukee Public Museum for providing access to their collections and records. Thanks are also due to the hardworking editors of this book and to the anonymous reviewers, whose suggestions significantly improved this work. Any imperfections are my own.

5
Arrangement of Human Remains and Artifacts in Scioto Hopewell Burials

Dramatic Rituals or Ritual Dramas?

Christopher Carr and Anna Novotny

In 1997, in the course of studying old field photographs of Scioto Hopewell burials in the archives of the Ohio Historical Society, Christopher Carr came across a surprise. Some skeletons of Hopewell people were laid out in peculiar body positions, including arms and legs akimbo (Figure 5.1a). Cremations were sometimes piled into distinct geometric forms. Artifacts sometimes embellished the cremation sculptures, as in the case of an arc of cremation remains with a conch shell at each end of the arc (Figure 5.1b). Artifacts with no or few accompanying human remains also were sometimes combined to create distinctive arrangements, as in the case of a grouping of a copper crescent with effigy hands, two copper breastplates, and a copper whistle (Figure 5.1c) and an arrangement of five copper celts and a pair of copper earspools (Figure 5.1d). Sometimes, artifacts and skeletons were combined into unusual layouts (Figure 5.1e).

Attention to such unusual layouts of human remains and artifacts under Scioto Hopewell mounds was first given by Henry Shetrone in his synthetic book, *The Mound-Builders* (1930). He included a couple of pictures of layouts (e.g., Figure 5.1f), but did not offer any description or interpretation of them.

In this chapter, we introduce the subject of ritual arrangement of interred human remains and artifacts by Scioto Hopewell peoples. We focus on a tight suite of burials that are positioned in the form of birds in flight, which suggest soul flight, among other interpretations, and related burial forms that suggest the journey of a soul to an afterlife. To guide our specific interpretations, we use the relatively new bioarchaeological methodology *anthropologie de terrain*, which provides insight into the natural and cultural taphonomy of burials. We also ask, more generally, whether the burials were the products of "ritual dramas"—that is, collective, theatrical performances that portrayed key characters and events in narratives comprising the mythology and social cosmology of Ohio Hopewell peoples—or whether the burials resulted from rites of some different social or personal nature. Toward this goal, we consider

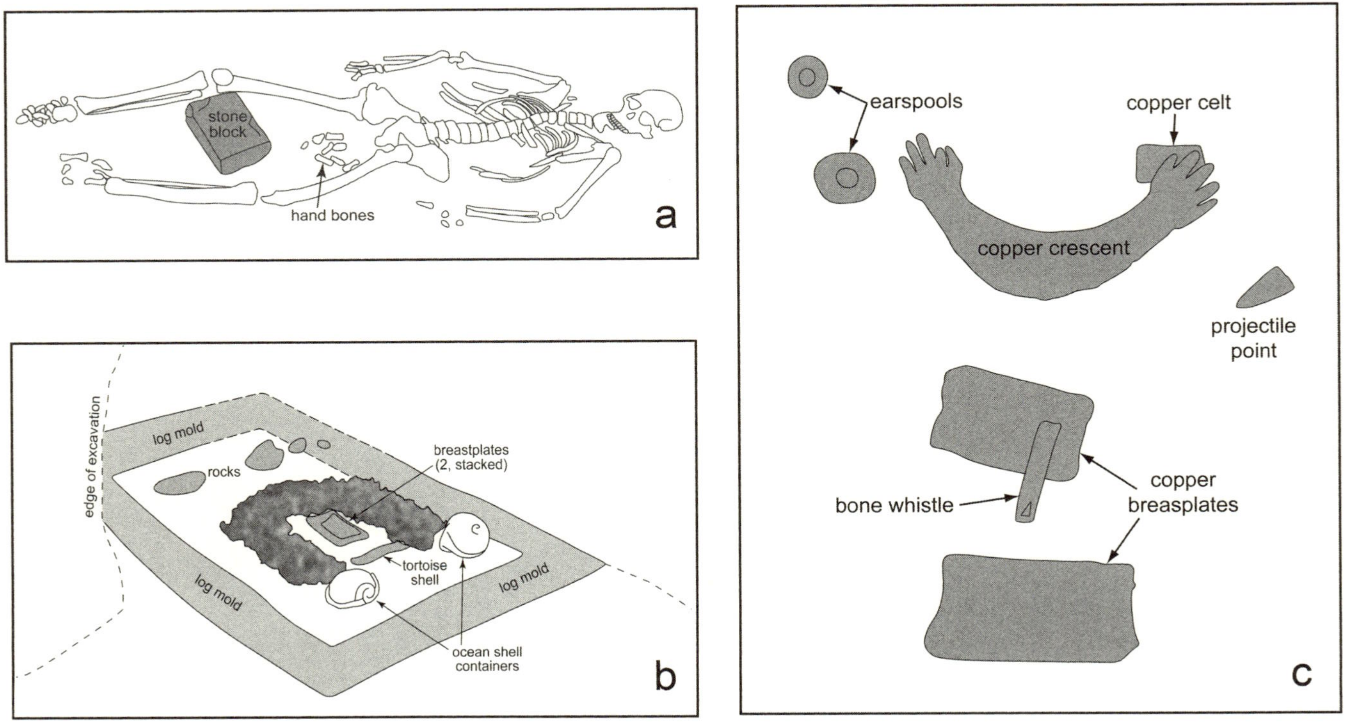
stone block
hand bones
a
log mold
rocks
breastplates (2, stacked)
edge of excavation
tortoise shell
log mold
log mold
ocean shell containers
b
earspools
copper celt
copper crescent
projectile point
bone whistle
copper breasplates
c

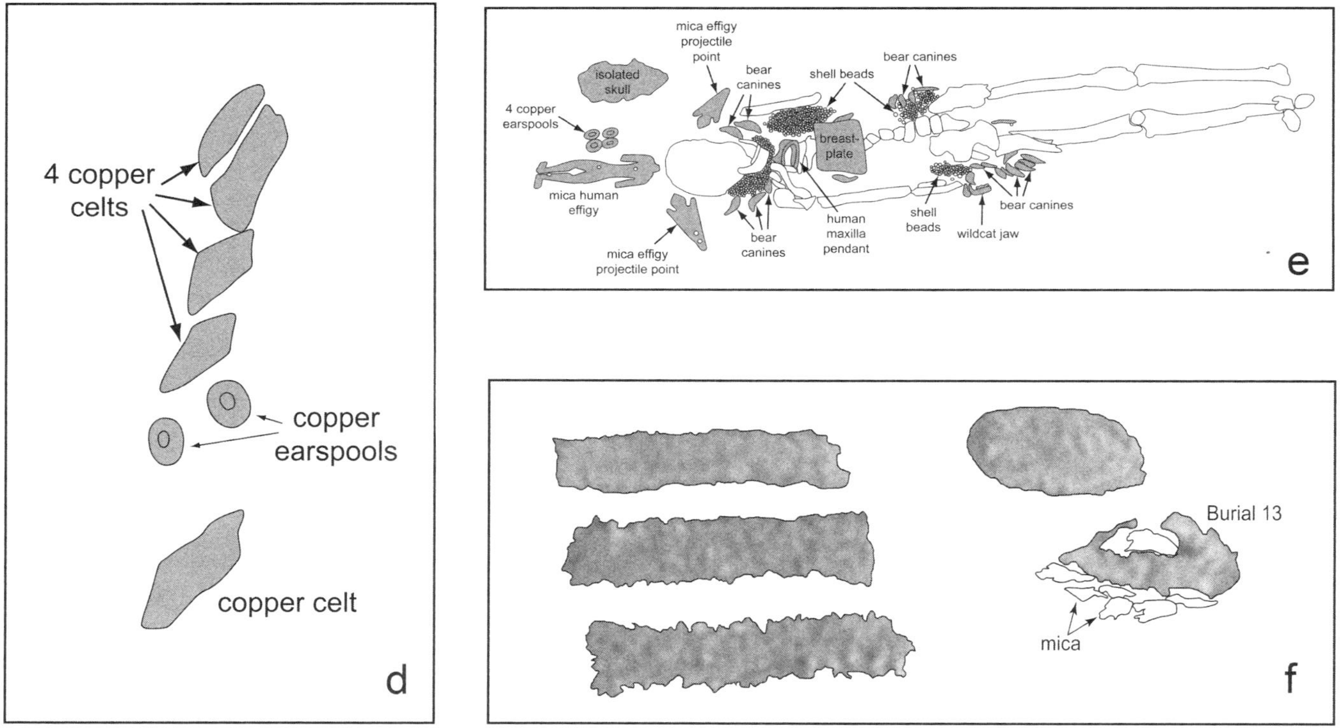

5.1. Unusual arrangements of skeletons, cremations, and artifacts in Scioto Hopewell sites, Ohio. (a) Hopewell site, Mound 4, Burial 3 (adapted from Shetrone 1926:34, Figure 9; and Ohio Historical Society, Prints 829, 830, AV17/3/1/E9/6). (b) Hopewell site, Mound 25, Burial 43 (adapted from Ohio Historical Society, Print 856, AV17/B3/F2/6). (c) Rockhold site, Burial 1 (adapted from Ohio Historical Society, Print 2339, AV17/B4/F7/E12/6). (d) Seip site, Pricer Mound, Burial 39 (adapted from Shetrone 1930:94, Figure 45). (e) Hopewell site, Mound 25, Burial 34 (adapted from Shetrone 1926:88, Figure 33; and Ohio Historical Society, Print 851, AV17/B3/F1/E3). (f) Mound City site (adapted from Ohio Historical Society, Print 2429-13, AV17/B3/F16/E6; see Shetrone 1936:99, Figure 49, for another view). (Drawings by Rebekah Zinser)

whether the rituals were large public events or restricted in their audience. In all, our studies reveal a tight spatial group of burials under Mound 25 of the Hopewell site that, taken together, comprised a narrative and served to orchestrate a ritual drama about the sequence of episodes in the death process and the journey to an afterlife that Scioto Hopewell peoples envisioned. The narrative corresponds closely to some historic Woodlands and Plains Indians understandings of death. We also establish the important basic fact that, at least occasionally, Hopewell peoples revisited tombs and manipulated corpses after their first layout and before interring them. Our analysis offers a more detailed look at the content and purpose of some kinds of Ohio Hopewell mortuary rites than previous studies have provided.

This chapter begins with a synopsis of the social and ritual lives of Scioto Hopewell peoples as the cultural context of creation of the arranged burials. We then introduce two innovative approaches and apply them to the study of Scioto Hopewell mortuary remains: the theoretical concept of the ritual drama and the methodology of *anthropologie de terrain*. With this foundation, we then describe the range of variation of unusual Scioto Hopewell burial forms, with a focus on skeletons that had arms and/or legs spread out like bird wings and/or tail feathers. Next, the broader charnel house and spatial contexts of the burials are employed along with their forms in order to posit cultural interpretations of the burials individually and as a set, leading to our conclusion that they are the product of a ritual drama of Scioto Hopewell peoples' understanding of death and a soul's journey to an afterlife. We then compare the formal qualities of the suite of burials to the definitional characteristics of a ritual drama as a collective, narrative performance, showing that the burials are likely the remains of this kind of ritual. Finally, we come full circle, placing the drama into the broader Scioto Hopewell context of local community creation and intercommunity alliance strategy.

Cultural Context: The Social and Ritual Lives of Scioto Hopewell Peoples

Native Americans who lived in the Scioto valley in south-central Ohio between approximately 50 B.C. and A.D. 350, whom we call Scioto Hopewell peoples, lived extraordinarily rich social and ritual lives. Together, the people built and gathered in monumental geometric-shaped earthworks up to 80 acres in size for ceremonies of many kinds. Among these were mortuary rites in which they processed and honored their dead, interring them with socially and cosmologically coded and masterfully crafted paraphernalia made of glistening metals, semiprecious stones, and bones of powerful animals. In some cases, the mortuary rites took place in huge community charnel houses up to two-thirds the size of a football field. These qualities of the Scioto Hopewell material record create awe and evoke images of large ceremonies that were "spectacles" in the comparative sociological sense (MacAloon 1984). However, their specific nature and in particular whether some were "ritual dramas" (e.g., Ortiz 1972; Raglan 2003) that had their own special and potent logic for attracting and integrating people have yet to be considered.

The concepts, ways, and material record of Scioto Hopewell peoples are now reasonably sketched out (Carr and Case 2005; Case and Carr 2008; Charles and Buikstra 2006; Dancey and Pacheco 1997; Pacheco 1996:References). At the structural foundation of Scioto Hopewell life was a rhythmic alternation between gatherings in ceremonial centers for large to small events and the relative isolation of routine domestic life. Scioto Hopewell peoples were mixed forager-swidden farmers who spent most of their time close to nature in small work groups and in residential groups composed of only one or two extended-family households with 5–25 people. Households were visibly hidden from one another and were dispersed fair distances over the densely forested floodplain and terraces of the Scioto valley and its tributaries. Countering this physical isolation, the lives of Hopewell peoples in the Scioto drainage were intricately interwoven socially, politically, ritually, and spiritually into larger groups of a variety of kinds, geographic scales, social compositions, and functions: local communities of households, clans, clan-specific ceremonial societies, sodalities, possibly a phratry, and multicommunity social-spiritual alliances. Diverse, complementary leadership roles filled by members of different households, clans, and sodalities also tied groups together. People in these various groups and roles assembled periodically and situationally at ceremonial centers and fulfilled in complement and in different combinations many of their life needs and social-spiritual obligations.

In the Scioto–Paint Creek area, households integrated themselves into three or so local communities, each situated in a different segment of the Scioto valley, the main Paint Creek valley, and the North Fork of Paint Creek valley, and their total number varied over time (Figure 5.2). Each local community was composed of a minimum of a hundred people and probably more, and had in its lands multiple large earthen-enclosure ceremonial centers with differentiated ceremonial functions. In turn, depending on the era, from two to several adjacent local communities created strong alliances with one another, forming a more encompassing, self-identifying network of several hundred people, who combined hands to build earthworks and to ceremonially meet the spiritual and earthly needs of their lives, and who exchanged mates and probably food and other material resources.

Alliances among local communities were social-spiritual in nature. The alliances involved communities burying some of their dead relatives together

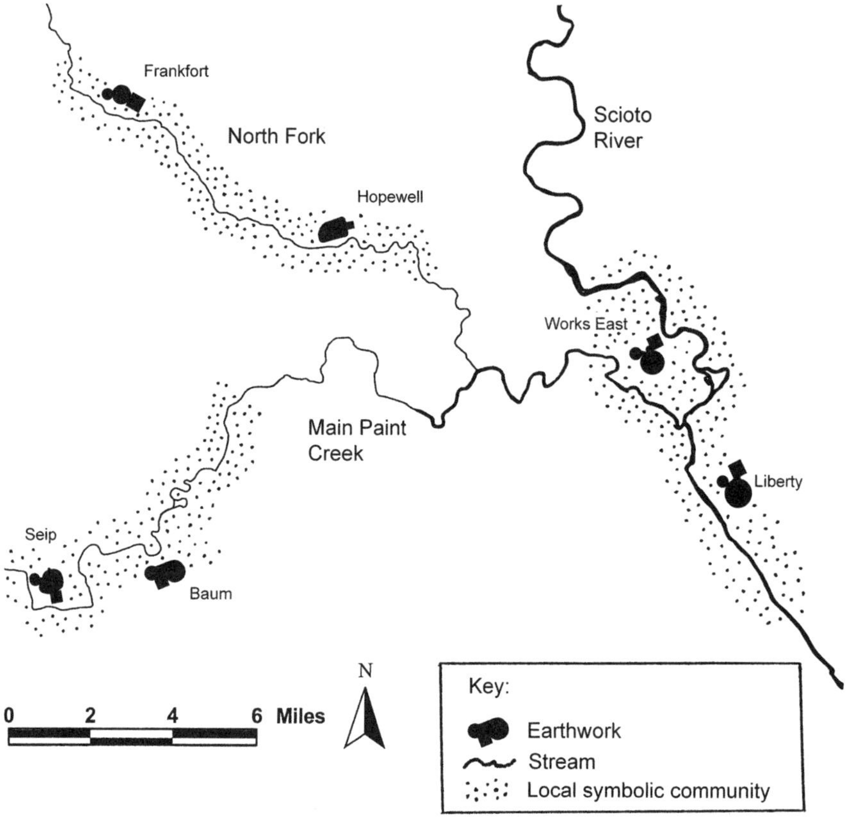

5.2. Three allied local communities in the North Fork of Paint Creek valley, the main Paint Creek valley, and the adjacent Scioto valley, ca. A.D. 250–325 in what is now Ross County, Ohio. (Drawing by Katharine Rainey Kolb and Christopher Carr)

in one to several shared cemeteries distributed across the communities (Carr 2005) and, in one instance, placing together the cremations of the deceased from multiple local communities in common ossuaries (Carr et al. 2005). These practices closely resemble the alliance-making efforts and ideology of historic Algonquian and Huron peoples, who believed that by mixing and burying the remains of their deceased relatives together, the souls of relatives, which were resident in their bones, were intermingled, creating strong, sanctified ties of cooperation among the deceased of different villages and tribes, and thereby among the living as well (Trigger 1969:103, 111). In this chapter, we focus on three allied local communities in the Scioto, Paint Creek, and North Fork valleys between about A.D. 250 and 325, and especially on one of the cemeteries in which the communities interred their dead: Mound 25 in the Hopewell earthworks (Figure 5.2).

Table 5.1. Minimum Number of Gift Givers for Largest Individual Burial Assemblages and Ceremonial Deposits, Scioto–Paint Creek Area[a]

Provenience	Size of Gathering (estimated number of gift givers)
Hopewell Mound 25, Altar 1	514[b]
Mound City, Mound 8, Depository	209
Tremper, Lower Cache	193
Hopewell Mound 25, Sk. 260–261 together	186
Hopewell Mound 25, Copper Deposit	127
Hopewell Mound 17, Offering 1	113
Hopewell Mound 17, Offering 2	111
Hopewell Mound 25, Sk. 260 by itself	93
Hopewell Mound 25, Sk. 261 by itself	93
Mound City, Mound 8, B2	58

[a]The number of gift givers who contributed to an assemblage or deposit is estimated by the methods of Carr, Goldstein, and Weets (2005:503–505). Essentially, in a given assemblage or deposit, each redundant artifact of a type that normally occurred (was owned) as one item per person in burial assemblages across Ohio is taken to represent the gift of one person for the assemblage or deposit. When an artifact class occurred typically two per burial (e.g., earspools), four per burial (e.g., bear canines), or some other unit number in burial assemblages across Ohio, then that unit is tallied instead of the individual artifacts for a given assemblage or deposit.
[b]This estimate conservatively assumes that the number of earspools deposited in Hopewell Mound 25, Altar 1, was 500 (250 pairs). If the number of earspools in the altar was 750–1,000 (375–500 pairs), per documentation summarized by Carr, Goldstein, and Weets (2005:488, Table 13.2, footnote a), then the estimated size of the gathering represented by this feature would be 643–768 people.

Ceremonial gatherings of Scioto Hopewell people in their earthworks were quite diverse in size and composition. Estimating the numbers of gift givers and their social roles by accumulations of artifacts of various kinds in burials or isolated deposits (following the methods of Carr et al. 2005:503–505) shows that most gatherings were small to moderate in size, with fewer than 25 gift givers. Much rarer were large gatherings of more than 90 gift givers (Carr et al. 2005:507, Table 13.6). The biggest documented gatherings ranged up to 500–700 gift givers (Table 5.1), and would have been larger if we include participants who did not give gifts. Large gatherings clearly involved the participation of multiple local communities. These occasions were ripe for the orchestration of ritual dramas or other formal spectacles.

The community organization and the political-ritual-mortuary system described here for Scioto Hopewell peoples were distinct from those of other Hopewellian peoples over the Eastern Woodlands (Brown 1979; Ruby et al.

2005). Our conclusions about ritual dramas and their functioning in Scioto Hopewell societies should not be extrapolated to other Hopewellian peoples without equal empirical study.

Sociocultural Theory and Bioarchaeological Method

Our approach to studying Scioto Hopewell peoples is innovative in two ways. The first is theoretical. We formalize the concept of the ritual drama in contrast to "ritual," "dramatic ritual," and "social drama," building on the work of Raglan (2003). Later, we apply these concepts to Scioto Hopewell arrangements of human remains and artifacts in burials in order to help interpret them. The second innovation is methodological. We apply the relatively new bioarchaeological methodology *anthropologie de terrain* to the burials in order to gain insight into their natural and cultural taphonomy and to enhance their cultural interpretation.

Rituals, Dramatic Rituals, and Ritual Dramas

The term "ritual drama" is reserved here for performances with a particular suite of characteristics, which we have drawn together from the works of other authors and cross-cultural comparisons.

First, a ritual drama is a performance—an act or proceeding. Second, as a ritual, the performance is largely set in form and content, being prescribed by social convention and usually repeated over time, either calendrically or situationally. Third, as a drama, by definition the performance relates a story. The story may be either mythic or historical, having a plot and characters of primeval time (e.g., Obeyesekere 1969:209) or of a remembered or not-too-distant past event (e.g., Metcalf and Huntington 1991:166). The myth or the historical narrative is acted out and structures the content and progression of the ritual. The myth is not simply told, or alluded to symbolically, during the course of the ritual but is a "charter" of the ritual, as defined by Malinowski (1954:144, 146).

Fourth, the story pertains to a collective: a village, a clan, a sodality, the state, and so on. Ritual dramas are expressions of "collective representations" in Durkheim's (1965:247–250, 253–255, 457) sense—collectively held ideas and sentiments about reality that are externalized/projected and materialized (e.g., Brown 2003:81–83, 94, 97, 2006:204–209). Fifth, in societies having small numbers of people, on the order of tens to a thousand or so, the performance involves all people in the band, village, clan, sodality, or society to which the rite pertains. The ritual is a collective effort, designed for individual and collective effects on the participants, rather than for observance by an audience. Some common collective purposes of ritual dramas, beyond their event-specific rationales, include releasing individual emotions (catharsis), channeling and regulating deviancy, reinforcing normative behavior, resolving tensions among factions, social integration and building collective identity, and mobilizing a community into action (Ortiz 1972:139). In larger, more complex societies, where not all can possibly participate in a single ceremony, the ritual drama can be transformed into an expression that includes an audience: civic ritual (Johnston and Hüsken 1997; Sudarsono 1984); cultic theater (Horn 1981; Nielsen 2002); pageants, mystery plays, and miracle plays (Cawley 1993; Holme 1987; Oakshott 2001); secular drama or theater (Miotshwa 1988; Raglan 2003; but see Rozik 2003); and opera (Omojola 2001–2002).

Sixth, in native North American societies, a ritual drama commonly concerns the cosmos at large. The rite may express the structure of the cosmos and the relationships among the beings within it, that is, the rite is a "cosmogram" (Brown 2003:93, 97). Renewal of the cosmos is a frequent theme (e.g., Ortiz 1972:153; Swanton 1928a:546–614). Emphasis on relationships at the expansive scale of the cosmos is encouraged by native North American concepts of personhood, which attribute it to many nonhuman animate beings and to inanimate things (e.g., Hallowell 1926, 1960; Harrod 2000; Morrison 2000; Overholt and Callicott 1982), and by native North American concepts of the self, which is conceived of and experienced as a human person in relationship with other human and nonhuman persons of the cosmos rather than as a separable individual (Diamond et al. 1994:22–24; Fogelson and Kutsche 1961; Morrison 1984:63, 2000:33–34, 2002; Peacock and Wisuri 2002:29; Peers and Brown 2000).

Seventh, the characters in a ritual drama, which the people of a society assume and in some instances become experientially, are commonly mythic heroes, other mythic or spirit beings, or "*personnages*" (Mauss 1938, 1985:31–33). By the latter is meant a role or character that is taken on by an individual in a ritual drama and/or in daily family and community life that is explicitly identified and experienced as the continuation of an ancestor who has reincarnated in that individual as the rightful successor. The role exists in perpetuity through the generations. In its equation with a reincarnated ancestor, a *personnage* is associated with a set of rights and duties, a title or name, a mask, other ceremonial paraphernalia, a badge or insignia, and/or a seat (Mauss 1938, 1985:31–33; see also Gillespie 2001:82–83). Masks, paraphernalia, badges, and insignia are commonly used in ritual dramas to identify specific *personnages* as the characters of the narrative.

In some ritual dramas, actors are stripped entirely of their social and personal identities in life and assume the roles of mythological characters. In other ritual dramas, the enactments blend mythic characters with earthly people and blend primeval time with current time in order to effectively connect earthly reality with the power of a mythic one (Sorensen 1986).

Prime examples of ritual dramas of native North Americans include those of the Puebloans and the Northwest Coast Indians, which involve the entire community or clan (Ortiz 1972; see also Cook 1976; Denman 1953; Frisbie 1980), and the medicine rite of the Winnebagos (Radin 1945), which includes the members of the medicine society.

Ritual dramas can occur as a part of rites of many kinds, including funerals. In a mortuary setting, the contents and layout of a cemetery, a cluster of graves, or a single grave, which are archaeologically visible, can indicate the narrative content and plot of the drama. This will be shown in our Scioto Hopewell case. Other examples of ritual dramas, their material correlates, or both include the layout of Cahokia's Mound 72 burials as a Mississippian cosmogram expressing the conquering of death through rebirth (Brown 2003, 2006); the funerary rites of the divine kings of the African Shilluk, during which the kingdom's unification is reenacted (Metcalf and Huntington 1991:166); a long Berawan funeral song that describes the geography that the soul of the deceased traverses on its way to an afterlife in the idyllic homeland from where the Berawan migrated historically (Metcalf and Huntington 1991:87–89); and the accession rites and funerals of Mayan aristocrats who, along with bundles of valuable heirlooms and memorializing tablets, represented the *personnage* of the founding head of their royal house (Gillespie 2001:96–99; Martin and Grube 2008; Schele and Freidel 1990).

The notion of the ritual drama and the term itself were first introduced, apparently, by Lord FitzRoy Richard Somerset Raglan (2003:279) in his work *The Hero: A Study in Tradition, Myth, and Drama.* His definition contains most of the seven characteristics given above. Mauss (1938, 1985:4–12) and Ortiz (1972) fleshed out some details, although Mauss used the term "sacred drama." A given ritual drama may be part of a larger cycle of dramas performed over the course of a year or years (Ortiz 1972:156). It also may be situationally determined but repeated (Metcalf and Huntington 1991:166) or, extending the definition, may be situationally determined and unique (e.g., Brown 2003, 2006).

In American archaeology, the term "ritual drama" was first used by Robert Hall (2000:249). He interpreted a quartet of headless burials in the Dickson Mounds Cemetery and a like foursome in Mound 72 at the Cahokia site in Illinois as the remains of a rite having elements similar to a Mesoamerican one in which an impersonator of the green corn goddess, Xilonen, was sacrificed. He also drew parallels to a Pawnee ritual drama in which an impersonator of Morning Star was sacrificed and to the Creek Green Corn Ceremony. Shortly thereafter, James A. Brown (2003, 2006) identified the "beaded burial" and surrounding corpses under Mound 72 as the result of a collective ritual about the conquest of death by Morning Star. Brown's conceptual framework and analysis for interpreting the Mound 72, Submound 1, burial assemblage fully accord with the notion of a ritual drama as defined here, although he did not use the term.

The concept of the ritual drama is distinct from the concepts "ritual" and "dramatic ritual" (Raglan 2003:279; see also MacAloon 1984). The latter two are more encompassing concepts that need not involve a narrative or a personification of mythic or historical figures, need not pertain to and be performed by a collective, and need not have a cosmological focus. A dramatic ritual is simply one that is "spectacular" (Raglan 2003:279; MacAloon 1984), such as a football game or a grand opening. Victor Turner's (1957, 1967, 1968, 1974, 1982) concept of the "social drama" is yet further removed from the notion of a "ritual drama."

Anthropologie de terrain

The bioarchaeological method *anthropologie de terrain*, or "field anthropology," as developed by the French anthropologists Henri Duday and Claude Masset (Duday 2006; see also Duday and Masset 1987; Duday et al. 1990), aims at identifying the intentions behind a mortuary ritual by reconstructing the original burial context (Roksandic 2002:101). How cultural and biological processes have transformed a burial is inferred by precisely documenting each skeletal element in a grave context and comparing their positions to those that normally result as the body undergoes a sequence of decomposition and decay events in a specific burial environment. Principles of archaeology, taphonomy, and forensic anthropology are used (Boddington et al. 1987; Duday 2006; Garland and Janaway 1987; Gifford 1981; Haglund and Sorg 2002; Mant 1987; Nilsson Stutz 2003; Rodriguez and Bass 1985; Roksandic 2002; Schiffer 1987; Tiesler Blos 2006). The skeletal analysis is most commonly done during excavation, but can be accomplished with photographs, notes, and drawings if they are clear and accurate (Nilsson Stutz 2003).

Anthropologie de terrain allows researchers to infer the nature of the burial (primary or secondary), the space of decomposition (open or filled with soil), whether grave furniture that has decayed (i.e., shrouds, biers, coffins, or other grave goods) was once present, the relative chronology of deposition of individuals in graves with multiple people, and postdecay manipulation of the body during revisiting of a tomb (Duday 2006; see also Duday et al. 1990; Nilsson Stutz 2003; Roksandic 2002; Tiesler Blos 2006). These inferences are made by considering, first, how far removed various skeletal articulations are from correct anatomical position (Roksandic 2002:102); second, that weaker, or labile, articulations, including cervical vertebrae, bones of the hands and feet, costosternal joints, and scapulothoracic junction, become disarticulated sooner than the lumbar vertebrae and sacrum, the femora and ilia, and the tarsals (Duday 2006); and third, that decomposition in an open space where bones are not supported by surrounding soil or a container allows opening of the pubic symphysis, lateral expansion of the iliac blades, and lateral movement of the bones of the legs, including the patellae (Duday 2006).

Scioto Hopewell Mortuary Ceremonies

In order to inventory the various ways in which Scioto Hopewell peoples ritually arranged human remains and artifacts prior to their final burial under mounds, we examined published and unpublished field photographs and drawings of 89 graves and artifact deposits in 18 Ohio Hopewell mortuary sites (Table 5.2). The sample includes most, if not all, extant field photographs and drawings from each of the 18 sites that are clear enough and close enough to have allowed us to identify bones to elements and artifacts to types.

We found that unusual arrangements of human remains and/or artifacts were common and not idiosyncratic in Scioto Hopewell cemeteries. The arrangements pattern into a suite of at least 10 definable forms with interpretable meanings grounded in Eastern Woodlands ethnohistory. The forms and meanings pertain broadly to the death process, the cosmos and its structure, and people from life or myth. They include (1) a skeletal-artifact arrangement and a cranial modification, each possibly depicting the soul of a deceased man leaving his body through his head; (2) human skeletons with their arms and sometimes their legs spread widely, which we interpret to represent a bird in flight with wings and tail feathers spread—a reference to the freed soul of the deceased in flight, the merger of the person in life or death with his or her bird tutelary spirit and metamorphosis into a bird, the human impersonation of birds or mythical birdpeople in ceremonies during life, or some combination of these; (3) skeletons and cremations sculpted into the form of heads of birds, possibly referencing soul flight or a person's metamorphosis into a bird in life or death; (4) layouts of cremated human remains or pearls in the form of an arc, which may represent the Milky Way—one of the paths in historic Woodland and Plains Indians' experience that souls of the deceased took to a land of the dead; (5) skeletons with artifacts implying the soul of the deceased at the edge of the earth-island, waiting to get onto the Milky Way path, and then the soul's encounters with beings along the path; (6) arrangements of skeletons or cremations that reference the four perpendicular directions of the cosmos; (7) skeletons and cremations surrounded by material symbols of

Table 5.2. Scioto Hopewell Sites, Graves, and Artifact Deposits

Site	Number of Graves and Artifact Deposits
Boyle's Farm	1
Porter Farm	1
Jesse Redman Farm	2
Glen Helen Mound	4
Hazlett Mound	2
Irvin Coy Mound	2
McKenzie Mound	1
Edwin Harness Mound	6
North Benton Mound	4
West Mound	1
Fort Ancient	1
Seip Pricer Mound	13
Hopewell	31
Mound City	9
Seip Mound	4
Purdom Mound	1
Rockhold Mound	1
Unknown, Scioto Hopewell	5
Total	89

Note: For locations of the sites in Ohio, see Case and Carr (2008:344, Figure 7.1).

ghost water barriers, which also probably represent the axis mundi in cross section, and a cremation set in a stump that likely represents the World Tree form of the axis mundi; (8) cremations and artifacts arranged to form human faces, which could represent the deceased, ancestors, or humans' impersonation of mythological characters; (9) cremations and artifacts made into bird-human composite faces and a human face with a bird mask, which possibly reference the soul flight of the deceased, shamanic metamorphosis, or mythological characters; and (10) combinations of skeletal parts, one or more cremations, or artifacts, or groupings of any of these kinds of items, arranged to create the extended body of a person/being.

We can give here only a small introduction to this diversity of forms and the beginning of an assessment of whether some of the arrangements were produced in the course of ritual dramas or rituals of a different social or personal nature. We also begin to evaluate whether some of the rituals were large public events or had a restricted audience. We concentrate on a tight set of

Table 5.3. Skeletons of the Scioto–Paint Creek Area Positioned or Modified to Resemble Birds

Site	Reference
Hopewell earthwork, Mound 4, Burial 3	Shetrone 1926:33–34
Hopewell earthwork, Mound 25, Burial 41A[a]	Shetrone 1926:92–93
Hopewell earthwork, Mound 25, Burial 41B	Shetrone 1926:92–93
Hopewell earthwork, Mound 25, Burial 41C	Shetrone 1926:92–93
Hopewell earthwork, Mound 25, Burial 42	Shetrone 1926:93–94
Hopewell earthwork, Mound 25, Burial 45A	Shetrone 1926:95
Hopewell earthwork, Mound 26, Burial 6	Shetrone 1926:103–105
Old Town (Frankfort) earthwork, Porter Mound 15, Skeleton R	Moorehead 1892:126–128
Seip earthwork, Pricer Mound, Burial 52	Shetrone and Greenman 1931:393–394

Note: [a]This individual had his foot bones modified to look like bird talons but did not have his arms or legs positioned like bird wings and tail feathers.

skeletons that were positioned with their arms, legs, or both spread out like the wings and/or tail feathers of a bird, and related burials, all of which depict a sequence of episodes in a death process and journey to an afterlife as understood by some historic Woodland and Plains Indians.

Skeletons with Arms and Legs Akimbo

Eight skeletons under five mounds in three geometric earthwork sites in the North Fork and main Paint Creek valleys were positioned with their arms and sometimes their legs spread like the wings and tail feathers of a bird (Table 5.3). As examples, consider Burials 41A, 41B, and 41C under Mound 25 in the Hopewell earthwork (Figure 5.3a). The skeletons of a male, a female, and a probable female, all of relatively old age for Hopewell peoples (36–49 years), were laid adjacent to one another in an unusually large log tomb. The two females (41B, 41C) had arms and legs akimbo in bird form. The male (41A) did not, but was missing all of his phalanges and some of his metatarsals on each foot. Three metatarsals were present on each foot, giving the appearance of the front three talons of a bird's foot. The bodies were laid out in the flesh, before any significant decay had occurred, as evident from the intact nature of labile costosternal articulations and the scapulothoracic junction. Phalanges of the hands and feet were excluded from consideration because they can easily be disturbed during tomb reentry and excavation. The three metatarsals on each foot of 41A were selected for retention or replaced after skele-

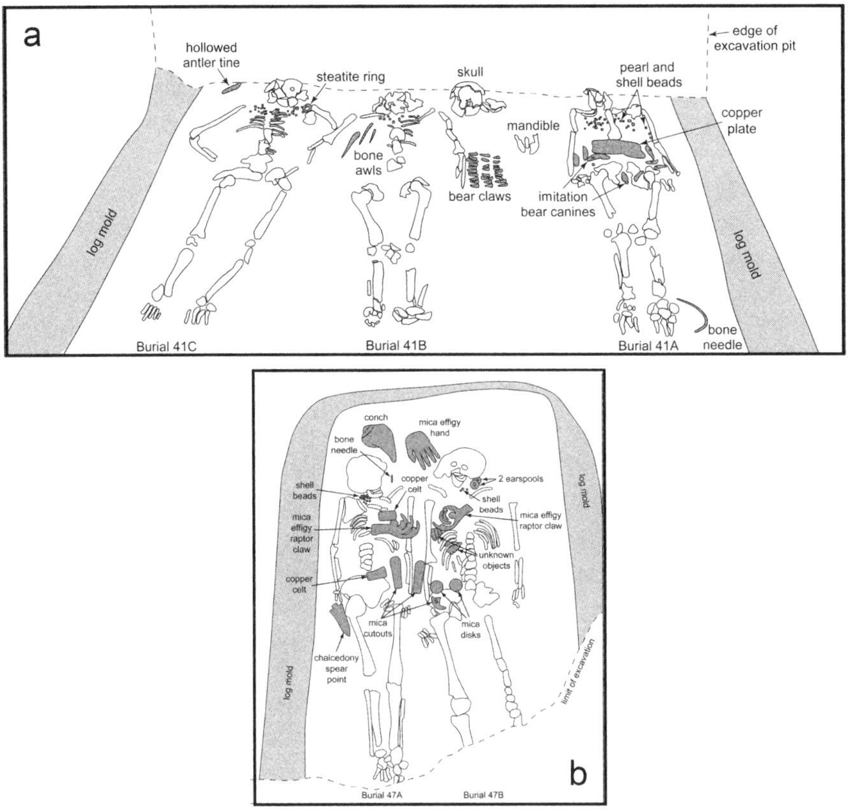

5.3. (a) Hopewell site, Mound 25, Burials 41A, B, C (*right to left*) (adapted from Ohio Historical Society, Print 855, AV17/B3/F2/E6/14). (b) Hopewell site, Mound 25, Burials 47A, B (*left to right*) (adapted from Shetrone 1926:96, Figure 35; and Ohio Historical Society, Print 859, AV17/B3/F2/5). (Drawings by Rebekah Zinser)

tonization, indicating tomb reentry. It is possible that 41B was laid out after 41C because the right arm of 41B overlaps the left arm of 41C. Such overlap does not occur, or occurs rarely, in other double burials at the Hopewell site. The length of time between the laying out of 41C and 41B is unknown; the superpositioning could have occurred in the same ceremony or significantly later, indicating tomb reentry. Both 41A and 41C have cut marks on their mandibles consistent with the removal of their mandibles for display or other purposes (Johnston 2002). Both mandibles were found in roughly correct anatomical position relative to the skull and the rest of the body. The mandible of 41C was missing an incisor—the tooth type first lost in both dental arcades when skulls and mandibles are curated and decay (Roksandic

2002:110). If the mandibles of 41A and 41C were removed and curated for some time, tomb reentry is again implicated. Consistent with all of the above evidence for tomb reentry and body manipulation, all three individuals decomposed in open tombs rather than in tombs filled in with dirt, as indicated by disarticulation of the pubic symphyses and expansion of the ilia laterally.

The workings of other taphonomic agents on Burials 41A, B, and C cannot be completely discounted. However, natural disturbance of bone positioning by rodents or other animals would have been discouraged by the burials' location on a clay platform within a closed tomb of heavy timbers, which in turn was within a larger charnel house. These observations support the interpretation of intentional manipulation of the bodies.

All of the five other individuals who were laid out with their arms, legs, or both akimbo (Table 5.3) were positioned while in the flesh and decayed in the open, whether they were placed in a log tomb (n = 3) or not (n = 2). None show evidence of postdecay body manipulation or other evidence of tomb reentry of the kinds cited above, save perhaps Skeleton R from Porter Mound 15 in the Old Town (Frankfort) works. Skeleton R's feet had only three metatarsals each, similar to Burial 41A's. However, some phalanges are present for both feet, making a representation of the talons of a bird's feet less apparent. Whether the presence of the three metatarsals with miscellaneous phalanges indicates the transition of human feet into bird talons—a kind of human-animal liminality common in Ohio Hopewell art—is unclear.

All but one of the eight individuals were interred with items that marked social and personal identities in life, including clan affiliation (drilled raccoon teeth), sodality membership (breastplates, earspools), public ceremonial leadership (barracuda jaw scratchers), personal importance (shell and pearl necklaces and bracelets), and personal domestic identity (bone needles, awls, antler tine, flake knives). All were older individuals who had time to achieve such positions during their lives. In these ways, the eight individuals do not appear on first impression to have been actors who were stripped of their social and personal identities in life and who played the roles of mythological characters in ritual dramas. Alternatively, more personal interpretations of the corpses, such as representation of the freed soul of the deceased in flight, or the merger of the person in life or death with his or her bird tutelary spirit and metamorphosis into a bird, might seem more reasonable. However, ritual dramas sometimes merge mythic characters with earthly identities, and primeval time with current time, to bring desirable qualities of a mythic reality (e.g., power, balance) into earthly life.

In order to evaluate whether any of the eight human skeletons laid out as birds were the product of ritual dramas that were performed by Scioto

Hopewell peoples in the course of their mortuary rites, or whether the layouts resulted from rites of some different kind, it is necessary to put the cases in their spatial context and in light of historic Woodland religious knowledge. Audience size and whether the rituals were large public events or smaller, perhaps more private occasions, can also be assessed contextually. For brevity, we consider only the five skeletons under Mound 25 at the Hopewell site—Burials 41A, B, and C; Burial 42; and Burial 45A—and the individuals with whom they were spatially associated.

Spatial Context: The Mound 25 Skeletons with Arms and Legs Akimbo

All five of the skeletons who have arms and legs akimbo and were interred under Mound 25 of the Hopewell site were located in the easternmost charnel house (C) (Figure 5.4) of the three main charnel buildings (C, D, E; Greber and Ruhl 1989:50, Figure 2.16, foldout) under the mound. The charnel house was elliptical to circular, with an interior area between 924 and 1,120 ft^2 of floor space, excluding graves and an altar. It easily could have accommodated a hundred individuals during a ceremony—in line with the sizes documented for large ceremonial gatherings in the Scioto–Paint Creek area (Table 5.1) and the equivalent of one to a few local communities (see Figure 5.2). Further, the eastern charnel house and its burials are inferred from mortuary studies to have been associated with one of the three allied local communities that resided in the Scioto, main Paint Creek, and North Fork valleys between A.D. 250 and 325 (Carr 2005:310–311). Both the size and the local community association of the eastern charnel house open the possibility that some of the ceremonies held in it were collective, community-wide affairs, perhaps augmented with participants from one or both of the other local two communities as well. The possible collective nature of the rites aligns with one defining characteristic of ritual dramas.

The fact that all five of the skeletons that had arms, legs, or both akimbo and that were interred under Mound 25 are restricted to the one (eastern) charnel building and missing from the other two suggests a style of mortuary rite tied to a local community. The community tie reinforces the interpretation of a collective, community ceremony but does not necessitate it.

A very specific reconstruction of the rites that were performed in the eastern charnel house is revealed by the nature of the burials with which the five individuals with arms and/or legs akimbo were associated spatially in the eastern end of the charnel building (Figure 5.4). The five burials and four near to them, taken together as a set, appear to depict a sequence of episodes commonly told by some historic Woodland Native Americans about the death process and journey from this life to an afterlife (Lankford 2007a:201–

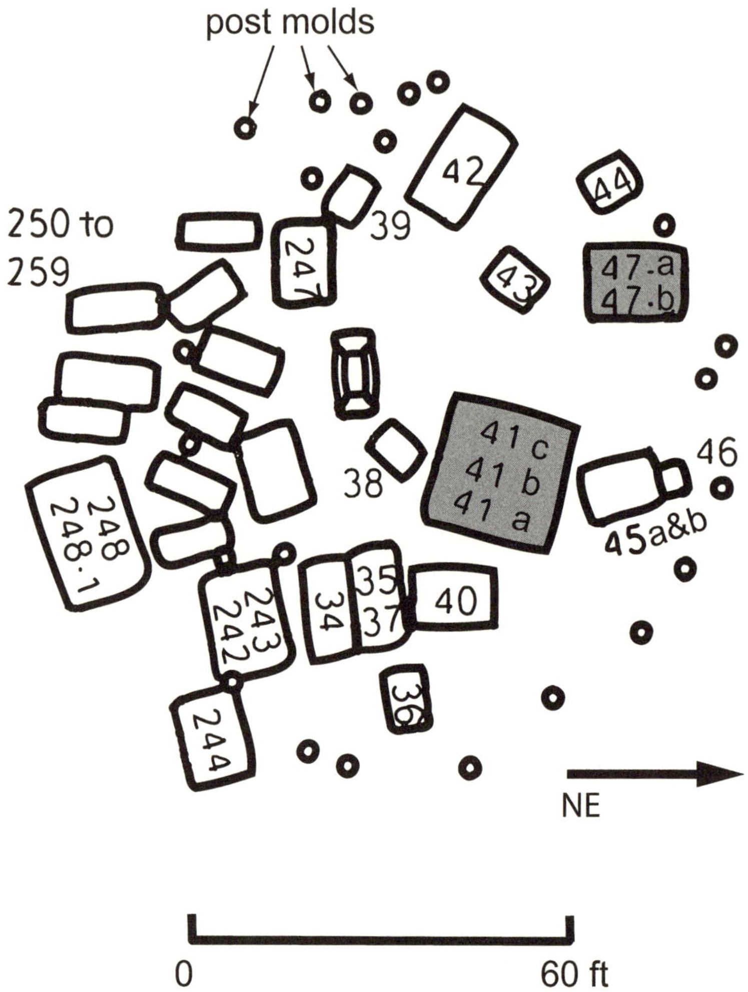

5.4. The easternmost charnel house (C) of the three main charnel houses, C, D, and E (Greber and Ruhl 1989:50, Figure 2.16, foldout), under Mound 25 in the Hopewell site. (Drawing by Christopher Carr)

256, 2007b, 2007c). The suite of nine burials seems to be the product of a collective rite orchestrated to a narrative having a cosmological plot—all defining characteristics of ritual dramas. Specifically, the nine burials can be interpreted to depict the release of a soul from the physical body, the flight of the soul as a bird, its arrival at the primal waters at the edge of the earth-island, its leap through a portal—the Hand constellation in Orion—onto the Milky Way path of souls that leads to a land of the dead, and the challenges the soul faces along the path, as described in historic Woodland Indian narratives (Lankford 2007a:201–256, 2007b, 2007c). The burials defining this sequence are as follows.

(1) Burial 34 (Figure 5.1e) is an extended skeleton with a mica cutout effigy of a headless human positioned as though emerging from the cranium of the deceased, feet first, with the cranium serving the dual role of head of the deceased and head of the cutout. We interpret the assemblage as a representation of one of the souls of the man leaving his head. The head is one of the parts of the body commonly thought by Woodland Indians to be the seat of a person's free soul, which sooner or later travels to an afterlife after death (e.g., Hewitt 1895:108–111, 114; Hultkrantz 1953:73–93). The mica cutout is an expectable way to represent a person's soul. The mica's flat, reflective, and watery-looking surface recalls the Woodland belief that one can see one's soul in the reflection of still water or in a mirror, including a mica mirror (Hall 1976:361), in which the soul looks flat. The same convention of a flat soul leaving the body of an individual for soul flight is used in another piece of Ohio Hopewell artwork (Carr 2008:183).

(2) Burials 41A, B, and C (Figure 5.3a), Burial 42, and Burial 45A, all with individuals having their arms, legs, or both akimbo, or their foot bones manipulated to look like bird talons, can be interpreted as expressing the bird-like free soul of the deceased in flight on its journey to a land of the dead. Birds are a common representation of the free soul across the globe and time (Eliade 1972:206, 392, 479–481; Vastokas 1974–1975:126, 130) because soul flight during trance is commonly experienced as being transformed into a bird that flies or as being carried by a flying bird (Balzer 1996:306; Butt 1967:56–58; Eliade 1972:477–482; Furst 1973–1974:34, 59; Halifax 1979:16–18, 156; Schultes and Hofmann 1979:122; Vastokas 1974–1975:130; Vitebsky 2001:70; Wilbert 1975:448). The trance experience of soul flight as being a flying bird is reported for historic Iroquois (Thwaites 1959:17:153, 26:267, 33:191, 39:19 [1896–1901], in von Gernet and Timmins 1987:39) and Lakota Sioux (Halifax 1979:74–75). The idea of the free soul of the deceased transforming into a flying bird or being carried by a flying bird was held by historic and contemporary Ojibwas (Hallowell 1940:38; Smith 1995:90), the historic Hurons (Thwaites 1959:10:143, 287 [1896–1901]), and Iroquois (Morgan 1901:167). Soul flight in bird form was also expressed specifically by Scioto Hopewell peoples in a hawk effigy that was carved with a human face on its head, found in one of the charnel houses under Mound 25 of the Hopewell earthwork (Altar 2; Moorehead 1922:160, 166, Figure 65). Later, late prehistoric peoples in the area carved a smoking pipe in the form of the body of a bird in flight with the head of a human. The pipe was found in an

earthwork near Chillicothe, Ohio (Squier and Davis 1848:247). Significantly, smoking the strong native tobacco of North America, *Nicotiana rustica*, can induce trance and the dissociational experience of soul flight (von Gernet 1988; von Gernet and Timmins 1987:38).

(3) Burial 43 (Figure 5.1b) consists of the cremation remains of an adult and a child sculpted into an arc, with a marine conch at either end. An elongated turtle-shell ornament spans the space between the two conchs. The layout is reminiscent of the arc of the Milky Way as conceived by many Woodland and Plains Indian tribes, with its two ends reaching down to the ocean waters (represented by the marine conchs) beyond the shore of this world, Turtle Island (represented by the turtle-shell ornament). The Milky Way was thought by many Woodland and Plains tribes of diverse regions and language groups to be the path taken by one of the souls of the deceased to a land of the dead: for example, the Hurons (Sagard-Théodat 1632, 1939:172; Thwaites 1959:6:181 [1896–1901]; Trigger 1969:103), Delawares (Kraft 1986:192), Shawnees (Howard 1981:167; Schutz 1975:95–97), Potawatomis (Skinner 1924:52), Menominees (Skinner 1913:85); Sauks (Skinner 1923:36), Cherokees (Hagar 1906:354), Creeks (Swanton 1928a:479, 1928b: 256), Omahas (Fletcher and La Flesche 1911:588, 590), and Pawnees (Fletcher 1903:13).[1] To the point, cremations of the deceased themselves were used in Burial 43 to make this path of souls. The same theme might have been rendered in the layout of two other individuals elsewhere in Mound 25 (Burials 6 and 24), who each had an arc of pearls over their heads.

(4) Burials 47A and 47B (Figure 5.3b)—a pair of side-by-side inhumations—complete the theme of a soul's journey to an afterlife. Burial 47A has a marine conch shell laid at its head—a place of entrance and exiting of the free soul known in many cultures around the world. The positioning of a conch shell at the head is a strong burial pattern at the Hopewell site, found in eight other graves under Mounds 25, 23, and 2. The arrangement can be interpreted as the journey of the soul across the earth-island to the ocean waters at its edge (represented by the conch), where the soul must wait for the right moment to get onto the Milky Way.

In line with this interpretation, above and in between the heads of Burials 47A and 47B and reaching downward, is a mica cutout of a human hand. It may correspond to the Hand constellation—the lower half of Orion with fingers reaching downward— recognized by some Plains tribes and possibly thought to be a portal through which the soul of the deceased must pass to get onto the Milky Way path of souls. The soul would have to leap from the earth through the portal in a brief moment before it sank below the waters at the edge of the earth-island or else miss its opportunity to journey on the Milky Way to an afterlife (Lankford 2007b:177). In Burials 47A and 47B, the waters into which the Hand constellation sinks are probably represented by the conch shell adjacent to the mica hand and above the head of Burial 47A.

The leap into the sinking portal would have been a critical, time-limited moment for a soul, and a dangerous one according to historic native Woodland peoples, when a soul might be crushed between the edge of the earth disk and the setting sky, that is, the Milky Way (Lankford 2007b:204). The moment would have also been of great concern to the living, for a soul that did not make it through the hand portal would eventually become unhappy and a threat to the living (Lankford 2007b:177). A ritual drama concerned with passing through the hand portal would not be an unexpected part of a mortuary ceremony.

Burials 47A and 47B each have on their chest a mica cutout of a raptor's claw. The claws may represent an eagle that a soul has to fight at one point when traversing the Milky Way. The Alabama and Seminole held this belief and prepared their dead for the fight by burying them with a knife or a burnt wood torch in hand (MacCauley 1887:522; Swanton 1946:724, in Lankford 2007b:210). Significantly, Burial 47A held in its right hand a seven-inch spear point or knife made of a rare amber chalcedony. Challenges of several kinds while traveling the Milky Way were widely described by Woodland and Plains Indians (Barnouw 1977:18–19, 136; Lankford 2007b:178, 182–187, 190–191, 207–211).

In sum, the nine individuals significantly buried near to one another at one end of the eastern charnel house under Mound 25 together likely depict a narrative of the soul's journey to an afterlife as held by Scioto Hopewell peoples. It is not hard to imagine a ritual drama of this journey, with its various episodes enacted in sequence at the graves that were arranged to express those events. The credibility of this reconstruction lies in the specific contents and internal layouts of individual burials, their spatial association, and the telling of the elements of the narrative by historic Woodland and Plains Indians.

Conclusion

The multiple lines of evidence presented here converge on the conclusion that Burials 41A, B, and C, with their arms and/or legs akimbo, were elements of a ritual drama in the formal sense defined in this chapter. The layout of Burials 41A, B, and C was *ritualistic*—it was repeated in a set way for eight skeletons under five different mounds in three different geometric earthwork sites in two different, neighboring valleys. The ritual that included Burials 41A, B, and C strongly appears to have been orchestrated around a *narrative*—the story of the journey that a soul makes to an afterlife. The grave of individuals 41A, B, and C, along with those of six other individuals nearby, expressed distinct episodes of the narrative. The narrative would most likely have been a *collective representation*—a cluster of ideas about death held collectively by Hopewell peoples who resided in one of the local communities in the Scioto–Paint Creek area and who used the eastern charnel house under Mound 25 in the Hopewell earthwork. At least some of the ideas were also held by people of the adjacent local Hopewell community in main Paint Creek valley, who interred at least one individual with arms akimbo—(Burial 52) in the middle burial cluster under the Pricer Mound in the Seip earthwork. The ritual that involved Burials 41A, B, and C and nearby burials may have been a *collective performance* that included many or all of the members of the local community that used the eastern charnel house under Mound 25, and perhaps participants from one or two other neighboring local communities. Collective participation is suggested by the large floor area of Mound 25's eastern charnel house, which contained the burials, and by conservative estimates of the maximum sizes of ceremonial gatherings that Scioto Hopewell peoples held (Table 5.1). The motive for performing the ritual drama was most probably collective: to guide and/or encourage deceased people in their journey to an afterlife and to aid them through the journey's challenges, both with empathy for them and/or with concern for keeping them from returning and causing problems for the living. Further, the ritual involving Burials 41A, B, and C was *cosmological* in its plot—the journey to an afterlife—and the burials in the eastern charnel house that together expressed this plot constituted a *cosmogram*. Finally, individuals 41A, B, and C and the others adjacent to them in the eastern charnel house, played roles of a cosmological nature and perhaps of mythic proportion, while retaining some of their more ordinary social and personal identities in life. The individuals could well have blended mythic characters with earthly people, and primeval time with current time, effectively bridging earthly and mythic realities. Whether the individuals were *personnages* in Mauss's (1938, 1985) sense is unknown.

In all these ways, it appears that ceremonies in the form of a ritual drama were part of the repertoire of the Scioto Hopewell peoples who gathered in their earthworks. Ritual drama was likely a fundamental means by which people in households dispersed across the landscape wove themselves together as a local community, and perhaps as allied local communities, in earthly and mythic time.

Acknowledgments

We thank the Ohio Historical Society, Columbus, for providing Chris Carr access to field excavation photographs of many of the Ohio Hopewell burials and artifact deposits analyzed in this chapter. We are very grateful to Rebekah Zinser for drafting the line drawings of the burials and artifact deposits.

Note

1. Most historic Woodland and Plains Indian groups held that a person has multiple souls rather than one (e.g., Hultkrantz 1953:15–126) and that only one of them went to a land of the dead. The Iroquois understood that a person has two souls, which went to different places at death, with only one soul following the Milky Way (Mann 2003:182–184; see also Howard 1981:166 vs. 167).

6

Phallic Batons Made of Bone in the Collections of the Ohio Historical Society

Anne B. Lee and Cheryl A. Johnston

Interest in artifacts emphasizing certain sexual characteristics of the female body (e.g., breasts, hips) has a long history and has spawned a large body of scholarly publications (Nelson 1993; Soffer et al. 2000:514 and references; Taylor 1996:115–125). Most often, these depictions of the female body are interpreted in terms of the fertility of women, society, or nature. Less common are artifacts representing male anatomy, particularly in North America. Two artifacts resembling human phalli, presumably made of human bone, were identified in the archaeological collections of the Ohio Historical Society (OHS). The approach of this chapter is intentionally atheoretical. Given the absence of any literature regarding such objects as phallic bone batons in the American Midwest, the goal of this chapter is to disseminate information about the artifacts and to open a dialogue in the archaeological community that may lead to the documentation of similar artifacts and the generation of meaningful and testable hypotheses regarding this artifact type.

The two artifacts are described and their respective archaeological and museum contexts are presented. An attempt is made to place these artifacts in a wider cultural context by presenting similar nonbone artifacts from regional and worldwide archaeological and ethnographic contexts. With so little known about the phallic batons of human bone described here, four possible lines of inquiry into their meaning and function are presented for consideration.

Phallic Batons in the Collections of the Ohio Historical Society

Terminology

The term "phallic baton" is derived from the Old World term *bâton de commandement* ("rod of command"), which refers to artifacts of a particular form (long, cylindrical, with both a tapering end and a wider end) and an unknown function. *Bâton de commandement* is applied to a wide range of Old World artifacts, from realistic to abstract representations of an erect penis. The term *bâton percé* ("pierced rod") is used for similar objects having a pierced end or a hole at the wider end; such artifacts are thought to have functioned as arrow or spear shaft straighteners.

The term "phallic baton" is used here to denote artifacts of a similar morphology (resembling a phallus) and similarly unknown function. These artifacts are longer than wide, cylindrical, and typically have a recognizable glans and sometimes a widening at the opposing end that resembles a scrotum. A conservative definition is used here since it would be quite easy to see phallic symbols in every long, narrow artifact.

Artifacts

Two artifacts resembling human phalli were identified in the archaeological collection of the OHS while we were conducting an inventory of human remains for federal Native American Graves Protection and Repatriation Act purposes in 1998–1999. Both artifacts were found in boxes containing only human remains; this museum/storage context suggested that these artifacts were made of human bone. Closer examination by a physical anthropologist and a zooarchaeologist indicated that the two artifacts were made of large mammal long bone shafts. It was determined that these artifacts were most likely manufactured of human bone based on three qualitative indicators: (1) the ratio of cortical bone thickness to cancellous bone thickness and the overall diameter of the long bone shaft; (2) the texture and density, which were most similar to human bone previously examined; and (3) at least for the item from a Hopewell context, the fact that bone artifacts were more commonly made of human bone than of the bones of other large mammals.

Artifact A283/131 is a calcined long bone modified to form a characteristic mushroom-shaped top resembling a glans with a straight, cylindrical shaft (Figure 6.1). Measurements for this artifact are listed in Table 6.1. It was recovered from Shetrone's Mound 17 (distinguished from Moorehead's Mound 17 by Greber and Ruhl [1989:17]) at the Hopewell Mound group, a Middle Woodland burial/ceremonial site in Ross County, Ohio. Hopewell is a cultural phenomenon that existed between 200 B.C. and A.D. 400 (Greber and Ruhl 1989) in the eastern half of the United States and is known for an elaborate material culture and the construction of numerous mounds and earthworks. It is strongly and richly expressed in south-central Ohio, where shared aspects of style, mortuary behavior, and certain raw materials suggest relationships of symbolism and ideology between contemporaneous groups. Depictions of human bodies and body parts and the modification of human skeletal remains are not uncommon in the context of Hopewell mortuary

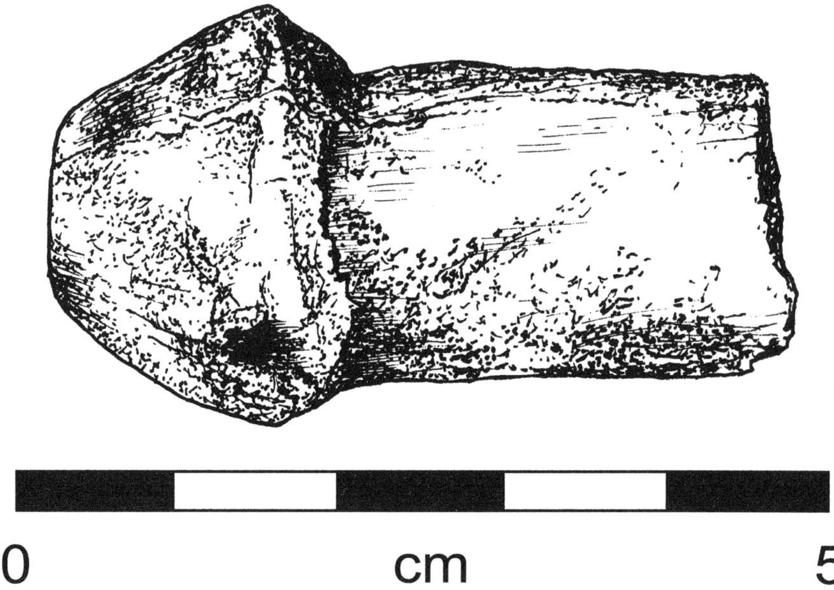

6.1. Phallic baton (A283/131) recovered from Cache 1, Mound 17, Hopewell Mound group, Chillicothe, Ohio. (Drawing by Julian Lee)

behavior. Artifacts of copper, mica, and clay representing human faces, heads, hands, and torsos have been documented in Hopewell mortuary and ceremonial contexts. Incised, drilled, ground, or cut human skeletal elements, such as long bones, crania, maxillae, and mandibles, have also been recovered from a number of Hopewell mortuary sites and represent a "chaotic" array of mortuary behaviors (Johnston 2002:5). Representations of human phalli in any media are, however, almost entirely unknown.

Beneath Shetrone's Mound 17 were three clay basins and two concentrated deposits of artifacts—identified as the Southern and Northern Deposits—associated with charred organic material, soil, and clay. The "phallic effigy" (Greber and Ruhl 1989:84) was recovered from the southernmost of the concentrated deposits. The Southern Deposit included objects made of copper, silver, meteoric iron, various lithic materials (including an assortment of pipes and points), and bone, as well as 49 stone celts or celt fragments (Greber and Ruhl 1989:83). Greber and Ruhl (1989, 2000) associated the Southern Deposit with maleness based on the phallic effigy and other artifacts thought to be masculine. Greber and Ruhl noted that the celts from the Southern Deposit mimic the phallic effigy in shape and that the pipes and points could be artifacts more likely to be associated with males than females. The comple-

Table 6.1. Measurements of Phallic Batons Made of Human Bone

Identifier	Total Length	Glans Length	Glans Width
A283/131	4.27 cm (1.68 in)	2.25 cm (.88 in)	1.7 cm (.67 in)
no label	8.5 cm (3.34 in)	2.7 cm (1.06 in)	4.2 cm (1.65 in)

mentary Northern Deposit was smaller than the Southern Deposit and represented femaleness by virtue of a lack of masculine artifacts; the Northern Deposit did not contain metal artifacts, pipes, points, or stone celts. Conversely, mica, bear claws, bone tool fragments, and bladelets of Flint Ridge flint were numerous in the Northern Deposit, yet were absent from the Southern Deposit. Also included in the Northern Deposit were over 60 cone-shaped objects (or partial objects) made of chlorite serpentine or limonite and approximately 20 rod- or bar-shaped objects made of chlorite serpentine (Greber and Ruhl 1989:83). None of the objects from the Northern Deposit (cones, bone tools, bladelets, and mica artifacts) are necessarily considered feminine. In fact, chlorite serpentine cones, rods, and bars were also present in the Southern Deposit, but in small numbers. In addition to the composition of the two deposits, the relative sizes of the two deposits can be interpreted as paralleling human sexual dimorphism in that the Southern Deposit, thought to be masculine, is larger than the feminine Northern Deposit. Greber and Ruhl (1989:81) argued that the deposits were placed at about the same time and that they represented a "cultural complimentarity [*sic*]." The inclusion of an abundance of some artifact types and certain raw materials in one of the Mound 17 deposits, but not in the other, is suggestive of a complementary duality, according to Greber and Ruhl (1989:275). If the two deposits represented complementary activities associated with the sexes, then the assumption must be made that the Northern Deposit represented the female contribution to the duality. Greber and Ruhl (1989:275–276) proposed that the deposits may reflect an acknowledgment of the two basic entities that contribute to the life force.

The other worked bone from the OHS collections is also a modified long bone, possibly a proximal human femur head, with a realistically shaped glans and a straight, cylindrical shaft (Figure 6.2). The measurements for this artifact are in Table 6.1. It did not have a catalog number associated with it, and the archaeological context is unknown. While it is possible that this artifact is Hopewell in origin, nothing in its museum context suggests this affiliation. Given the occurrence of culturally modified human remains from other temporal and cultural contexts in Ohio and given the wide range of time

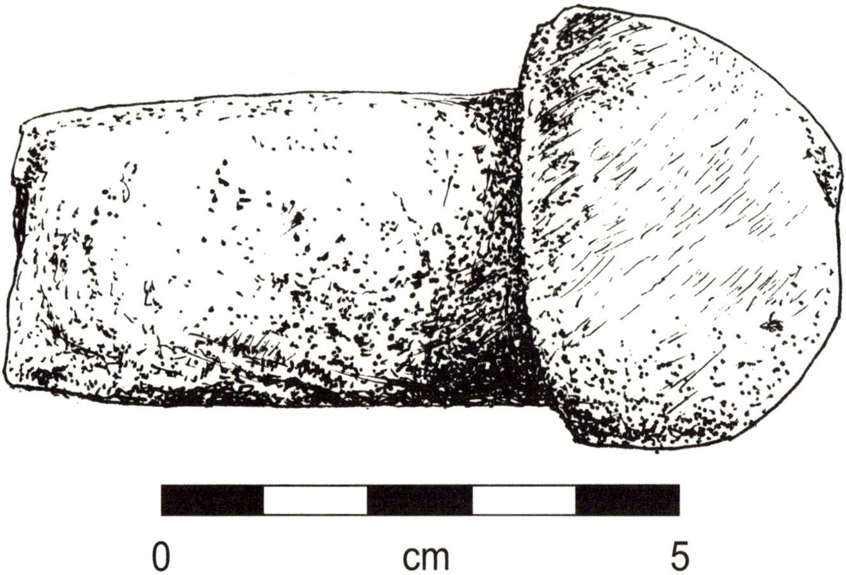

6.2. Phallic baton in the collections of the Ohio Historical Society (no identification number, unknown archaeological provenience). (Drawing by Julian Lee)

periods and cultures represented by human remains in the OHS collections in 1998, it is equally likely that this second, unprovenienced phallic baton of human bone is affiliated with an archaeological context other than Hopewell.

Phallic Batons in Regional and Worldwide Contexts

In order to place these two phallic batons of human bone in an appropriate cultural context, a search was conducted to find similar artifacts from archaeological and ethnographic contexts. Material type was not restricted to human bone. Archaeological correlates were found in private collections and in the archaeological literature dealing primarily with Old World contexts. Few clear correlates were found in the ethnographic literature.

The private collection of Frank Otto of Ohio provided the most examples of phallic batons from North America to date; information on other examples may be buried in the literature. Otto's collection contained three ground stone phallic batons collected from various locations in Ohio, including Crawford, Adams, and Hocking counties (Figures 6.3, 6.4, 6.5). Three additional ground stone phallic batons in Otto's collection were recovered from Kentucky, Tennessee, and Nebraska. The ground stone double phallus from Madison County, Tennessee, is shown in Figure 6.6. Geographic pro-

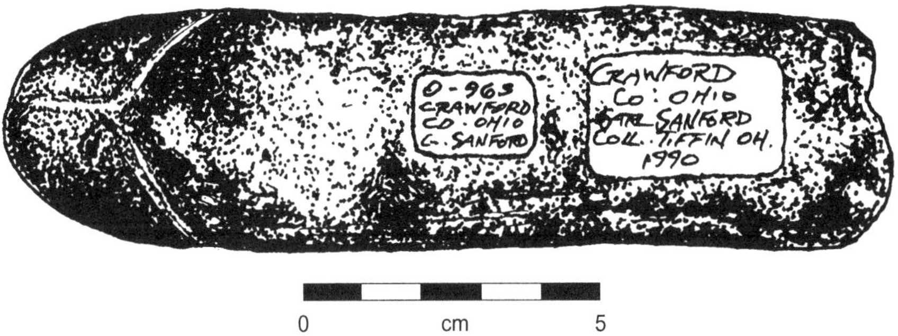

6.3. Ground stone phallic baton from Crawford County, Ohio. Frank Otto collection. (Drawing by Julian Lee)

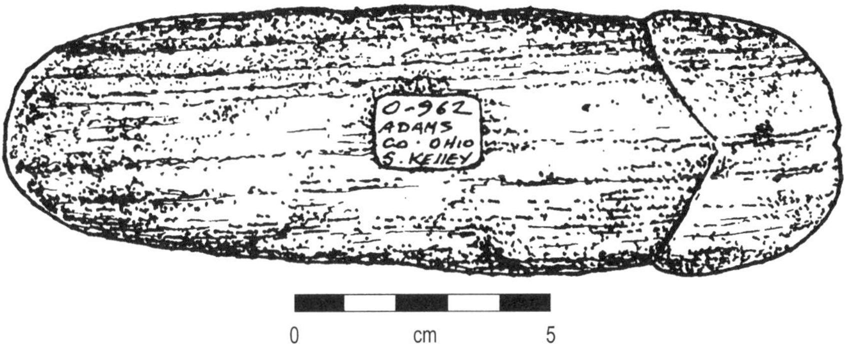

6.4. Ground stone phallic baton from Adams County, Ohio. Frank Otto collection. (Drawing by Julian Lee)

venience, measurements, and any additional information for these six artifacts are summarized in Table 6.2. The ground stone phallic batons from Ohio and the Midwest are all similar in size and have realistic proportions within the range of modern, erect penises (Ansell Research 2001; Wessells et al. 1996). An example of a similar midwestern phallic artifact has recently come to light (Douglas Jackson, personal communication 2013). That artifact, a sandstone pipe in the collection of Edmund Butkus, was recovered in southwestern Cook County, Illinois, on the surface of a low ridge south of the Sagaunashke Swamp (now the Cal-Sag Channel). The sandstone pipe is comparable in size and proportion to the phallic batons of human bone curated at the OHS and to the ground stone phallic batons in the Frank Otto collection. The existence of this artifact extends the geographic distribution of phallic artifacts in the American Midwest.

Farther afield, there is an example of a double phallus in the Frank Otto

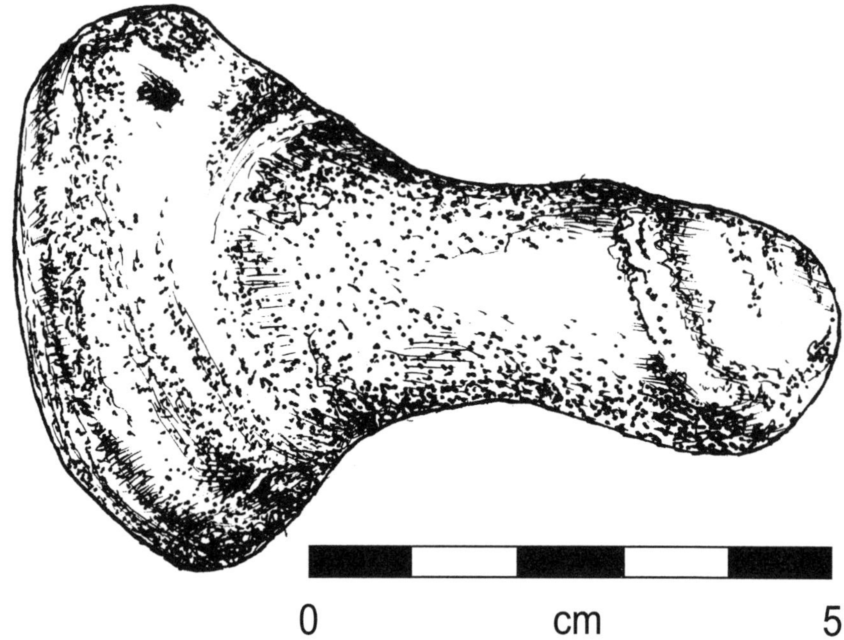

6.5. Ground stone phallic baton from Hocking County, Ohio. Frank Otto collection. (Drawing by Julian Lee)

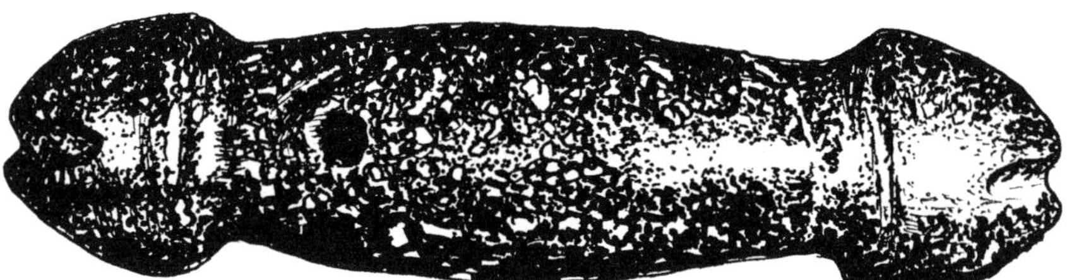

6.6. Ground stone double phallic baton from Madison County, Tennessee. Frank Otto collection. (Drawing by Julian Lee)

collection that was recovered in California (Figure 6.7), and even farther abroad there are examples of Roman and Egyptian carved stone phalli (Scott 1996:39, Plates 6, 7). Examples of phallic batons have been reported from the Neolithic and Mesolithic periods of Europe and Asia. Parker Pearson and the Stonehenge Riverside Project (2012:66–68) presented the discovery of a flint phallus in a pit below the Neolithic Durrington Walls in England; this object was found near two "testicle-sized" flint balls (Parker Pearson and the Stone-

Table 6.2. Otto Collection Ground Stone Phallic Baton Attributes

Geographic Provenience	Length	Width	Notes
Crawford County, Ohio	14.48 cm (5.7 in)	3.81 cm (1.5 in)	
Adams County, Ohio	15.75 cm (6.2 in)	4.57 cm (1.8 in)	
Hocking County, Ohio	6.35 cm (2.5 in)	2.54 cm (1 in)	base is perforated as if to allow for a suspension cord
Mason County, Kentucky	14.73 cm (5.8 in)	3.81 cm (1.5 in)	
Madison County, Tennessee	17.78 cm (7 in)	4.32 cm (1.7 in)	double phallus with "spear straightener" hole in center
Gage County, Nebraska	13.97 cm (5.5 in)	3.81 cm (1.5 in)	

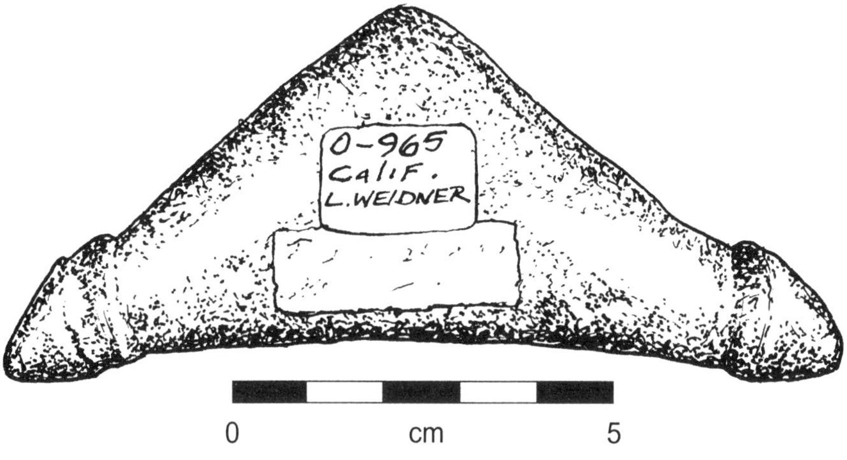

6.7. Ground stone double phallic baton from California. Frank Otto collection. (Drawing by Julian Lee)

henge Riverside Project 2012:68). In connection with this discovery, Parker Pearson and the Stonehenge Riverside Project (2012:68) also mentioned the existence of other Neolithic carved phalli from England, including one from Stonehenge. In 2010, a phallus carved from antler, measuring 10.5 cm (4 in) in length and 2 cm (.8 in) in diameter, was recovered from the Swedish Mesolithic site of Motala (Moskowitz 2010). One of the archaeologists involved in the Swedish investigation commented that this type of artifact was previously unreported from northern Europe or Scandinavia, and that the function was as yet undetermined (Moskowitz 2010). In the northwestern autonomous Chinese region of Xinjiang, "life-sized wooden phalluses" were found lying on or next to the bodies of females interred in the Small River Cemetery No. 5, which dates to approximately 3,980 years ago (Wade 2010); researchers linked these phalli to the cultural importance of fertility. The oldest known phallic batons, including double phalli, date to the European Upper Paleolithic (Marshack 1972; Taylor 1996:127–129). According to Taylor (1996:128), the European Upper Paleolithic phallic batons are rarely published with measurements and are frequently interpreted as ritual objects.

A preliminary review of the Electronic Human Relations Area Files Collection of Ethnography (eHRAF) yielded few clear correlates. The closest match was a figure reproduced from Karsten's 1955 work on Saami religion, which depicted the tree seidis of the Saami (eHRAF 1987). Seidis represent a form of animism in which inanimate objects of stone and wood are thought to contain spiritual beings and hence to have supernatural powers. The tree seidis shown are reportedly made of stone; no scale is given. Scott (1996) described numerous examples of large phalli among historic cultures, but in each case the phalli are depicted in two-dimensional iconography, are attached to human figurines, or are so large as to be far outside the realm of modern human variation. These representations of the phallus are not the detached, life-sized, independent entities represented by the examples from the Ohio Historical Society and the Frank Otto collection.

Meaning and Possible Lines of Inquiry and Explanation

Given the dearth of archaeological and ethnographic examples of phallic batons and their meaning, arriving at an understanding of the bone phallic batons from the OHS collection appears to lie far in the future. A review of the available literature suggests four broad categories of possible explanations for the prehistoric meaning and function of phallic batons: phallicism and fertility rituals, initiation and defloration rituals, symbolic male substitutes, and utilitarian uses. Each of these lines of explanation is discussed here briefly.

Phallicism and Fertility Rituals

Scott (1996:15, 37) argued that phallicism, worship of the penis, has its origins in the recognition of the duality of males and females in nature and the pleasure associated with sexual activity, rather than an understanding of the organ's role in reproduction. Thus, phallic worship, at its core, is nearly universal. Connotations of male power, authority, and virility appear to be particular to phallicism in patriarchal societies. Regardless of the meaning behind the phallus and phallic worship, the phallus appears cross-culturally in fertility rites applied to plants, animals, and humans. Phallic deities, such as the Egyptian god Osiris, the Roman and Greek god Priapus (see Knight 2006 [1865]), the ithyphallic god of nature, Shiva, in the Indian traditions (Daniélou 1995), and Bo of the Dahomeys of Africa, are common cross-culturally and across time. Similarly, the worship of the "generative powers" (the ability to sexually reproduce) is found across cultures and time (Wright 2006 [1865]).

In the context of fertility rites and phallicism, the phallic baton would serve as a symbol of whatever beliefs a particular culture held about the phallus and the powers it contained. In the majority of cases, the phalli associated with fertility rites and phallicism are of extremely exaggerated proportions. While the objects discussed here from the Ohio Historical Society and the Frank Otto collections are not of large or exaggerated proportions, they may still have served a function in the context of phallicism or fertility rites. This is especially true given the apparent dualistic, male-female nature of Shetrone's Mound 17 at the Hopewell Mound group. Although discussions of Hopewell fertility symbolism are uncommon, Greber and Ruhl's work (1989, 2000) is an exception. In one of the largest scholarly collections incorporating the study of symbolism into a discussion of the Hopewell, analyses of sociopolitical and ritual differentiation dominated the topics (Carr and Case 2005). Chapters discussing males and females were confined to analyses of gender roles in Hopewell society (Field et al. 2005; Keller and Carr 2005; Rodrigues 2005). Similarly, Carr (2008) discussed gender relations in Hopewell based on mortuary evidence and concluded that males played the dominant roles in sociopolitical and ritual activities. Other works analyzing Hopewell symbols have focused on the broader topic of Hopewell cosmology (e.g., Giles 2013).

Initiation and Defloration Rituals

Phallic batons also may have played a role in initiation and defloration rituals, either as symbolic objects intended for demonstrative or instructional purposes, or as objects physically used in a rite. However, a search of the eHRAF yielded no clear ethnographic examples of the use of phallus-shaped objects in defloration or initiation rituals.

Symbolic Male Substitutes

A third line of explanation for some phallic batons is that female leaders, warriors, and/or transgender individuals used the items as public (and perhaps private) representations of male genitalia and, hence, male power and status. A display of male power and status may have been particularly important for women taking on nontraditional or atypical gender roles in a culture. Taylor (1996:180) suggested this line of explanation for archaeological phallic batons that have some means of being attached to a strap or clothing, particularly if found in the graves of females or individuals of indeterminate sex (see Taylor's [1996:179–182] discussion of Grave 43 at the Neolithic Varna Cemetery in Bulgaria).

Utilitarian Uses

Finally, one of the most obvious, yet perhaps most often overlooked, explanations for phallic batons is that they are what they appear to be—items that were used for sexual stimulation, both self-stimulation and as part of heterosexual or homosexual sexual behavior. Numerous cultures have depicted the use of such items in art and iconography (e.g., Greek and Roman art), and there is even the modern correlate of the "sex toy." Despite evidence indicating the use of such items in a utilitarian fashion, western scholars seem to avoid exploring the utilitarian line of explanation/inquiry, perhaps because of our deep-rooted Puritan backgrounds or because many disciplines exploring the topic have been, until recently, male-dominated. However, the utilitarian explanation may be the most parsimonious, especially for items whose size falls within the range of known human variation.

Conclusions

Intentional cultural modification of human bone is a documented phenomenon in the precontact American Midwest, particularly as part of the elaborate Hopewell mortuary complex. Modification of human bone suggests that there was no cultural prohibition on handling human remains, at least under specific circumstances (Johnston 2002:113). Also not unique in the midcontinent was the creation of three-dimensional phallic effigies, or phallic batons, as demonstrated by examples made of ground stone. More unusual is the use of human bone to create an effigy of a human body part, especially a human phallus. The two artifacts discussed in this chapter present a double mystery then: why a phallus, and why sculpted from human bone?

The explanations for why certain skeletal elements were modified and why the bone was modified in specific ways have long eluded scholars, and this chapter does not pretend to solve the puzzle. However, one fact highlighted by the artifacts described here and by the various explanations of the meaning and function of phallic batons is that there are variations in phallic batons morphologically, contextually, and in terms of meaning cross-culturally. All phallic-shaped items cannot be lumped together under one overarching explanation. Clearly, much remains unknown about the two bone phallic batons found in the collection of the Ohio Historical Society—especially the one that is not cataloged. In order to gain a more comprehensive understanding of what these items may represent, there are many areas yet to explore. For instance, what is the prevalence of phallic batons, both those made of bone and those made of other materials, in Ohio and the greater Midwest? How many of these items are in private and museum collections and, to date, remain unreported? More important, in terms of placing the phallic batons of human bone within a broader framework of meaning, what are the archaeological contexts of these items? How does context vary by time? Does context vary by raw material, size, or morphology? In the case of the phallic baton from the Hopewell context, what, if anything, separates this artifact from other Hopewell artifacts made from human bone? That is to say, what significance does this artifact have in Hopewell culture? Is it part of a fertility rite, a larger worldview, or something else entirely? Once there is a better understanding of prevalence and context, attention can be focused on the two artifacts presented here and the more specific question regarding the significance of creating phallic batons from human bone can be addressed.

Acknowledgments

We would like to thank the Ohio Historical Society (OHS) and Martha Potter Otto for kindly granting access to the collections housed at the OHS and providing workspace for the identification process. Gratitude is also extended to Frank Otto for bringing his collection of ground stone phallic batons to our attention and allowing these artifacts to be examined and photographed. Thanks also to Edmund Butkus for allowing us to include a description of the ground sandstone phallic pipe in his collection, and to Kristin Hedman for bringing this sandstone pipe to our attention. We are also grateful to Julian Lee for creating the illustrations included in this chapter. The comments of an anonymous reviewer are appreciated. Finally, we wish to thank the editors of this volume for their suggestions and assistance during the final stages of revision. All errors and omissions remain our responsibility.

7
Excised and Drilled Human Bone from Eastern Iowa Woodland Sites

Shirley J. Schermer and Robin M. Lillie

Examples of culturally modified human skeletal remains have been found across the state of Iowa, with most dating to the Woodland or late prehistoric periods (see Lillie and Schermer, this volume). Examples of excision—the deliberate removal of a portion of bone from a larger whole—and drilling of bone are associated primarily with Woodland sites. The alterations characteristic of these examples are very different from those commonly associated with warfare, violence, or burial preparation (see Chacon and Dye, ed. 2007). Rather, these modifications more likely relate to the ornamental or ritual use of human bone, although we recognize that these uses are not always mutually exclusive.

Human bones as cultural objects may have been used to ritualize claims to particular territories "by identifying with their ancestors and, in turn, with traditionally used village sites and resources" (Simon and Steffian 1994:97). Veneration also needs to be considered, not necessarily in the sense of ancestor worship but in terms of respect and remembrance. Weltfish (1965:83), in discussing the Pawnee creation story and ceremony, described a special ceremonial bundle made by the "Chief of Center Village" to denote his chieftainship: "To commemorate his creative intellectual powers, he directed that when he died his skull was to be attached to the outside of this bundle. Thus it came to be known as the Skull bundle, although it was also referred to as the bundle of the Wonderful Person. . . . This bundle presided over the meeting of the chiefs late in the spring as well as over other rituals. When the original skull was accidentally broken, it was replaced with another." What is unknown is whether this replacement suggests a symbolic role as a continuing remembrance of a specific individual ("Chief of Center Village") or if the use of any skull simply became an integral part of the group's bundle.

Use of modified human bone may also have played a role in widespread mourning practices and releasing of the soul. Hall (1997) noted at least one account of a historic observance of a soul bundle containing bones to represent the soul, and he discussed the beliefs of other ethnographers that bone bundles they observed were actually soul bundles. He stated that such bundles likely would have been respected after the soul release ceremony, possibly retained and passed on as heirlooms, but at some point the bones might no longer be considered sacred or objects of veneration (Hall 1997:26).

The modified bones described in this chapter are, for the most part, portions of bones, excised from a complete bone element. The deliberate modifications created objects with cultural meanings and roles, possibly in one or more of the contexts mentioned above. It is also possible that their meaning evolved over their "life history."

Bone Rondelles

Rondelles, or bone disks—circular pieces of bone removed from the cranium—may be formed by drilling or cutting repeatedly through cranial bone, which often results in a circumferentially scalloped border. The rondelle is then punched or cut out of the larger piece. In Iowa, rondelles occur only in mortuary contexts as isolated fragments. They show minimal modification with the exception of some marginal and surface polish, with no or only nominal evidence for suspension or attachment to something else. Rondelles or evidence of their manufacture have been found at three Middle Woodland mound groups in eastern Iowa (ca. 200 B.C.–A.D. 300), all on landforms overlooking the Mississippi River.

Deppe Mound Group

The Deppe Mound group (13JK11) consists of a string of eight conical mounds along a bluff spur in Jackson County. In 1935, Ellison Orr conducted excavations in three of the mounds (Logan 1976:12; Marcucci 1997; Orr 1935:54–73; Schermer et al. 1998). An additional three mounds may have been dug into prior to Orr's excavations. Little information is available on these earlier explorations of the mound group, other than mention that "Dr. Hanske of Bellevue, with other boys . . . found besides skeletons and some other relics, a thin copper plate on which were scratched some characters" (Orr 1935:56).

Orr investigated Mounds 6, 7, and 8. No human remains or artifacts were found in Mound 6, and no artifacts were found in Mound 7. The interior of Mound 7 contained rows of limestone slabs, oriented southwest to northeast and described as "low irregular walls" (Orr 1934:57). Five bundle burials representing a minimum of 21 individuals were found under and adjacent to the

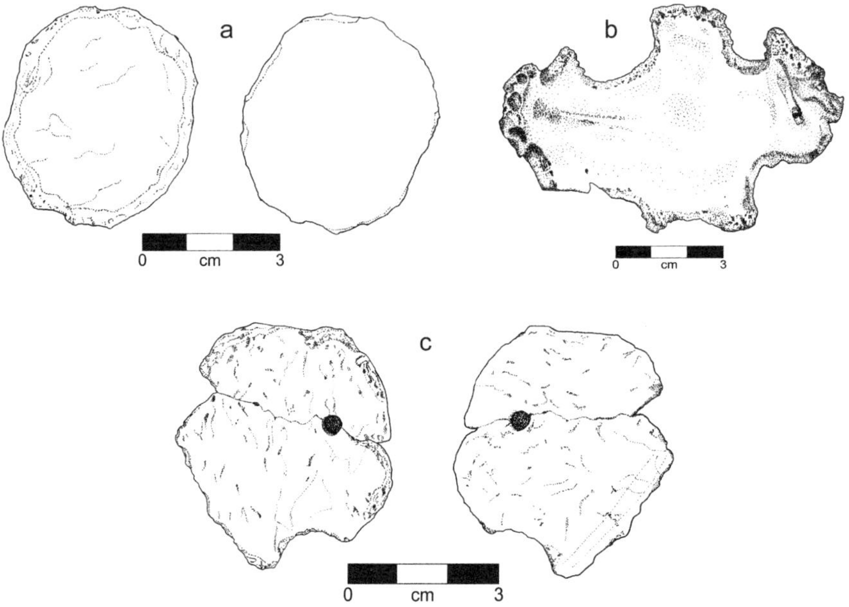

7.1. Human bone rondelles and examples of rondelle manufacture: (a) excised bone disk recovered from Mound 8, 13JK11; (b) calvarium from 13MC4 with multiple disk-shaped portions of bone excised; (c) perforated cranial fragment from 13AM104. (Drawings by Liz Niec, courtesy of University of Iowa Office of the State Archaeologist)

stones, but Orr does not appear to have collected any of the remains (Lillie 1998; Orr 1935). Limestone construction in Mound 8 consisted of two discrete slab-covered areas in the southwest quadrant of the mound and a more widespread slab-covered area in the remainder of the mound (Orr 1935:56). Incomplete human remains were scattered throughout the mound, adjacent to and below the limestone slabs. Orr's notes mention five crania and miscellaneous bones and fragments, including two "round pieces" of human cranial bone. One, or possibly both, of the cranial "disks" were found in the northeast portion of the mound adjacent to a limestone slab along with a freshwater mussel shell, but no other human remains were immediately adjacent. The remains collected by Orr from Mound 8 represent minimally an older middle-aged to older adult male; a young adult, probably female; and an adult of indeterminate age and sex (represented by the two rondelles) (Lillie 1998:1). Both rondelles were probably cut from a parietal (though not necessarily the same one), side undetermined, and possibly came from the same cranium. The larger rondelle measures 47 mm by 40 mm (Figure 7.1a), the smaller rondelle measures 28 mm by 22 mm, and the thickness of both ranges from 4 mm to 6 mm. The edge of the smaller rondelle suggests excision by cutting and snapping. Both rondelles show slight smoothing along some portions of the margins, possibly resulting from handling or use-wear.

Cook Farm Mound Group

The Cook Farm Mound group (13ST82), now destroyed by urban development, consisted of 11 mounds located on a terrace in current-day Davenport, Scott County. Members of the Davenport Academy of Sciences and local residents conducted numerous excavations in the mounds during the late nineteenth century (Farquharson 1876, 1880; Gass 1877a, 1877b; Harrison 1878; Tiffany 1876). Starr (1895:110–114) provided a brief description and summary of the mounds' contents, which included primary burials, bundle burials, scattered human skeletal fragments, copper implements, chipped stone tools, stone effigy pipes, pottery vessels, marine shells, bear canines, and mica.

The construction of Mound 5 included several strata of stones separated by loose shells. In addition to mortuary features, "a rondelle 1 inch in diameter" (Starr 1895:112; also see Farquharson 1876:120–121) was recovered from Mound 5, but no specific location was described. The rondelle was described as human and illustrated by Farquharson (1876:121, Plate VII, Figure 8). The squamous portion of a right temporal has been culturally modified so it is generally circular in form, measuring 24 mm by 25 mm (Lillie 2002a:122). The thickness is comparable to that of adult temporal bones. Most of the margins of the cranial rondelle are somewhat irregular, although straight-sided rather than beveled. Slight scalloping of the margins suggests that breakage was caused by repeated strikes with a small awl or chisel-like tool. The smoothed edges suggest long-term handling or use.

Lowry Farm Mound Group

The Lowry Farm Mound group (13MC4) consists of nine mounds located on a bluff in Muscatine County (Starr 1895:104–105). Archaeological investigations of two mounds took place in the late nineteenth century. Witter (1878) described Mound 4 as having numerous flat limestone slabs set on edge in a circle. Within this circle he noted burned earth or stone, two large marine shells, a cluster of shell beads, two pottery vessels, and human teeth. Members of the Davenport Academy of Sciences excavated a second mound (Pratt 1876:109–110), revealing large quantities of crushed charcoal mixed throughout the mound fill, a small scattering of human bone fragments (2–3 ft below the mound surface), a modified cranial bone (7 ft below the mound surface), and one shell bead (6 ft below the mound surface).

The modified partial cranium, consisting of the superior portion of the frontal and anterior portions of the parietals, suggests a possible method of rondelle production (Figure 7.1b). Seven semicircular sections had been drilled or cut around the outer margins of the bone (Pratt 1876:Plate VII, Figure 9). The modified margins are beveled inward from the ectocranial edge to the endocranial edge and display polishing (Hodges 1989:58–59; Schermer and Owsley 1989–1990a).

Drilled and Perforated Bone

"Drilling" is defined here as a circular hole or incomplete perforation of bone or tooth resulting from the intentional use of a stone or bone tool. The absence of crushing or bone fragmentation in the modified area distinguishes these drilled perforations from punctures, chopping marks, or postdepositional taphonomic factors. In Iowa, drilled human elements were found in burial and habitation contexts from the Middle and Late Woodland periods.

Lane Farm Mound Group

The Late Woodland Lane Farm Mound group (13AM104; ca. A.D. 750–1000) is located on the Hartley Terrace overlooking the Upper Iowa River in Allamakee County, northeastern Iowa. In addition to the mound group, a Late Woodland habitation site, a late prehistoric Oneota village, and an earthen enclosure are located on the terrace. Part of the later Oneota village overlays the Woodland mounds.

Orr conducted excavations in 10 mounds at this site in the 1930s and recorded burials in all but two mounds. As many as 52 burials were uncovered, including extended and bundled interments and isolated bone fragments (Logan 1976:39–48; Orr 1934:21–66, 1937:1–12, 1942:149–152; Schermer et al. 1998:132–145). Excavations conducted in 1970 in Mounds 14 and 50 revealed additional burials (Fisher 1977a, 1977b; Lillie 2002a; McKusick 1973). Mound 50 burials consisted mostly of isolated fragments or very incomplete remains, except for a possibly rearticulated skeleton labeled Burial S (McKusick 1973:77). Burials C and D from Mound 14 consisted of a single subadult cranial fragment each. The Burial C fragment was from the central portion of an unsided parietal. This fragment had broken postdeposition, but it was possible to reconstruct the portions. The maximum diameter of the fragment is 45 mm, and it measures 40 mm at a right angle to the maximum diameter. The thickness of the bone suggests a subadult. The fragment had split at the point where a 3.2 mm diameter hole perforated the bone (Figure 7.1c). There is no beveling to the edges of the perforation on either the ectocranial or endocranial surfaces, and the diameter appears to be consistent through-

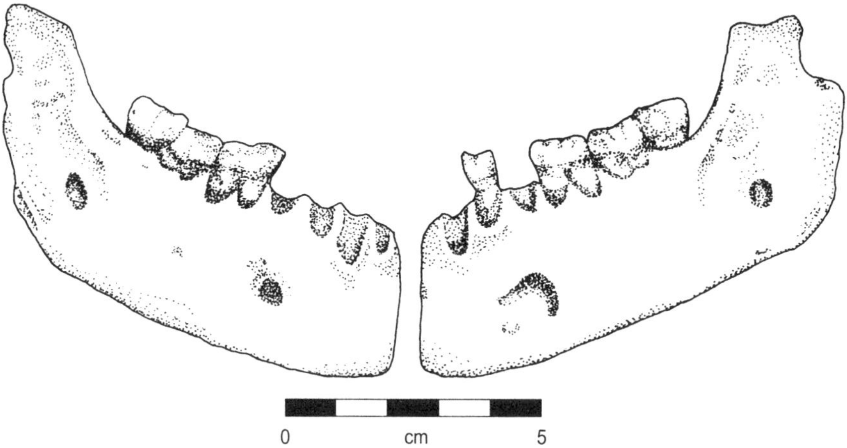

7.2. Cut, ground, and drilled human mandible from the Quandahl rockshelter. (Drawing by Liz Niec, courtesy of University of Iowa Office of the State Archaeologist)

out the depth of the perforation. There are no fractures radiating from the hole and no discernible cut marks or animal gnaw marks (Lillie 2002a). Although the fragment is roughly circular in shape, the margins are more ragged and irregular than the rondelles described above.

Quandahl Rockshelter

The Quandahl rockshelter (13WH35) is located along North Bear Creek, Winneshiek County, northeastern Iowa. The rockshelter was utilized from the Archaic period through the Oneota, with the most intensive occupation during the Late Woodland (Mallam 1978, 1979). The rockshelter had been extensively looted over a long period.

A local amateur conducted limited test excavations in the 1940s and early 1960s. During the latter testing, he found a modified mandible in an undisturbed portion of fill underneath a large section of roof fall. While there is some evidence of occupation during the Middle Woodland period, no association of the mandible with any specific cultural horizon is possible. However, most known modified mandibles from elsewhere in the Midwest are from Middle Woodland contexts (see Cobb, Johnston, and Nawrocki and Emanovsky, this volume). The remains represent an adult male, approximately 30–40 years of age, and were described in detail by Mallam (1979). Cut at the symphysis, the cut edges of both sides of the mandible are heavily ground (Figure 7.2). The ascending rami also have been cut and ground, removing the condyles and coronoid processes. A hole has been drilled in the body of each half, posterior to the third molars and superior to the gonial angle. Mallam (1979:33) described these perforations as biconical, probably produced with a tapered drill. The mental foramina on each half have been intentionally enlarged but do not penetrate the interior surface.

Mallam (1979) experimented with ways that the Quandahl rockshelter mandible could have been suspended. He felt the only way the sections could have been joined would have been "by passing a cord through the ramus perforation from the medial surface to the lateral surface and then along the body to the mental foramen. At this point the mental foramen perforation intersects the mandibular canal. The cord was then passed through this opening and into the mandibular canal of the other section through the openings exposed by sectioning of the symphysis. In this fashion the two sections were joined together" (Mallam 1979:33).

H. P. Field Collection

A drilled tooth and hand phalanx were at one time included in the H. P. Field Collection, Luther College, Decorah, northeastern Iowa. Provenience and cultural affiliation are unknown, but both had been stored in the same container as the skeletal remains of two individuals, suggesting their association with burials.

The human single-rooted tooth, probably a maxillary canine, has a 1.3 mm diameter hole drilled in a mesial-distal direction just inferior to the root tip (Lillie 1996b:12) (Figure 7.3a). Most of the crown had been lost through postdepositional damage. The tooth is burned, with evidence of polishing on the buccal surface of the root. The degree of burning ranges from moderate at the crown end of the root to slight at the root tip, suggesting the tooth may have been in situ in the maxilla at the time of exposure to fire. Drilling appears to have occurred at some point after the tooth was burned.

The hand phalanx from the same collection has a 3 mm diameter hole drilled near the proximal end, running anteroposteriorly (Figure 7.3b). Microscopic examination of the perforation found no evidence of tool marks. The margin on the anterior surface is jagged and irregular, while the margin on the posterior surface is smooth. The hole may have been partially drilled and then punched out with an awl or similar tool, breaking small fragments at the point of exit (Lillie 1996b:13).

Woodland Examples from Outside Iowa

Examples of excised human bone from eastern Iowa Middle Woodland sites have been found only in mortuary contexts. While Iowa was on the fringe of Middle Woodland Hopewell, the Iowa bone rondelle examples bear similarities to those seen in classic Hopewell sites in other areas of the Midwest.

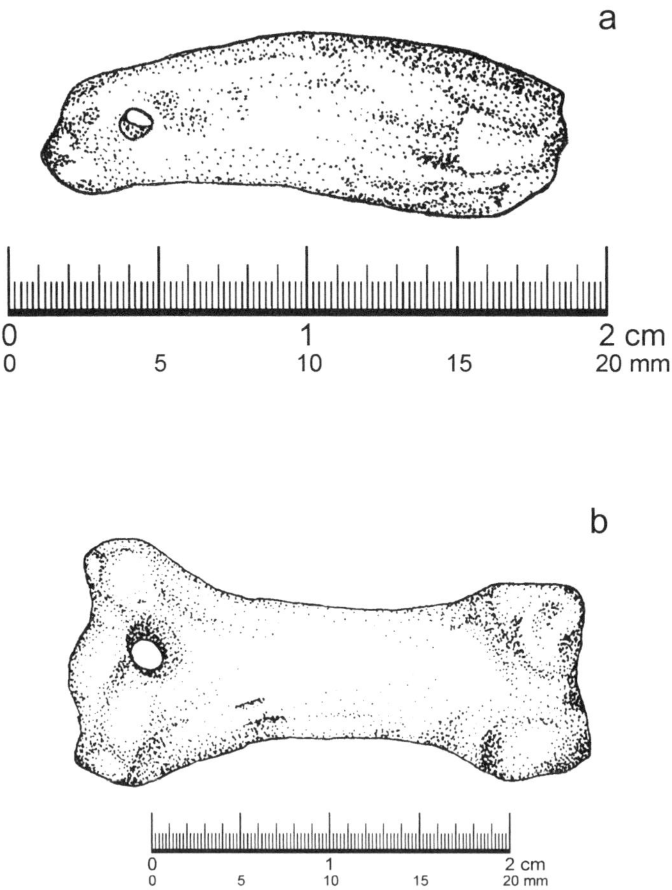

7.3. Drilled elements from an unknown context in northeastern Iowa: (a) drilled human canine, most of crown missing; (b) drilled human phalanx. (Drawings by Liz Niec, courtesy of University of Iowa Office of the State Archaeologist)

An elaborately incised human parietal disk was recovered from an altar in a mound at the Turner Mound group in Ohio (Willoughby and Hooton 1922:57–58). The disk had been broken and partially destroyed by burning. Also recovered were an elaborately incised human femur and ulna. Five crania from the site have 1–4 perforations, ranging in diameter from 5 mm to 9 mm, while a sixth has 11 perforations (Willoughby and Hooton 1922:124, 61). Willoughby suggested that the perforations may have been for suspension by a cord or for the insertion of feathers or other decorations.

The multiple burials recovered from the Younge site in Michigan fell into seven categories—extended, flexed, bundled, torso, cremated, fragmentary, and single unassociated crania (Greenman 1967:55). Crania with perforations, crania with openings where circular disks had been excised, and cranial bone disks were found. Greenman (1967:57) also noted that several postcranial bones had been perforated, cut, or grooved. A pipe was the only artifact found with a burial (Burial 56), excluding the bone disks and bark or charred wood (Greenman 1967:58).

Two modified cranial bones were recovered from a burial discovered in an inundated multicomponent site, 40KN23, on the Tennessee River. Williams (1975) described the burial as similar to Woodland burials found throughout the eastern Tennessee region. Charred skeletal remains had been placed in a pit along with the two modified cranial bones. Neither of these modified bones showed any evidence of burning. One, a portion of a frontal, had a 3 mm diameter hole drilled in the approximate center of the bone. The other was a bone disk cut from a right parietal and measuring approximately 73 mm by 77 mm. Both had evidence of edge grinding and surface polishing.

Webb and Baby (1957:94, Figure 44) described an ornately incised bone disk with two drilled holes from the Florence Mound. Excised from a child's frontal bone, the disk was deposited with an infant burial. Blue (this volume) mentions cranial disks or rondelles from a burned house feature at the Bryan site (21GD04) in Minnesota along with the two "trophy skulls" from which the rondelles were derived.

Discussion

Modified and drilled human bone, found in both Woodland and late prehistoric sites, may have fulfilled or been part of necessary rites or rituals related to belief systems or a cosmology important to individual or group relationships. Curated objects, ornamentation, and bone ritualism have been posited to explain drilled holes in crania, mandibles, and long bones similar to those seen in the Iowa examples (Urcid 1994). The bone rondelles excised from human crania and recovered exclusively in Woodland mortuary contexts may also have served as curated or ritual objects related to burial ceremonies or may be imbued with special significance or power.

It may not be possible to determine the exact cultural significance of rondelles made from human cranial bone. If they were "preforms" for drilled disks, then one would expect to find them in midden or feature contexts. Schermer and Owsley (1989–1990a) posed the question of whether the cranial rondelles were the byproducts (discards) or if the bone disks were the primary products. What represents the object of design, the skulls with their perforations or the disks themselves? The recovery of both rondelles and crania with disks removed (as well as perforated crania) from culturally defined mortuary contexts suggests the use of both disks and crania in burial rituals or their possible retention in sacred bundles prior to ceremonial reburial in mounds. This would suggest that both items, the source crania and the individual rondelles, were considered important.

The exclusivity of the rondelles to Woodland mortuary contexts may indicate a strong link to death and rebirth. The presence of such objects in a mound context implies that they were still viewed as having some significance—ritual or otherwise—and, as such, needed to be carefully disposed of (in contrast to simply being tossed into a general habitation feature or midden), or that they were an integral part of a mortuary event. Perhaps these were significant objects used by a single individual or were somehow tied closely to the identity of an individual or group—so much so that when the individual died, the object had to be taken out of commission. Perhaps their power was such that they could only be used by or were of significance only to one individual.

Burials in mounds at the Lane Farm Mound group included primary and secondary burials as well as isolated bone fragments. Two "burials" consisted of a single cranial fragment each, both from subadults. One fragment had been drilled and the other had not. Soul keeping and spirit keeping by eastern Plains tribes were common when mourning for a child (Hall 1997:26–27). The drilled bone disk may have been retained from a spirit bundle or drilled for wear as a pendant as a symbolic remembrance or representation of a lost child. Or perhaps, since it was treated differently from the other isolated fragment, there was a stronger link to the group, and the bone disk possibly held some power related to the circumstances of death or to the group's identity.

The examples described at the beginning of this chapter focused on eastern Iowa Woodland sites. However, an example of ornamental use of culturally modified bone from the Larson site (13PM61), a late Late Woodland Great Oasis to early late prehistoric Mill Creek village site in northwestern Iowa (ca. A.D. 1050–1100; Stephen C. Lensink, personal communication 2011), provides a possible explanation for the drilled cranial bones described here. A human cranial fragment found in a midden had been deliberately cut and the edges and surfaces smoothed, forming a circular piece with a small endocranial surface (17.7 mm), a larger ectocranial surface (24.8 mm), and a hole drilled through the center (4.9 mm) (Figure 7.4). Numerous cut marks are visible on the endocranial disk surface. This fragment was illustrated by Henning (1982, 1996) and described as a "pulley" type "ear spool" with a circular groove, 4.5 mm in width, over which the ear lobe was pulled (Henning 1982:192). Its similarity to an object made from fish bone suggests that

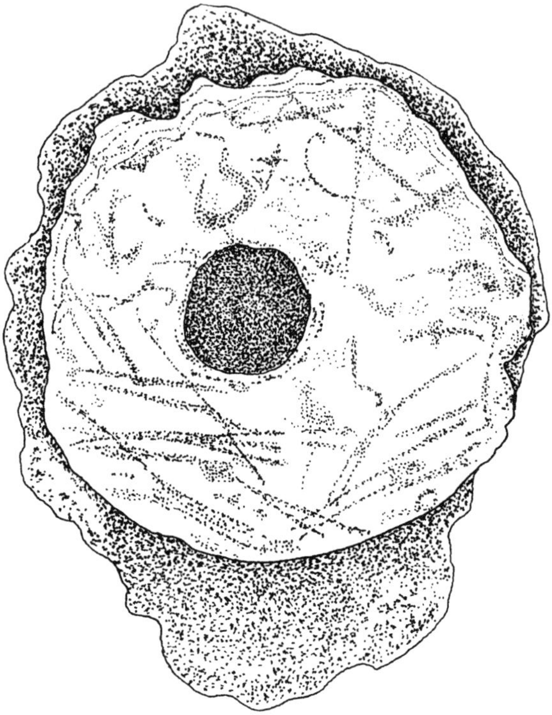

7.4. Possible ear spool made of human cranial bone, from a late prehistoric northwestern Iowa village, 13PM61. (Drawing by Liz Niec, courtesy of University of Iowa Office of the State Archaeologist)

the switch to human bone for the manufacture of these earspools was possibly for more than ornamental purposes. The completely drilled holes in the previously described examples could have allowed suspension of the modified elements. That human bone was used for their manufacture is of significance, suggesting a role beyond simply ornamentation.

In his article on the modified human mandible, Mallam (1979) discussed the modification of nonhuman mandibles throughout the Archaic and into the late prehistoric in the Midwest, as well as the modification of human mandibles in the Middle Woodland period (also see Cobb, this volume; Nawrocki and Emanovsky, this volume). Deuel (1952:169–170) noted that mandibles of powerful animals were chosen for modification, so the specific selection of *human* mandibles could have been from brave enemies, or, "if the jaws had a protective quality or religious significance, they might rather represent friendly relationships and hence the human jaws might be those of dead friends, patrons, or relatives."

The drilled elements described in this chapter suggest the manipulation of elements for suspension or the construction of some object for a specific purpose (e.g., mask, rattle, rearticulated remains). Possible motives for selecting human elements include veneration (remembrance), the control of spirits through possession of parts of a known individual, inclusion as part of a prolonged mortuary program, or the construction of objects for use in personal or civic ritual functions. The cut and drilled mandible was modified similarly to masks or ornamentations made from animals. "The symbol somehow comes to possess the power of that which it symbolizes. Indeed, the symbol, being the communicator of power, may be thought of as the essence of that power" (Wallace 1966:67). Whether used as ornamentation or as part of a ritual, curated alone or as part of a sacred bundle, the use of human bone and the types of modifications suggest that these objects took on symbolic roles for the cultural group.

Most of the modified bone discussed in this chapter, like most of the modified bone discussed in this volume, comes from the skull. Sundstrom (this volume) notes that the head is seen almost universally as a source of power. The rondelles found exclusively in Middle Woodland burial contexts support a spiritual, ritual, or mortuary function of the objects related to either the individual or group. The purpose of drilled or other modified bones found in both burial and habitation contexts is less clear and may have been more utilitarian (i.e., ornamentation), may have been for ritual, may have been a combination of the two, or may indicate a shift from one to the other. Perhaps there was something about these various objects that dictated, or allowed, disposition in one context or another. With better temporal control, one could look for shifts through time, such as a shift in perception of what modified bone signifies. Or, possibly, differences in modification technique and subsequent use account for the contexts of the ultimate disposition.

Ornamentation, curation, and personal or civic ritual use are not mutually exclusive. These objects have individual use histories that presumably changed with succeeding generations or acquisition by different groups or individuals. At some point, a deliberate decision was made to discard the object (e.g., in a habitation context) or to place it in a mound or other mortuary context, possibly reflecting a change in the role, importance, or significance of that object over time.

II

MISSISSIPPIAN PERIOD

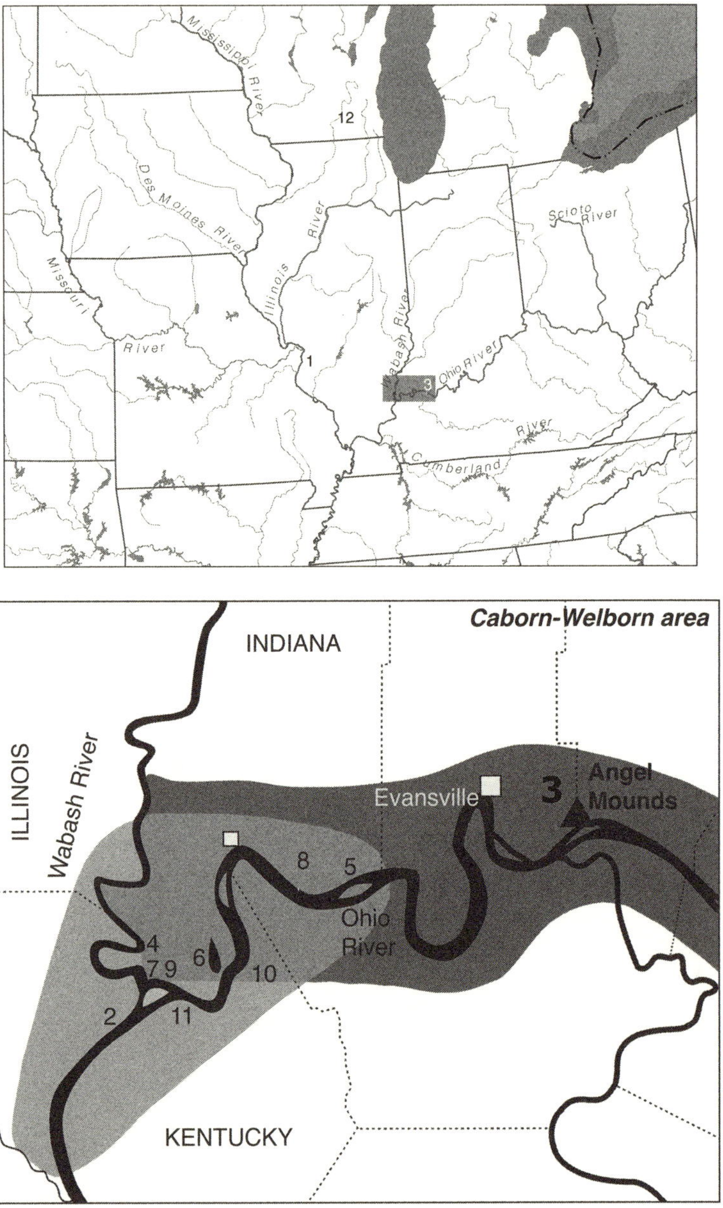

Mississippian sites. *Illinois*: (1) Cahokia, Submound 51 (chapter 8); (2) Galt (chapter 11). *Indiana*: (3) Angel (chapter 10); (4) Bone Bank (chapter 11); (5) Caborn (chapter 11); (6) Hovey Lake (chapter 11); (7) Leonard (chapter 11); (8) Mann (chapter 11); (9) Murphy (chapter 11). *Kentucky*: (10) Mulligan (chapter 11); (11) Slack Farm (chapter 11). *Wisconsin*: (12) Aztalan (chapter 9). (Courtesy of Illinois State Archaeological Survey, University of Illinois)

8
Life after Death

A Brief History of Human Bone Tools in Submound 51 at Cahokia

Eve A. Hargrave and Della Collins Cook

Human remains have been manipulated for a multitude of purposes ranging from worship of ancestors, demonstration of political power, war trophies, ritual obligation to kin, embodiment of magico-religious energies, and linkage to the spirit world (e.g., Beck 1995; Chacon and Dye, ed. 2007; Chapman et al. 1981; Chesson 2001; Geary 1990; Metcalf and Huntington 1991; Rakita et al. 2005; Sullivan and Mainfort, ed. 2010). Most examples found in the literature attribute such modification to instances of trophy taking, mortuary manipulation, or alterations to the human body (e.g., teeth, cranial modification) during life. Modified human elements that do not conform to these characteristics tend to be represented by isolated, often single, elements and are often ornamental, utilitarian, or practical in nature. Modifications include incised designs on bone, cutting and smoothing of long bones for pipes or musical instruments, cut bone circles, drilled teeth for ornaments or suspension, cut and polished cranial portions that functioned as a container or mask, and polish on the broken edges of long bones, which is attributable to use as a tool. Despite their limited visibility in the archaeological literature, such objects are fairly common, which is abundantly illustrated in the contributions to this volume.

The biography of objects is an analytical approach that is particularly relevant to the interpretation of modified human remains (Gosden and Marshall 1999; Holtorf 2002; Joy 2009; Kopytoff 1986; Spector 1993). This approach focuses on the fluid interactions between objects and people, beginning with the "birth" (production) and ending with the "death" (discard) of the object. Unlike Schiffer's (1976) behavioral theory, which focused primarily on the physical characteristics of an artifact, object biographies aim to place an object within the unique social setting for which it was used and to acknowledge that the reciprocal relationships between objects and people are always changing. It recognizes that the meaning and significance of objects are dependent on the particular way the object is perceived by individual members of a social group at particular points in time.

This chapter focuses on several modified human long bones from the late prehistoric Cahokia site located just east of present-day East St. Louis. The Cahokia site is a Mississippian (A.D. 1050–1350) mound center with over 100 platform, ridgetop, and conical mounds (Fowler 1997). The core area of the site consists of a large constructed plaza surrounded by platform and conical mounds. The largest mound, with a height of over 100 ft—Monks Mound—is located on the north end of the plaza. Multiple subsidiary mound centers are also present in the American Bottom floodplain and surrounding uplands (Ahler and DePuydt 1987; Fortier 2007; Fowler 1997; Kelly 2000; Milner 1998; Pauketat 1993, 1998a, 2005; Porter 1974). Together, these sites comprise the largest built environment in prehistoric North America.

Cahokia's rise to preeminence in the region occurred during the Lohmann phase (A.D. 1050–1100), which has been characterized as the "big bang" due to the abrupt changes that occurred in this relatively short period of time (Emerson and Pauketat 2002; Pauketat 1998a, 1998b, 2003; Pauketat and Emerson 1997). In particular, increases in population density were accompanied by the sudden appearance of large population centers, large-scale projects such as mound and plaza construction, clear status distinctions in communities, and an increase in the use of exotic materials as symbols of power and authority.

Mound 51 is located directly southeast of Monks Mound and on the northeastern edge of the plaza. In 1961, as Mound 51 was slowly being destroyed by local residents, who used the mound fill for building projects, Charles Bareis and James Porter from the University of Illinois initiated salvage excavations on the remainder of the mound. In the course of this work, they identified a large feature at the base of the mound that clearly predated the mound construction. This feature—identified as Submound 51—was 3 m deep, over 56 m long (north-south), and 19 m wide (east-west) (Pauketat et al. 2002). Bareis excavated a total of 10 units (each 3 m^2) over the course of five field seasons, 1967–1971. Located on the northern and middle sections of Submound 51, these units represent an estimated 13 percent of the total feature fill; roughly 87 percent of the feature remains intact to this day.

The large size of Submound 51 indicates that it was initially one of several borrow pits from which soil was removed prehistorically to be used in the construction of the surrounding mounds and plaza. It is unclear just how long this feature may have remained open to the elements, although the presence of well-preserved marsh grass at the bottom suggests that it was open for at least a year (Pauketat et al. 2002). At some point, large quantities of refuse were deposited rapidly over the marsh grass, thereby sealing this organic material and its accompanying insects and creating an anaerobic environment. Multiple depositional episodes followed, during which large quantities of refuse and materials were discarded across the entire surface of the feature, burying the previous layer completely. A total of seven strata—some with subzones—were identified through the course of the excavations. Pauketat and colleagues (2002) examined the different material remains excavated during the 1967–1968 excavation. A summary of this research (Pauketat et al. 2002) identified these deposits as residues from feasting events that occurred at Cahokia, presumably in the large central plaza or very close by. The rapid filling in of these deposits is indicated by the presence of well-preserved uncarbonized insect and floral remains. One of the lower zones, Zone F, contained large quantities of carbonized and uncarbonized thatch (presumably from a structure) that was burned in situ at a very high temperature as indicated by the vitrified fragments of plant silica. Additional materials identified in the submound deposits include large quantities of tobacco seeds; carbonized and uncarbonized pieces of red cedar and bald cypress; debitage from tool production using exotic materials, such as quartz crystals and nonlocal cherts; pigments, such as hematite, galena, and kaolinite; unusual painted ceramic fragments (some with distinctive icons sketched on the surface); a terra cotta figurine of a seated person; faunal remains; and isolated human remains. Surprisingly, little maize was recovered from the portion of the feature analyzed by Pauketat et al. (2002). Given the significant increase in maize consumption that occurred in the American Bottom at this time, the absence of this key food item is notable.

More recent osteological analysis of the human skeletal remains recovered from all of Bareis's Submound 51 excavations, including portions of this massive feature that were not discussed in Pauketat et al. (2002), identified several unusual examples of postmortem bone modification. The isolated human remains found in this feature represent 28 individuals (8 subadults, 3 adolescent/young adult females, and 17 adults: 2 males, 4 females, and 11 of unknown sex). Most of the elements are associated with Zones G and H—two of the lowest zones underneath the layer of burnt thatch. With one exception (Burial 60, an adult of unknown sex), none of these elements appear to have resulted from intentional primary burials in this feature.

Many of the human elements in Submound 51 exhibit both taphonomic and cultural modifications. For example, carnivore gnawing is clearly evident in the form of tooth groove furrows and tooth punctures on seven long bone fragments, indicating that these particular remains had been exposed to the elements for an indeterminate period of time prior to being deposited in the feature. The carnivore gnawing could have occurred when the remains were stored in a mortuary facility, such as a charnel house, or when they were left exposed prior to or after deposition in the Submound 51 feature.

Cut marks are also found on a number of cranial and postcranial elements. The location of the cut marks on most of these elements near muscle attachments suggests that they resulted from postmortem processing related to mortuary treatment. However, several elements exhibit cut marks that differ from defleshing marks, reflecting modification for a different purpose. For example, multiple scores are located perpendicular to the axis of the midshaft diaphysis of a right radius. Immediately superior to these cut marks, the diaphysis had clearly been deliberately snapped sometime shortly after death, when the bone was still fresh.

Polishing is present on several elements. The distal diaphyses of a left femur and a left fibula each display a linear patch of polish with linear striations characteristic of sand abrasion. Given the high sand content in the Submound 51 feature and in the surrounding soils, the presence of such linear patches of striated polish along the diaphyses is probably due to taphonomic forces.

Human Bone Tools

Two long bones exhibit patterns of postmortem modification that are clearly distinct from the types of alterations discussed above. We argue that these elements most likely functioned as tools.

Modified Ulna

The first example is the diaphysis of a right ulna from an adult of unknown sex (Figure 8.1), associated with Zones E and F. Evidence of a healed infection is provided by the remodeled surface of the bone. The distal end is missing, and the medial surface of the diaphysis is split longitudinally halfway up the diaphysis, tapering to a point distally. The tip is missing, although whether this occurred during use or after final discard is difficult to determine. The smoothed and polished broken edges identify the function of this object as a bone awl. Numerous perpendicular scrape marks are present along the polished edges, primarily in the upper areas of the modification.

Nonhuman ulnas were commonly used as awls in the Americas and elsewhere; their functions included perforating materials (skins, cloth) and basket weaving. Human ulnas are less well suited for this task. They require more modification, are less strong, and have much more trabecular and less compact bone than do the nonhuman alternatives, so the manufacture of this tool may well represent a conscious choice and carry some symbolic meaning. Some

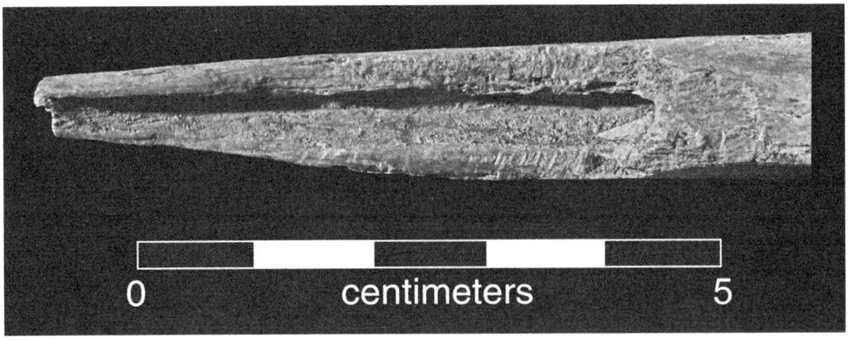

8.1. Cahokia Submound 51 (Zones E–F): awl made from a human right ulna diaphysis. (Courtesy of Illinois State Archaeological Survey, University of Illinois)

sense of the wealth of potential meanings is suggested in Janet Spector's ethnographic reading of a Dakota awl handle (1993), but unlike the Dakota example and like most other prehistoric ulna awls, the Cahokia example is undecorated. Perhaps this tool was used during the production of special ritual objects, such as clothing, mats, or containers. Certainly the presence of this unusual object among other discarded ritual materials in the Submound 51 feature suggests a unique function beyond that of awls recovered from a general habitation feature.

Modified Femur

The second human bone tool is a right femur of an adult male, which was also recovered from D1, one of the higher zones. The element is fractured at midshaft. The characteristic beveling and angle of the fracture suggests that the break occurred while the bone was still relatively fresh, or perhaps in the perimortem interval (Figure 8.2). The edges of the break are very smooth, rounded, and highly polished, both on the outer edge and on the inner or medullary edge of the fracture. At some point during use, a small vertical portion of cortical bone at the utilized edge snapped off from the posterior portion of the femur. Continued use of the element after this event is indicated by the presence of polish over the surface of the newly exposed bone. This sequence of events is illustrated by the high amount of polish on most of the broken edge of the midshaft except where this secondary fracture occurred. The surface of the newly exposed bone has much less polish than the rest of the midshaft edges.

On the superior portion of the diaphysis, additional modification is indicated by a line of discoloration just inferior to the femoral head that extends just below the lesser trochanter and encircles the diaphysis (Figure 8.3). The

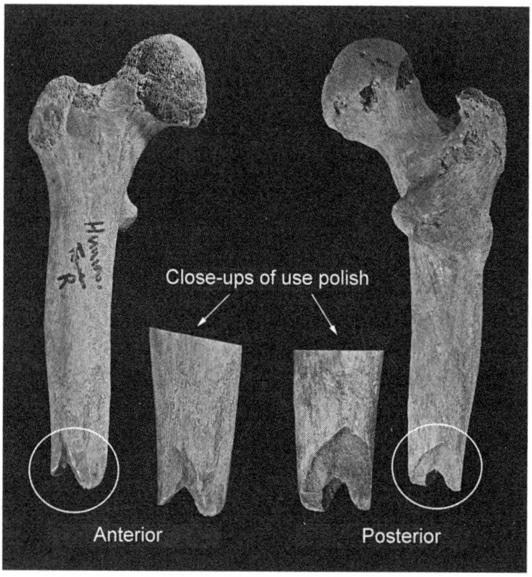

8.2. Cahokia Submound 51 (Zone D1): digging tool made from a human right femur. (Courtesy of Illinois State Archaeological Survey, University of Illinois)

coloration of the bone surface in this area appears darker, more mottled, and exhibits more patina than that of the superior portion of the neck or lower diaphysis. The discrete nature of this discoloration suggests that this element was bound with some type of material, such as sinew or hide. This interpretation is supported by the clearly worn appearance of the linea aspera surface and the lesser trochanter, which are within this discolored area. The absence of any impressions in the bone surface within the confines of this discolored area indicate that the purpose of this modification was to facilitate a grip on the object while it was being used rather than to haft it to another component, such as a handle.

The distinctive nature of the polish on this particular element clearly indicates that this femur was used as a tool. Such localized high polish and smoothing of the broken midshaft edges are not commonly found on bone that has been altered by taphonomic processes, such as friction with sand, as is seen on several other isolated human elements in this feature. The polish shown on the right femur lacks linear striations, is present on all surfaces of the fractured edges, and is more continuous than what we see in examples of sand abrasion.

Given the evidence presented above, it is safe to say that this element was

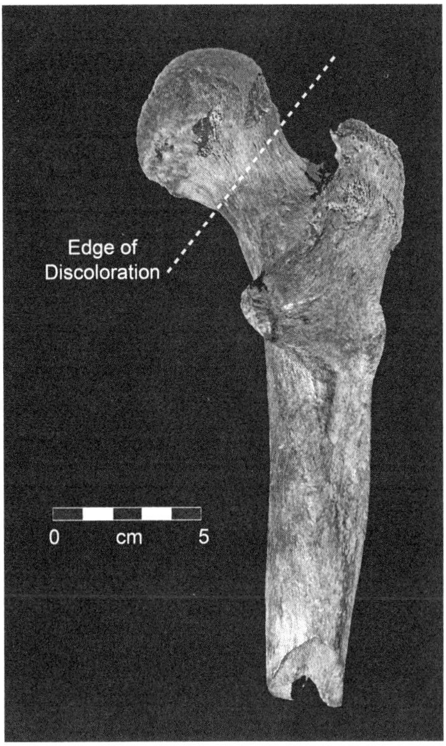

8.3. Cahokia Submound 51 (Zone D1): close-up of discoloration on proximal diaphysis of right femur. (Courtesy of Illinois State Archaeological Survey, University of Illinois)

utilized as some type of tool. But what was its function? The smooth, polished edges of the midshaft fracture suggest that it may have been used as a digging tool. The sharp beveled edges of the fractures are perfect for digging in the ground. The unique characteristics of this modification call to mind a planting tool commonly referred to as a dibble. A dibble is a pointed tool used to make holes in the ground when planting seeds, bulbs, or young plants (Figure 8.4). Alternatively, if the brown stain is evidence for more substantial hafting, as we have argued, the femur may have functioned as the bit of a compound digging stick. However, we find no direct evidence for similar objects in the literature.

Experiments

To test this hypothesis, Cook conducted an experiment using a cadaver femur from an anatomy lab to punch holes in the ground to aid in planting squash seeds. Using a hacksaw, Cook cross-sectioned the modern human femur above the midshaft. The soil used in the experiment was a damp, friable

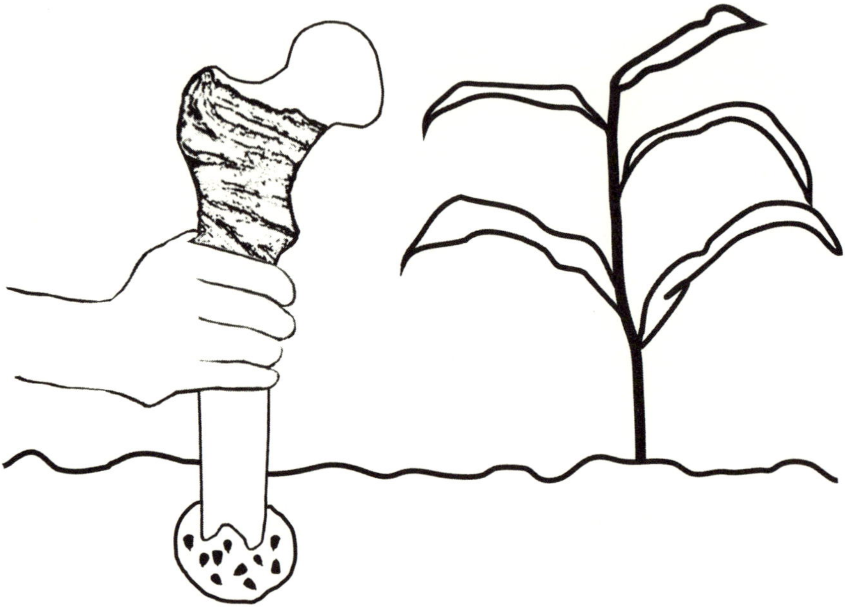

8.4. Example of a dibble. (Drawing by Eve A. Hargrave)

clay soil that had been plowed the previous year and spaded into a 65-ft-long hilled row over manure six months previously. Using the cut midshaft of the modern modified femur, an approximately 2-inch planting hole was placed every 4 inches along the row, and a squash seed was set in each hole. This was only slightly more difficult than using her usual implement, a large eye bolt, and the proximal femur fit comfortably in the hand. This limited one-time use resulted in slight polish on both the cut surface and the adjacent shaft. The opening of the medullary cavity became packed with soil, but the edge did not fracture or spall, despite a preexisting longitudinal crack.

The inference from this experiment is that it would take a great deal more use (or a more abrasive soil) to produce the high polish present on the Submound 51 modified femur. Upon close examination of the modified femur, it was noted that the medullary cavity contained soil with a high sand content. However, it is difficult (if not impossible) to determine whether this represents soil impacted during use, postdepositional taphonomic processes, or both. Clearly the tool was used much more intensively than in Cook's one-time experiment based on the high polish on the edges of the primary fracture. Polish along the edges of the secondary fracture on the anterior surface suggests that even after the element was damaged, it continued to be used for an indefinite period of time.

Milner and colleagues (2010) conducted an experiment focusing on the effectiveness of chert hoes in moving soil for agricultural and earth-moving purposes. Several of their results are pertinent for our study. First, they noted that a fairly uniform polish formed on the edge of the hoe after four hours of continuous use. Second, chipping of the hoe edges increased significantly in the more rocky soils. The implications of these results are that, although the amount of polish on the femoral edges of Cook's experimental femur was minimal, it might not have taken much longer to form the polish on the Submound 51 femur tool. Milner and colleagues' (2010) results also suggest that the Submound 51 femur was used to dig in a softer soil, such as would be typically found in the ridge and swale sand ridge system of the American Bottom floodplain.

Discussion

The biography of these modified human elements presents intriguing insights into the worldview and relationships with the dead among the early Cahokia inhabitants. Let us assume that the "birth" of the elements occurred at the time of an individual's death. Upon death, the individual was probably placed in a nearby cemetery or charnel structure, where the body was allowed to decay. Such mortuary facilities typically would have housed human remains in multiple stages of decomposition ranging from primary, fully articulated bodies to secondary deposits of bones that had been cleaned according to the prevailing mortuary rites. Charnel houses have been identified at numerous Mississippian sites in the American Bottom and surrounding areas and are often believed to represent the mortuary houses of specific kin or community groups (Alt 2006; Emerson 1997a; Emerson and Hargrave 2000; Emerson and Jackson 1984; Emerson et al. 1983; Fowler et al. 1999; Goldstein 1980; Holley et al. 2001; McElrath et al. 1987; Milner 1983, 1984). Ethnographic accounts suggest that a secondary burial or disposition of remains often accentuates group membership, since individual identity is lost, deemphasized, or transformed (Metcalf and Huntington 1991).

The deposition of the materials in Submound 51 occurred primarily during the Lohmann phase (A.D. 1050–1100) based on ceramic analysis and radiocarbon assays (Pauketat and Emerson 1997; Pauketat et al. 2002). During this period of time we also see the dismantling of charnel structures associated with the earliest construction phases of Mound 72, located approximately 300 m south of the grand plaza and the large Submound 51 borrow feature (Fowler et al. 1999; Goldstein 2000). We propose that the remains present in the lower zones of Submound 51 represent the cleaning out of one or more charnel structures—perhaps even the earliest one from Mound 72—and that the burned thatch covering these lower zones may have come from one of these charnel structures or from a temple, as suggested by Pauketat and colleagues (2002). As part of this process of dismantling existing charnel structures, at least one femur and ulna were retained for a special purpose. It is at this point that these remains entered a new stage of "life," where they became simultaneously symbols and functional tools. Thus would begin the ongoing interactions between the person(s) who, through use, modified this particular object (a.k.a. the modifier) and the individual whose body part was modified. Each time the tool was used, it would have reinforced the significance and importance of the ritual act to the participants and observers. The question is, how was this tool used? What was the significance of using this human bone as a tool? What was the context in which it was used?

A common theme attributed to Mississippian ritual at Cahokia is death, renewal, and rebirth (Emerson 1997a, 1997b, 2003; Pauketat and Emerson 1991). Evidence for rituals associated with this theme at Cahokia includes elaborate mortuary facilities, as seen in Mound 72, which also functioned as a focus for political and social affiliation; the incremental layers deposited in the construction of certain mounds; and agricultural symbolism, reflected in features such as corn and gourds on figurines (Brown and Kelly 2000; Emerson 1997a, 1997b, 2003; Emerson et al. 2003; Emerson et al. 2000; Fowler et al. 1999; Goldstein 2000; Hall 2000; Kelly 1997; Pauketat and Emerson 1997; Porubcan 2000). After the cranium and mandible, the proximal femur is surely the next most distinctive element of the human skeleton; hence, we think it unlikely that this bone was selected expediently from an array of disturbed human remains. The element was chosen deliberately and must have been laden with symbolic meaning.

Frazer, in the classic anthropology text *The Golden Bough* (1922), addressed the relationship between death and rebirth on a number of different levels. In particular, one chapter focused on the association of death and rebirth with agriculture. In many cultures around the world, sacrifices of humans or effigies of humans are made during the planting season (Frazer 1922:478–518). A common feature is the belief in the power imbued in the various components of the sacrificed individual: bone, flesh, bodily fluids, ashes after cremation, teeth, hair. The power contained in the object can then be transferred to the soil through subsequent burial in the field or the scattering of ashes. Such actions ensure the rebirth of the corn gods and result in a good harvest. We propose that the modified femur from Submound 51 was used in just such a way.

The evidence provided by Pauketat and colleagues (2002) clearly indicates that most of the deposits from Submound 51 were directly tied to ritual community events that occurred in the vicinity of the feature—presumably in the adjacent grand plaza. Several lines of evidence, including botanical, faunal, and entomological, indicate that the feasting that may have been tied to these rituals occurred during the growing season, from late spring to fall. The timing of these events correlates well with the interpretation of this modified femur's function as a ritual tool tied to the agricultural cycle of the Cahokian population. The characteristics of the polish on the fractured edge of the Submound 51 femur, combined with the possible binding as a grip, clearly support the interpretation of its use as a tool—probably a digging tool. This femur would clearly have represented death both symbolically and literally. An additional level of significance could also have been present if the element came from a known person, such as a leader, shaman, war captive, or sacrificial victim. Alternatively, the femur may have symbolized the social group(s) to which the individual belonged in life.

Perhaps these elements, particularly the femur, represented the spirit of an earlier leader—one whose lineage, although no longer prominent at the time the charnel house was dismantled, remained important in a historical sense. The use and modification of human remains from a powerful individual who lived in the critical period leading up to the development of Cahokia would have aided in legitimizing both the spiritual and political authority of the existing rulers. Given the increased prominence of agriculture in the Mississippian economy, the linking of the ancestral lineage (via the human remains) directly to the land and to a key source of food could potentially have played a role in legitimizing the existing ruling lineage(s). What better way to emphasize the close relationship between death and life than through the use of human bone to facilitate the growth of crops?

In biographical terms, the "death" of these human tools occurred later in the Lohmann phase, as indicated by their deposition in the upper levels of Submound 51. Perhaps these objects had served their purpose in mediating between the old sociopolitical order and the new Cahokia world order. Alternatively, other types of material objects may have been developed that better suited the aims and goals of the individuals involved in rituals. The association of these tools with the feasting debris in the Submound 51 feature suggests that they played a role in the events and rituals that occurred during community events in the nearby areas, possibly in the central plaza.

Conclusions

We have shown that these two worked human bones likely had special meaning and that the femur was likely used as a hand-digging tool, such as a dibble. The association with tobacco seeds in the Submound 51 deposits and the striking lack of archaeobotanical evidence for maize may well point to its use during the planting season for maize or squash, both of which are readily planted using a dibble. The salience of squash/gourd symbolism at Cahokia (Emerson et al. 2003; Emerson et al. 2000) is particularly interesting in this regard. Alternatively, it is possible that the tools were connected to tobacco. The prehistoric cultivation of tobacco is largely a mystery, but we imagine that starting seedlings in a sheltered plot and then transplanting them in late spring may well have been an ancient innovation in growing this crop in temperate regions, such as the American Bottom (Rafferty and Mann 2004; Winter 2000).

Acknowledgments

We would like to acknowledge the support of Thomas Emerson, the director of the Illinois State Archaeological Survey, Prairie Research Institute, University of Illinois; John Walthall at the Illinois Department of Transportation; and the Bioanthropology Laboratory, Department of Anthropology, Indiana University, for their support in this research. Additional thanks go to the following individuals, who contributed their expertise and knowledge during conversations regarding the identification and function of the modified elements discussed here: Kristin Hedman, Dawn Cobb, Shirley Schermer, Robin Lillie, Stephen Nawrocki, Cheryl Munson, Steve Kuehn, and Timothy Pauketat.

9
Opportunity Knocks
Nonritual Use of Human Bone at the Aztalan Site, Jefferson County, Wisconsin

Katie J. Zejdlik

The Aztalan archaeological site, located on the west bank of the Crawfish River in Jefferson County, Wisconsin, has been heralded as one of the largest and most significant archaeological sites in the state (Barrett 1933:74; Ritzenthaler 1958:1). Materials recovered from the site show evidence of repeated occupation since the Paleoindian period (Goldstein 1987:251; Sampson 2008); radiocarbon dates suggest that the most substantial occupation of the site was from A.D. 1000 to 1200 (Richards 1992). During this time, a palisade with square bastions enclosed and subdivided 9 ha of a mound-village complex. This included three flat-topped pyramidal mounds at the northwest, northeast, and southwest corners; a natural gravel knoll on the southeast corner; a central plaza; and domestic structures, including houses, hearths, storage pits, and midden deposits (Figure 9.1). The majority of materials recovered from the site represent components of Late Woodland and Middle Mississippian cultures.

I utilized the archaeological context, museum records, and archaeological and ethnographic reports to interpret the function of an unidentified implement made from a modified human tibia recovered from Aztalan and curated at the Milwaukee Public Museum (MPM). A literature review suggested that the Aztalan tibia is an implement style common to the Plains and that it either pre- or postdates the main occupation of the Aztalan site. The archaeological context implies that despite being a modified *human* bone, this tool was used opportunistically rather than ritually.

Human Remains from Aztalan

For over a century, beginning as early as 1837 (Richards 2007), human osteological material has been excavated from the site's mortuary and nonmortuary contexts (Barrett 1933; Goldstein and Gaff 2002; Lapham 2001 [1855]; Maher 1958; Richards 2007; Rowe 1958; Somers 1920; Sterling 1920). Although considerable research has been conducted on Aztalan's human skeletal

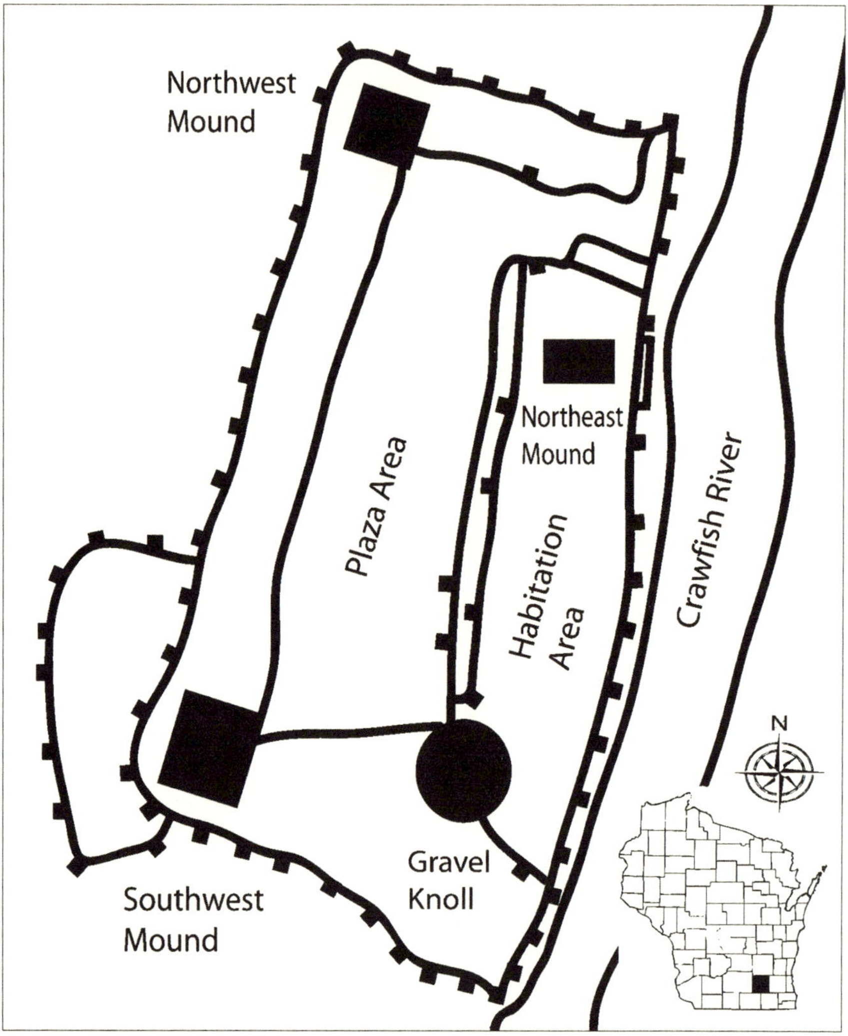

9.1. Map of the Aztalan site. (Based on a drawing by E. Paulsen, University of Wisconsin, Milwaukee, Department of Anthropology)

assemblage, many questions are still unanswered. Interpretation of Aztalan's human osteological material is complicated by the use of diverse mortuary programs at the site and skeletal evidence of violence on isolated, informally buried human remains. Additionally, Aztalan was occupied by various groups with different traditions since the Paleoindian period. The lack of available radiocarbon dates on human remains and the loss of field notes and provenience information further add to the interpretive conundrum.

Human remains at Aztalan have been recovered primarily in four known contexts: primary, in-flesh inhumations; secondary bundle burials; charnel structure cremations; and scattered, isolated remains—some with cut marks—in refuse pits, in fire pits, along the palisade, and strewn across the habitation area (Barrett 1933; Goldstein 2010; Rudolph 2009).

Primary, in-flesh inhumations at Aztalan occurred in a variety of forms, a few of which are demonstrated in the following examples. The primary interment of a 20- to 25-year-old female, supine and fully extended, was found on a natural layer of white sand and gravel in a conical mound overlooking the site. She had been wrapped at the chest, hips, and lower legs in a garment that included 2,000 round and square shell beads (Barrett 1933:241–243). Near the gravel knoll at the southeast corner of the site, two children, both approximately six years old, had been placed next to each other and interred under a cone of gravel (Rudolph 2009). One child was prone and extended with a turtle carapace on its legs. The other was flexed on its side. Its lower body had been placed on the right torso of the extended child (Barrett 1933:137–138). At the southwest corner of the site, an adult female was found truncated by a portion of a palisade bastion. She had been buried supine and headless. No grave goods were included (Maher 1958:99).

Secondary bundle burials found in the "largest oval mound in the enclosure" (Sterling 1920:18) consisted of 6–12 forearm bones, wrapped around once with a three-strand cord tied in a bow knot. The bones were broken in two places and burnt black; the thermal alteration had cemented the bone and cord together (Sterling 1920:19).

Cremations were recovered from a semi-subterranean charnel structure on the west side of the northwest mound. The structure was 12 ft long, 5 ft wide, and 4.8 ft–5.3 ft high. Inside were the highly burnt and fragmented remains of 10 extended, supine individuals and one bundle burial, which had been placed on a large mat of woven bulrushes (Johnsen 2003:143; Rowe 1958). All interments were adult men and women, as indicated by Rowe (1958). A Mississippian seed jar, a textile fragment, and a loosely woven bag containing five hickory nuts were found with them (Johnsen 2003; Richards 2007; Rowe 1958).

In addition to the variety of formal burials, large quantities of isolated human bone showing cut marks, chop marks, and perimortem fractures were recovered from refuse pits, fire pits, the palisade, and across the habitation area (Anderson 1994; Barrett 1933; Goldstein 2010; Holcomb 1952; Richards 2007; Rudolph 2009; Somers 1920). Most of these were found in conjunction with other broken materials, such as shell, ceramics, lithic debris, and processed faunal material. Interpretations of these isolated remains include warfare or other violence (Lapham 2001 [1855]; Richards 2007; Richards and Jeske 2002; Rudolph 2009; Sullivan 1990), cannibalism (Barrett 1933; Freeman 1966; Holcomb 1952; Somers 1920), and mortuary ritual (Anderson 1994; Goldstein 2010).

Context of the Aztalan Modified Tibia

The first major excavation of Aztalan was conducted by Samuel Barrett of the MPM during the years 1919, 1920, and 1932. A detailed description of his findings, titled *Ancient Aztalan*, was published in 1933 by the MPM. During his three seasons at the site, Barrett uncovered a series of post molds; remains of houses; thousands of pieces of human and animal bone; food remains; storage and refuse pits; stone, bone, and shell tools; shell, bone, and copper ornaments; and a variety of Late Woodland and Mississippian pottery sherds.

The modified tibia was recovered during Barrett's excavation and is the only modified human bone implement reported from the site. It was recovered from Pit 31, a refuse pit located on the south side of a small gravel ridge that runs east-west through the river midden. The pit was approximately 6 ft deep and of "unusual and irregular form," was used strictly for refuse, and consisted of a "great mass of usual black earth mixed with broken bones, deer teeth, shells, and a few small potsherds" (Barrett 1933:132). There are no plan or profile drawings available for Pit 31. The only items recovered from Pit 31 and listed in the MPM records were an Aztalan collared rim sherd, a Cahokia Red-Slipped rim sherd, and an unidentified, thick-rimmed, shell-tempered sherd exemplary of wares from both the Late Woodland and Mississippian periods (Milwaukee Public Museum 1921:79–80; John Richards, personal communication 2008).

Pits 27–30, located immediately adjacent to Pit 31, contained refuse such as sherds, animal bone, shell, and some floral remains (Barrett 1933:127). In addition, Pit 27 held a concentration of discarded bone tools, and Pit 28 had an unusually large amount of processed animal bone (Milwaukee Public Museum 1921:78–79, 83). The most interesting is Pit 29, which contained a few pieces of sheet copper, a brass ring, a small piece of iron, and Late Woodland and Mississippian ceramics (Milwaukee Public Museum 1921:83). The ceramics were located stratigraphically higher than the historic objects, indicating mixing within the pit (Barrett 1933:129). Pit 29 is located near other pits with historic period objects, possibly indicative of a postcontact village site (Barrett 1933:107; Bruhy and Goldstein 1981; Hudson 2004; Warwick 2002). The proximity of this historic material to Pit 31 is important in the interpretation of the Aztalan tibia.

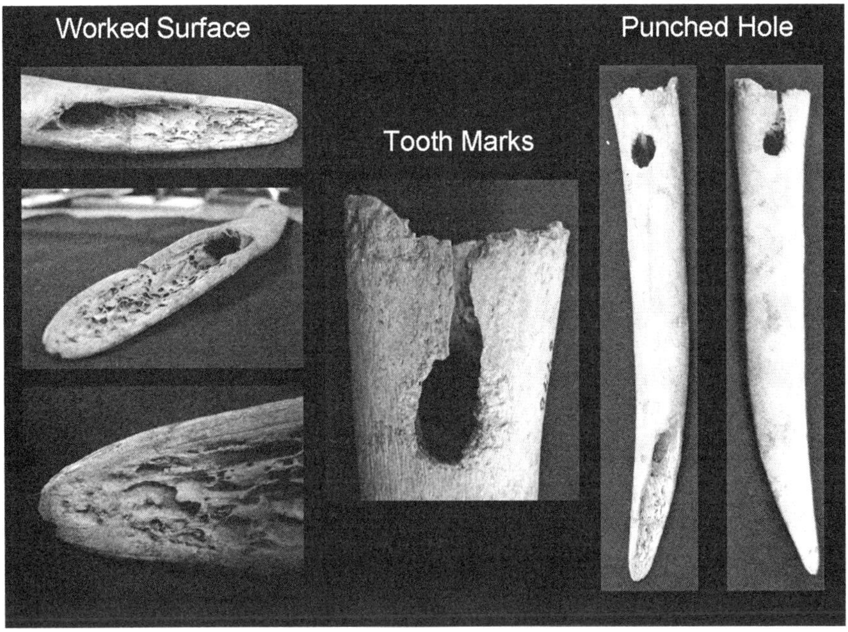

9.2. Types of modification to the Aztalan tibia. (Courtesy of Katie J. Zejdlik)

Description of the Aztalan Tibia

The implement is composed of the proximal 268 mm of the tibia shaft and is 80 mm in circumference at the nutrient foramen. The tibia's worked surface is 88 mm long, located just distal to the midshaft, and has been modified to an approximate 20 degree angle of shear relative to the shaft. The angled surface shows a moderately shiny, smooth polish with long striations that run parallel to the long axis of the bone. The proximal end of the tibia exhibits a quantity of wide, U-shaped tooth marks and appears to have been gnawed off by a large carnivore. The proximal end contains a punched hole extending mediolaterally through the bone. The hole is approximately 18 mm long and 12 mm wide on each side (Figure 9.2).

The wear on this implement suggests that it was used to work soft materials, such as hides or wood (Johnson 1989:438; LeMoine 1991, 1994; Runnings et al. 1989:264–265; Shipman 1989). In addition, wear around the margins of the perforation on the proximal end consists of small scratches that radiate in every direction except on the most distal aspect. This pattern of wear indicates that something was attached to the tibia through the perforation holes and moved in a swinging, anterioposterior direction.

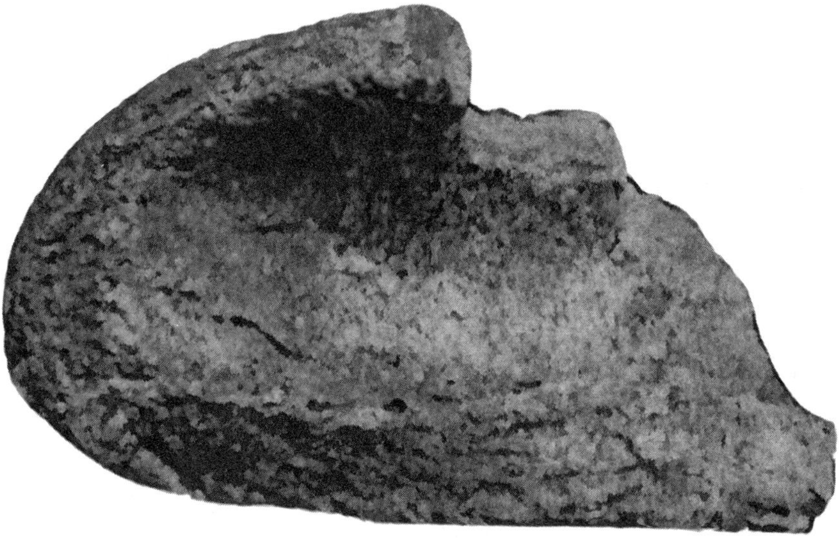

9.3. Worked tip of modified human femur from the Price III site, Wisconsin. (Reprinted with permission from *Wisconsin Archeologist*)

Barrett originally identified the tibia as an "elk antler dagger (?)" (Barrett 1933:530–531) with the following description: "an implement, 266 mm. in length, made of an elk antler prong and provided with a cutting (?) edge at the point and a perforation at the base. Such an instrument might well have been used as a weapon, the perforation at the base serving for the attachment of a weapon by a thong to the wrist of the wearer or elsewhere. It is not unlike daggers made of bone or antler by some of the west coast tribes in more recent times" (Barrett 1933:291). Barrett compared the tibia to the daggers used by Pomo bear doctors, which have a very similar size and shape as well as a hole for attaching a handle (Barrett 1917, 1952).

Nevertheless, the implement is clearly a human tibia. When accessioned into the MPM's collection, it was listed as "1 implement made of human leg bone (sketch) polished at end" (Milwaukee Public Museum 1921:79–82). The date on the entry is July 26, 1921, suggesting that the implement had been identified as a human bone prior to Barrett's publication of *Ancient Aztalan* in 1933. We do not know whether the Aztalan items were accessioned after the publication of *Ancient Aztalan* and the records backdated with the date of excavation, or if there was simply a lack of communication between the cataloger and Barrett.

There have been no similar implements recovered from Aztalan, and a review of midwestern archaeological literature found that only one other object like this has been identified in the region. A modified human femur was recovered from the Price III site in Richland County, Wisconsin (Freeman 1966). The Price III site is an Archaic cemetery with 37 burials containing 88 individuals. The implement had been interred with a middle-aged adult female. The written description matches that of the Aztalan tibia, and the published photograph of the worked distal surface appears nearly the same (Figure 9.3). Freeman (1966:45) identified the worked femur as a defleshing tool. The Aztalan tibia also appears to be a defleshing tool. Based on the size, shape, and use-wear pattern, the tibia best matches a style of hide flesher common to the late prehistoric or historic period in the Plains.

Bone Hide Fleshers

Bone hide fleshers were used to scrape away soft tissues from the inside of a hide. Wissler (1910:63) observed Blackfoot people stretch the hide out on the ground, hair side down, and hold it in place with wooden stakes. The flesher was then used to remove the remaining soft tissue. After the flesh side was completed, the fur side was processed in a similar manner. Steinbring (1966:576) observed a similar process among the Black River Band of Ojibwas. After enough decomposition had taken place to loosen the hair, the hide was tied to a frame. A flesher was then used to scrape off any excess tissues still present on the skin side. A separate tool, a scraper, was used to remove the hair.

Archaeologically in the Plains, fleshers appear around A.D. 1000 (MacNeish 1958; Matwychuck 1980:3) and carry over into the Coalescent period (A.D. 1000–1500) (Lehmer 1954:153). Accounts describe the utilization of fleshers by tribes in the northern Plains and, as mentioned above, by the Black River Band of Ojibwas in Manitoba (Kehoe 2005; Steinbring 1966).

Flesher descriptions vary only slightly. Fleshers are made from the long bones or metapodials of large mammals—usually moose, bison, deer, elk, or caribou. The bone is split at the midshaft, and the inner surface is worked until there is a sharp excurvate edge where the inner and exterior surfaces meet. Sometimes, this edge is serrated. The implement can vary from 60 mm to 250 mm in length (Kehoe 2005; Lehmer 1954:68; MacNeish 1958:135–136; Matwychuck 1980; Steinbring 1966). Many reports combine fleshers with scrapers, noting that some of the fleshers are entirely made of bone and others had stone or metal blades attached to them (Kehoe 2005; Lehmer 1954; MacNeish 1958; Matwychuck 1980; Steinbring 1966). Alternatively, fleshers and scrapers are documented as two separate tools. Fleshers are noted as being made only of bone while hide scrapers had a blade attached to them (Schultz 1992:337–338; Steinbring 1966:576). Fleshers and scrapers also had wrist straps attached to them on one end via a perforation in the bone (Grinnell

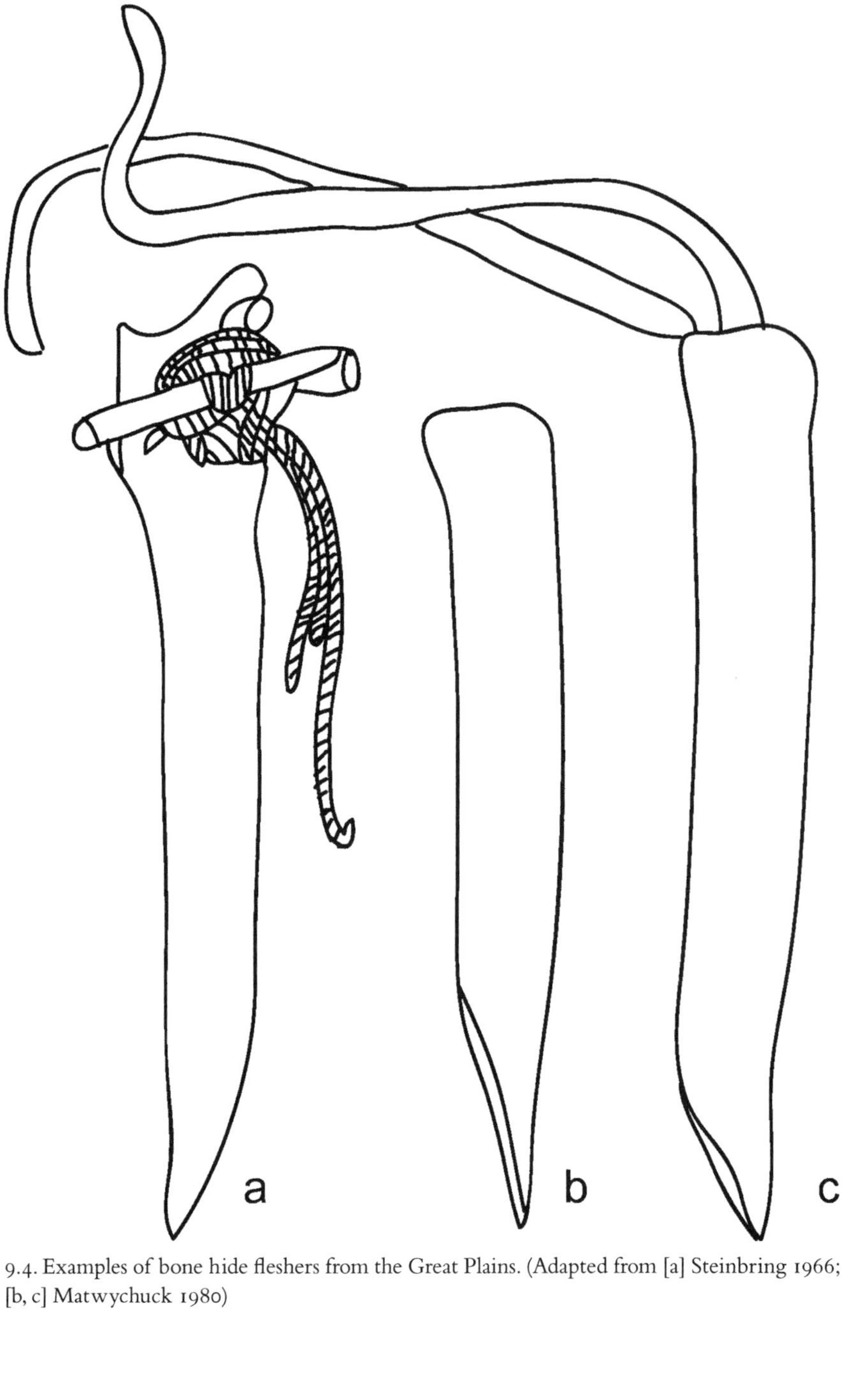

9.4. Examples of bone hide fleshers from the Great Plains. (Adapted from [a] Steinbring 1966; [b, c] Matwychuck 1980)

1923:214; Matwychuck 1980:12; Steinbring 1966:579–580; Weltfish 1965:369) (Figure 9.4).

Discussion

The Aztalan tibia flesher is problematic. It is made from human bone, in a style more common to the Plains, and may pre- or postdate the main occupation of Aztalan based on its deposition in both a prehistoric and historically occupied portion of the site. There are no other implements like it at Aztalan or among other Late Woodland or Middle Mississippian sites in the area (e.g., Black 1967; Finney and Stoltman 1991; Green and Rodell 1994; Rodell 1991).

The presence of a human femur flesher at the Archaic Price III site suggests that fleshers were being used in the area as early as the Late Archaic period. However, archaeological and ethnographic reports of this flesher style indicate that it likely occurred during the late prehistoric or early historic period. The archaeological context of the Aztalan tibia shows that it is not likely to be an Archaic object based on the presence of Late Woodland and Mississippian ceramic sherds in the pit. Additionally, several other pits adjacent to Pit 31 show postcontact mixing (Barrett 1933:82). Although there were no postcontact objects found in Pit 31, a diachronic study of the Aztalan faunal remains indicates that a postcontact village was present at that location (Hudson 2004; Warwick 2002). Furthermore, Bruhy and Goldstein (1981) found evidence of six Winnebago camps and one camp of unknown affiliation at the site.

Many researchers have speculated about migrations of people from east to west through this region via sites like Aztalan (Fugle 1962; Griffin 1946, 1960; Ives 1962). Wilford (1945:39) found direct links between Aztalan and the Mill Creek culture of northwestern Iowa. Sampson (2008) found that a quantity of lithic material at Aztalan originated in the western portion of Wisconsin, indicating contact between the two areas.

There appears to be a lower standard for the manufacture of fleshers and scrapers in the postcontact period (Matwychuck 1980:14; Steinbring 1966:581). The energy and time spent on production of these tools "waned considerably" as the need for hides decreased and the availability of steel tools increased (Steinbring 1966:581). "Possibly, as a partial result of the new ease of manufacture, less 'value' is placed on the article. When one is chipped or broken, it is discarded, not repaired" (Steinbring 1966:581). Matwychuck (1980:14) stated that fleshers were made from the remains of the first kill at a new site and then discarded when the camp moved on.

The taphonomic modifications and archaeological context of the Aztalan tibia suggest that it was a tool of opportunity. The hole for the wrist strap is broken on one side. The fracture goes through tooth marks, indicating that the bone had been discarded and gnawed on prior to being fashioned into a tool. Perimortem fracturing and/or gnawing is present on 36 percent of the recovered isolated tibiae, making this a common taphonomic modification to human remains processing at the site (Rudolph 2009). A spiral fracture would have left an edge, which could be worked into a flesher. With the long bone already split at the midshaft, like the fleshers discussed in the archaeological and ethnographic literature, the tibia would have been an attractive potential tool. Additionally, the Aztalan tibia was broken in two places: at the scraping edge and at the hole for the wrist strap attachment. Other tools at Aztalan also appeared to be tools of opportunity and possibly were expedient. Of approximately 61 animal bone awls recovered from the site, the majority were made from splinters of bone (Barrett 1933:286).

The femur hide flesher found at the Price III site may suggest ritual use since it was interred with a burial; however, grave goods do not always signify ritual use, and the flesher may have been viewed merely as a tool. Mensforth (2007) examined 38 Archaic artifacts from the eastern United States that were made from human bone and recovered from both grave and nongrave features. He argued that the style of manufacture and pattern and the degree of use-wear present on many of the human long bone tools are equivalent to what has been found on animal bone tools, suggesting utilitarianism (Mensforth 2007:260). There is nothing in Pit 31 to indicate that this tool was used in a ritual context. Unlike the human remains in the Submound 51 borrow pit at Cahokia, where materials demonstrated ritual feasting (Hargrave and Cook, this volume; Pauketat et al. 2002; Richards 2007:12), Pit 31 was so typical of a refuse pit at Aztalan that Barrett did not even provide a profile sketch. Additionally, none of the archaeological or ethnographic literature that I reviewed suggested that fleshers/scrapers were used ritually or found in ritual contexts (Kehoe 2005; Lehmer 1954; MacNeish 1958; Matwychuck 1980; Steinbring 1966).

Last, the individual using the Aztalan tibia may not have identified it as human. The proximal end had been gnawed off and the distal shaft had broken into a spiral fracture, leaving only the shaft available to identify it as human. Furthermore, it was likely recovered from a refuse pit mixed with other habitation debris, as were many of the processed human remains from Aztalan. The condition of the bone combined with the context may not have led to a conclusion that it was human. Barrett's seemingly keen eye misidentified it as an elk antler dagger (Barrett 1933:530–531), and he went as far as saying that "in no case was any implement encountered which was made from human bone" (Barrett 1933:286).

Conclusion

The presence of a modified human bone implement at the Aztalan site leads to a range of interpretations related to the use of the tool and of human bone. It also offers an opportunity for additional insight into the cultural milieu at Aztalan. The majority of the human osteological materials collected from Aztalan were recovered as isolated bones from refuse pits. Of the isolated bones, 7.3 percent show some form of perimortem processing, likely as a result of intergroup hostility (Rudolph 2009). The spiral fracture present on the distal shaft of the human tibia flesher may be the result of this primary process. However, secondary modification to the tibia into the form of a tool is another example of human remains processing at Aztalan that deviates from the pattern of culturally modified human bone at the site.

The Plains-like style of the flesher provides information about its function and may indicate cultural influence, even migration, between Aztalan and the Plains.

As a modified human bone, it offers an example of an opportunistic tool. It might be easy to assume that the Aztalan tibia is related to ritual or trophy taking; however, there is no evidence available to support that conclusion. The tibia may not have been recognized as human by whoever collected or modified it. Yet, if the tibia was recognized as human, then a variety of questions can be posed. Was it selected because it was human? If so, is this because of who or where the bone came from? Do the remains of an unknown individual mean something to someone else? How do economy and the need for a tool factor into the opportunistic use of human vs. nonhuman bone? Was this tibia used in a ritual where, after having served its function, it was discarded? Is it possible that this tool served both utilitarian and ritual functions?

This single artifact from Aztalan raises questions about the treatment of human remains, migration, interaction, and occupation of the site—thereby illustrating the vast and varied information available from the analysis of culturally modified human remains. Additional inquiry will lead to additional questions and research, further impacting our knowledge of Midwest archaeology and, more important, the people who created these implements.

Acknowledgments

I would like to thank the Milwaukee Public Museum, the *Wisconsin Archeologist*, and the University of Wisconsin, Milwaukee, for the use of their resources and for their support of this project. I would also like to thank Eve Hargrave, Kris Hedman, Shirley Schermer, and Robin Lillie for organizing the symposium that led to this publication.

10

Vessel, Ornament, Mask, or Rattle?

Reconstructing a Mississippian Worked Bone Object from the Angel Site

Della Collins Cook and Cheryl Ann Munson

A worked human skull fragment (X11C/5) was described in the Angel site report as a portion of a container with a "stepped-fret" rim. We describe this artifact more completely, emphasizing tool mark evidence for defleshing and decoration. The object was broken while the bone still had fresh fracture characteristics, suggesting considerable force. Several plausible reconstructions are consistent with the evidence, including rattle, mask, and headdress ornament. The iconography of similar designs in both historic and prehistoric containers, ornaments, textiles, and other objects is used to evaluate these alternatives.

The Mississippian Angel site, located in the Ohio River valley of southern Indiana, was occupied for several centuries prior to A.D. 1400. In Glenn A. Black's final report on the Angel site, a worked human skull fragment was described twice: first, Black wrote snarkily, "A trowel man [from the Works Progress Administration crew] came up on the first day of work in X-11-C, with a specimen in hand which he 'thought' was a piece of human skull. It was that, but more, it had been worked! As can be seen in Fig. 123, an adult calvarium had been cut, probably in the form of a cup or vessel, and the edge adorned with a stepped-fret motif. These edges were smoothed and polished" (Black 1967:152–153).

Second, James Kellar also described this bone artifact from the Angel site: "A fragment of parietal was undoubtedly part of a container made from a human cranium. The exterior surface is polished, probably from much handling, and it retains some remnants of a red pigment. The edge (lip) has been cut in the form of a stepped fret: a regular pattern of castellations separated one from the other by a horizontal section and a narrowed square depression" (Kellar 1967:455).

A container? What type of container? We revisit this interesting object, describe it more completely, and review other worked human bone objects from the Angel site.

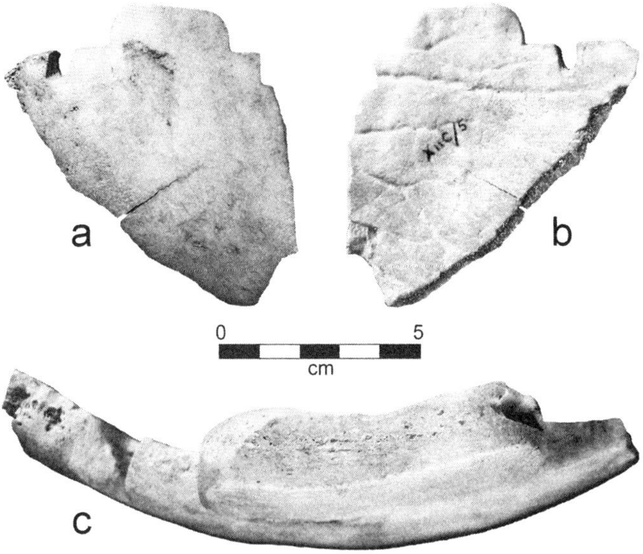

10.1. Modified human cranium X11C/5, Angel site: (a) exterior, (b) interior, (c) enlarged view of worked edge. (Courtesy of Glenn A. Black Laboratory of Archaeology, Indiana University)

Description

The Angel site is the political and religious center of the Angel phase. Archaeologists have explored this fortified town and its multiple mounds since the 1930s (Black 1967). The Angel phase dates to cal A.D. 1050–1400 (Green and Munson 1978; Hilgeman 2000). Excavations have revealed deep midden deposits and numerous wall and post features for residential and public buildings. All modified human bone comes from midden deposits.

The fragmentary object (Figure 10.1) is 6.5 cm long on its worked edge, or "rim," and 8.3 cm on the longer of the two broken margins. There is a partial fracture nearly perpendicular to the worked margin. The inferior and superior temporal lines are visible from the center of the most projecting element of the rim to the end of the fragment. Despite the polishing that Black describes, the outer surface retains the fine striations characteristic of the origins of the temporalis muscle as well as the pinpoint foramina that are usually visible in the portion of the vault that lies under the galea aponeurotica between the two temporal lines. At the intersection of the longer broken edge and the rim, this texture is particularly pronounced and the surface is dense and irregular, reflecting healed minor trauma or inflammation under the scalp. A small segment of open suture is visible in two places. Traces of red pigment are most extensive near the temporal lines.

The location of the suture remnants and the temporal lines show that the object consists of a left frontal with a small portion of the fused anterior margin of parietal. The worked rim lies close to the coronal suture, and the broken edges converge near the frontal boss. The suture cannot be the lambdoid suture because the temporal lines do not intersect the lambdoid suture. The inner surface confirms the assessment that this fragment is a frontal (Figure 10.1b). There are many meningeal vessel impressions, the largest one corresponding to the coronal suture. These impressions may have led the person Kellar consulted to identify the bone as a parietal, but some people have well-developed blood vessel impressions anterior to the coronal suture. There is fine polish on the elevated areas of the internal surface and a trace of red pigment near the suture remnant.

The temporal lines show fine cut marks that indicate defleshing. Preparation of this object required cutting away the fascia and muscle tissue of the temporalis. The artisan began this work on a more or less fresh head with soft tissue still attached, not a dry skull. The person's head had thick internal and external tables and little diploic bone, as well as a fused coronal suture (Figure 10.1c). The artisan may have chosen carefully, seeking a skull suitable for manufacturing the object. Tellingly, this skull broke through the thinner bone inferior to the temporal line.

The partial fracture and the character of the broken edges indicate that the object was broken while the bone still had plastic, fresh fracture characteristics. The broken edges bent before breaking and retain their plastic deformation, indicating that the bone collagen was still quite strong. Depending on the conditions of preservation, this is consistent with an interval of perhaps several years after death (Wieberg and Wescott 2008).

Following manufacture, the object was broken. The fracture along the longest edge is beveled, with the external table extending as much as 5 mm beyond the internal table. Through the cross section there are several plastic or bending fracture lines. The other, thinner broken margin has fractured more or less perpendicular to the surface. Near the frontal boss is a hinge fracture of the internal table. These fractures together suggest considerable blunt force applied in the region of the frontal boss. The manufactured object broke with a radial fracture pattern converging on the frontal. We suggest that the object was intentionally broken, or "killed," as has been occasionally found in Mississippian contexts (cf. Emerson 1982:3; Emerson et al. 1983; Prentice 1986; Webb and DeJarnette 1942:227–228, Plates 242, 251).

Despite these characteristics, nothing about the object's depositional rec-

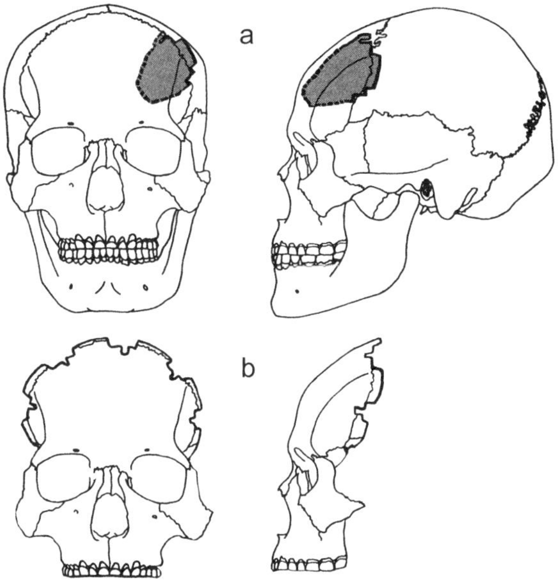

10.2. Reconstruction of X11C/5: (a) fragmentary cranial artifact placed in relation to anatomical features (solid lines on artifact are the modified edges, dashed lines are the fragmentary edges); (b) our conjectures regarding the shape of the whole artifact. (Drawings by Della Collins Cook, adapted from Neumann 1950)

ord (excavation unit X11C/5R4) suggests a ritual association. It was found in the uppermost excavation level (plow zone) above defined wall trenches and postholes (Black 1967:Figure 89). No burials are present in the vicinity. Other artifacts found in the same square are typical of domestic refuse.

Figure 10.2 shows the relationship of what remains of the object to the textural and contour features that allow the precise anatomical location of this skull fragment. We have considered several plausible reconstructions of the artifact of which it was a part. It may have come from a small, shallow container; a rondelle or similar decorative element; a mask; or a rattle. Perforations for attachment in the missing portion would support the idea that the object was a decorative element attached to some larger item. A wearer of a mask made from the facial bones and frontal could look out through the superior orbital fissures. Alternatively, if this object were a rattle, then a backing, perhaps of perishable material, would have been needed, and the fissures would have required closing with caulk or other material.

The placement of the apex of the terrace along the coronal suture allowed the artisan to polish this surface nicely. Had it been placed away from the suture, much of the surface would have been trabecular. If we assume that the upper limit of an agnathous mask or rattle element followed the coronal suture, we can approximate its height using an unconventional skull measurement, alveolare-bregma chord (the straight-line distance between bregma—the intersection of the coronal and sagittal sutures—and the most distant point on the alveolar bone between the maxillary central incisors). We measured Mississippian crania from Schild Knoll A, Greene County, Illinois, to estimate this distance. The results are 177.4 mm in males (n = 20) and 169.3 mm in females (n = 17), with a combined range of 161 mm–188 mm, which approximates the height of the object as reconstructed here. If the upper margin of an agnathous mask crossed the frontal bosses instead, the height would be about 30 mm less, and if the mandible were included, about 30 mm more.

Thus we have reconstructed the osteological origin of the Angel bone object based on morphology. Its stylistic features allow other comparisons that may elucidate the object's function and—more broadly—Angel site's relationship to other Mississippian sites. Comparisons of style may help us to choose among our conjectures about the artifact of which it was a part.

Possible Analogues for the Terraced Object

If the X11C object was a cup or vessel, it was not a calotte, the most usual form of bowl made from the frontal, parietals, and occipital of a person with fused or tightly knit cranial sutures. The reader may want to compare examples of modified human skulls in Jacobi (2007), Webb and Haag (1947), and Willoughby and Hooton (1922), and of a modified deer skull in MacLean (1931). A container with this rim would have been quite small and shallow, a saucer of sorts made from a human frontal. A saucer-like container is a possible reconstruction, but such a small object is more likely to have been a gorget resembling the Florence Mound Early Woodland frontal with an engraved raptor that accompanied the burial of an infant (Burks 2009; Converse 1979; Cheryl Johnston, personal communication 2008). Several similar Woodland objects made from human crania are known from Ohio, both decorated and undecorated, perforated and unperforated (Mills 1917; Webb and Baby 1957). Eve Hargrave (2005) described a circular rondelle made from a parietal with a central perforation produced by drilling from both surfaces from the St. Thomas site near Cahokia; this suspended ornament dates to the Mississippian Stirling phase. At the Armstrong site—an Oneota Silvernale occupation in west-central Wisconsin—excavations recovered a human vault fragment with sutural interdigitations cut away, suggesting that modifications resembling the Angel object may have been more widespread (Savage

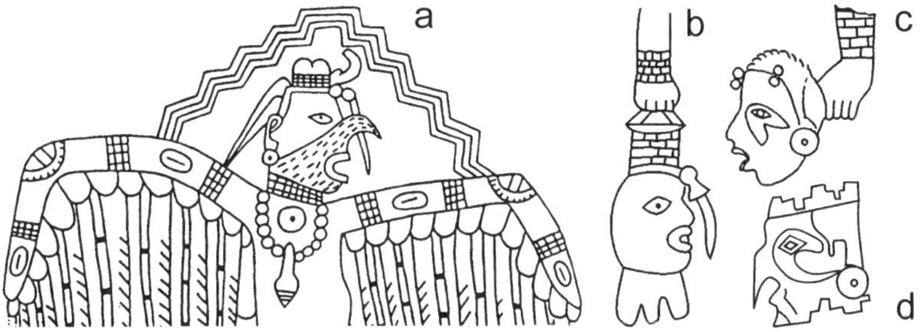

10.3. Terraced crowns and necks: (a) terrace above birdman, engraved shell cup, Spiro site (from Phillips and Brown 1978:Figure 189; Reilly 2007:Figure 3.3); (b) severed head with terraced neck, engraved shell cup, Spiro site (from Phillips and Brown 1978:Plate 153); (c) detail of head held in hand, embossed copper plate, Etowah site (from Willoughby 1932:Figure 14); (d) headdress ornament (or human head rattle) with terraced head and neck, copper plate, Malden, Missouri (from Howard 1968:Figure 8). (Drawings by Della Collins Cook and Cheryl Ann Munson)

1978). A human vault two-hole gorget and a singularly drilled irregular segment of a frontal have been reported from what may be Mississippian Dallas phase contexts in Tennessee (Williams 1975).

The shaped margin of the Angel object—its stepped or terraced motif (following Phillips and Brown 1978:156)—is the basis for our inquiry. Terraced motifs occur on shell, bone, copper, stone, ceramic, and wooden Mississippian artifacts, as well as on woven, beaded, and quilled ethnohistoric artifacts from the Eastern Woodlands and beyond. Collectively, these occur on containers, ornaments, palettes, rattles, masks, bags, belts, and saddles, and they depict headdresses or crowns, snakes, maces, and abstract designs having no known symbolic representation.

Artifacts that immediately come to mind as analogues are engraved conch shell cups, like one from Spiro's Craig Mound that depicts a birdman, or "falcon dancer," with a terraced superstructure above the head (e.g., Brown 1975: Figure 15, 2004:Figure 1; Phillips and Brown 1978:Figure 189, 1980:Plate 203; Reilly 2007:Figure 3.3). From casual reading we initially thought that there were several similar artifacts, but the multiple published images actually represent *one* Spiro shell cup depicting a terraced crown or nimbus above the human-bird figure with outstretched wings (Figure 10.3a). About this engraving, Phillips and Brown (1980:Plate 203) said: "The broad terraced motif framing the head of our bird-man demands attention if only because it is unique for Spiro and does not occur elsewhere in the Southeast so far as we know. Its very rarity adds interest to the question of possible relationship to the 'cloud-terrace' of the Southwest."

While we have not found a terraced crown above the head of a birdman occurring on other Mississippian artifacts, Phillips and Brown compared it to a Zuni war shield originally illustrated by Holmes (1883:Plate 76), which has a birdman with outstretched wings and a terraced headdress. Other southwestern artifacts illustrate this association (see Time-Life Books 1992:120), and we find Phillips and Brown's (1980) conjectures about the meaning of this iconography fascinating because of their wide-ranging command of the ethnographic literature.

Eastern Ethnographic Examples

Several ethnographic specimens from the nineteenth-century Eastern Woodlands that similarly depict terraced superstructures over thunderbirds with outstretched wings are twined bags (Figure 10.4). These include bags for Menominee sacred bundles (Berres 2001:Figure 15; Ourada 1990:18; Wilson 1982:Figures 3a, 4a, 5a) and a twined Winnebago storage bag (Berres 2001: Figure 18; Penney 1992:Figure 22). In other bags, such as two from the central Great Lakes (Phillips 1984:Figures 19, 20) and bags of the Meskwaki (Penney 1992:Plate 20), Chippewa (Phillips 1989:Figure 3), Potawatomi (Phillips 1989:Figure 5), and Sauk-Fox (Phillips 1989:Figure 7), the terraced crown is only partly depicted or abbreviated. A similar terrace composition occurs in a small, glass-beaded, twined Winnebago charm bag (Lurie 1989:Figure 7).

Other ethnographic examples of the seventeenth to nineteenth centuries show geometric terrace motifs that may carry the same meaning as the crown. These are widespread but remarkably rare compared to other geometric shapes. Examples include a Lenape wampum belt, given to William Penn (Figure 10.5) (Hill and Hill 1994:17; New York Times 1916); a Wyandot (Huron) wampum belt (Harrison 1987:Figure W45); and Huron or Iroquois wampum armbands (Harrison 1987:Figure W48). Glass-beaded objects and clothing with terrace motifs have diverse functions, but the motif is still rare in the Eastern Woodlands: a Great Lakes region sash (Penney 1992: Figure 16); Iroquois or Huron burden straps (Phillips 1984:Figures 23, 24); a Mohawk prisoner halter (Harrison 1987:Figure W55); a Chippewa shoulder bag (Penney 1992:Figure 38); and a Potawatomi charm bag (Lurie 1989:Figure 12). Decoration in other media even more rarely employed the terrace: a Cree *rogan* (birch bark container) (Harrison 1987:Figure W143); an Ottawa rush mat (Harrison 1987:Figure W144); a twined bag from New England (Abenaki?) (Drooker and Hammell 2004); and Micmac quill work on various objects (Harrison 1987:Figures E101, E102, E105, E106).

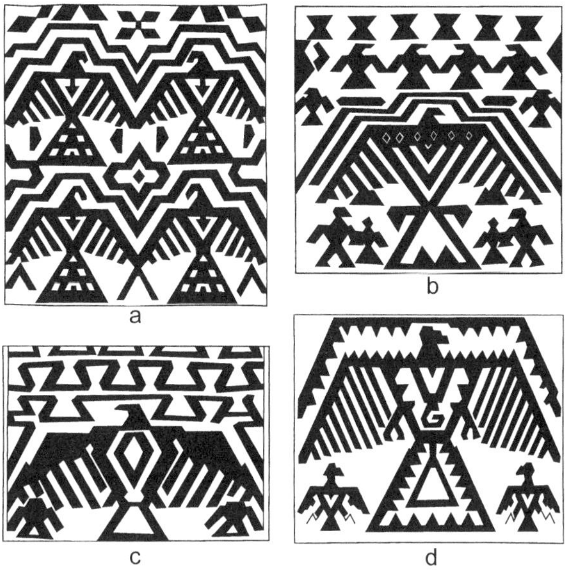

10.4. Historic examples of terrace and thunderbird motifs on twined bags: (a) Menominee (from Berres 2001:Figure 15); (b) Menominee (from Wilson 1982:Figure 4a); (c) Sauk-Fox (Meskwaki) (Penney 1992:Plate 20); (d) Chippewa (Phillips 1989:Figure 3). (Drawings by Della Collins Cook and Cheryl Ann Munson)

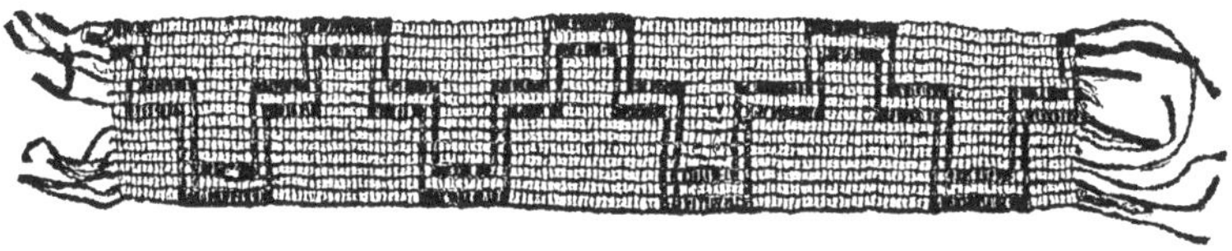

10.5. Lenape (Delaware) wampum belt with terrace motif (from Hill and Hill 1994:17 [NMAI catalog no. 053151]). (Drawing by Della Collins Cook and Cheryl Ann Munson)

Prehistoric Examples

In the prehistoric Eastern Woodlands, the terrace motif is similarly rare in both figurative art and geometric designs of the Mississippian period, but these examples have the potential to give hints about the meaning of the Angel terraced object. The engraved shell containers and ornaments from the Craig Mound at Spiro provide the largest body of comparative information, but other sites have painted, modeled, or cut objects that are potentially informative. Figurative art includes human heads, decorated clothing, birds, human-bird figures, and serpents.

Severed Heads

Related to a terrace motif above a human head might be one that is positioned below. Several Spiro shell cups depict what looks like a terrace beneath "severed" human heads (Figure 10.3b) (Phillips and Brown 1978:119–120, Plates 61, 63; Phillips and Brown 1980:Plate B-5), in which case the terrace stands for the serrated neck motif and has stepped rather than sawtooth or scalloped neck margins, as found on other Spiro cups (Dye 2007: Figure 7.1b; Phillips and Brown 1978:119–120, Figures 163, 164, Plate 17, 1980:Plates 153, 154). Severed heads also occur on a Moundville shell gorget (Moore 1907:Figures 96, 97) and a sandstone tablet from near Monks Mound at Cahokia (Fowler et al. 1999:189, Figure 15.5). A terraced line at the neck is obviously not a crown or a cloud, but perhaps positioning beneath a human head conveyed the opposite meaning: a collar, a garotte, a flow of blood, or some other postmortem emanation.

Cobb and Drake (2008) have called attention to the association of the color red with ceramic representations of severed heads in the lower Mississippi valley. This association may be echoed in the pigment traces on the Angel object.

Birds, Birdmen, Men

Other examples of figurative art on Spiro shell cups that use a terrace include a bird (rather than a birdman) in which the motif is repeated on the shoulders of the outstretched wings (Phillips and Brown 1978:Figure 189, Plate 85). There are also multiple examples of images of humans wearing decorated kilts and belts in which the engraving may depict a motif that was woven into fabric (Phillips and Brown 1978:Figures 127, 128, Plate 9, 1980:Plates 125, 126, 127, 158, 189, 190). In some cases, terrace-decorated clothing is associated with a birdman (e.g., Phillips and Brown 1980:Plates 205, 206).

Serpents and Related Figures

Serpents occur broadly on what might be considered to be a wide variety of Mississippian display containers and occasionally the terrace motif depicts scale patterns. Spiro shell cups provide numerous examples (Phillips and Brown 1978:Plates 8, 20, 72, 79, 110, 111, 1980:Plate 197), as do engraved ceramic bottles with the winged serpent motif at Moundville (Figure 10.6a)

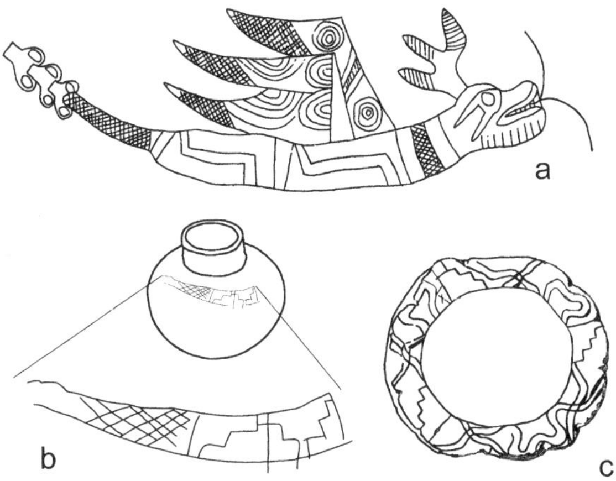

10.6. Serpents, some with terraces: (a) engraved ceramic bottle with winged serpent, Moundville site, Alabama (from Moore 1905:Figure 152); (b) partial serpent design engraved on a bottle, Bone Bank site, Indiana (from photo by Cheryl Ann Munson, courtesy of National Museum of the American Indian, catalog no. 5/5732); (c) stone palette, Moundville (from Moore 1907:Figure 88). (Drawings by Della Collins Cook and Cheryl Ann Munson)

(e.g., Moore 1905:Figure 152; Steponaitis and Knight 2004:Figure 4). On pottery vessels in the Mississippi valley, engraved or painted serpents seem to be limited to the Late Mississippian period (e.g., Hathcock 1988:Figures 160, 234; O'Brien 1994:Figure 7.15). The one known ceramic example from the Ohio valley comes from the Bone Bank site near its confluence with the Wabash, just 50 km west of the Angel site (Figure 10.6b) (Munson 2003; Munson, Munson, Bush, and Henderson 2004). Two stone palettes with terraced serpents were found at Moundville, one with careful engraving (Moore 1905: Figure 7; Steponaitis and Knight 2004:Figure 1) and one with crude (Figure 10.6c) (Moore 1907:391–392, Figure 88).

Not unexpectedly, serpent-like figures also incorporate the terrace motif. The Perino Piasa jar from the Mississippi valley is one example (Phillips and Brown 1978:200–201, Figure 262). Spiro shell cups are another, with the composites snake-bird (Phillips and Brown 1978:Plate 32) and snake-human (Phillips and Brown 1980:Plate 197). Winged serpents engraved on Moundville jars are well known to archaeologists (Moore 1905:Figures 151, 152; 1907:Figures 52, 53, 55).

None of the figurative art presents good analogues for the Angel object, but most examples point to terraces in association with other symbols of importance.

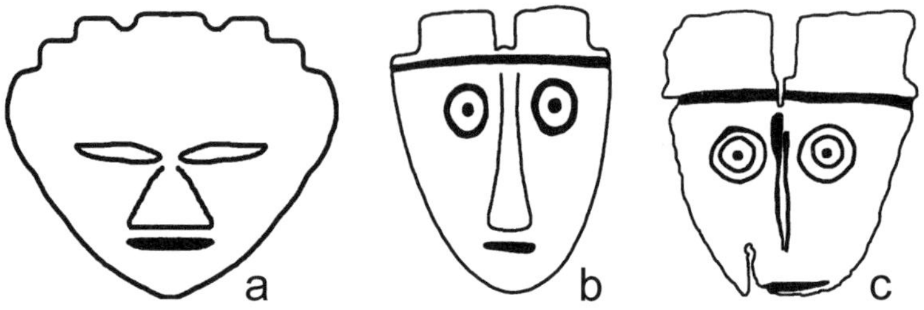

10.7. Adornos and maskettes with terraces on heads: (a) crowned human head effigy attachment on Mississippian bowl, unknown site (from Dye and Wharey 1989:327); (b) short-nosed god maskette ear ornament of shell, Booker T. Washington site, Illinois (from Reilly 2004:Figure 14); (c) god maskette of copper, Calhoun County, Illinois (from Lithics Casting Lab 2012). (Drawings by Della Collins Cook and Cheryl Ann Munson)

Terraced Hair Ornaments

Hair ornaments of sheet copper in the form of maces sometimes incorporate the terrace motif on one or both sides. These have been found at multiple Mississippian sites, including Moundville (Moore 1905:Figure 105), Kogers Island (Webb and DeJarnette 1942:Plate 253-1), Etowah (Willoughby 1932:42–43, Figure 18), and Lake Jackson, Florida (Brain and Phillips 1996:372–373). Maces with terraced margins are also depicted on shell cups from Spiro (Phillips and Brown 1978:Plate 110). We cannot rule out the possibility that the Angel object might be part of a stepped hair ornament.

Representational Ceramics

Ceramic containers incorporate terrace motifs on modeled adornos. In the Mississippi valley two bowls with effigy attachments are reminiscent of the Spiro crowned birdman figure because they have terrace motifs modeled atop human heads. One bowl is from Turk Mound in western Kentucky (Hathcock 1988:Figure 95). The other bowl having a crowned human head adorno (Figure 10.7a) lacks reported provenience information (Dye and Wharey 1989:327).

Ceramics with Geometric Terraces

The most widely known ceramic vessels with terrace motifs are the rare rectangular bowls discovered at Moundville (Figure 10.8g). These have distinctive stepped rims created by modeling that are combined with engraved or painted designs (Moore 1905:Figure 76, 1907:Figures 22, 23; Steponaitis 1983:69, Figure 63 c–f). An incised terrace motif also was used on a bowl without a modeled rim (Steponaitis 1983:Figure 51n). Examples with mod-

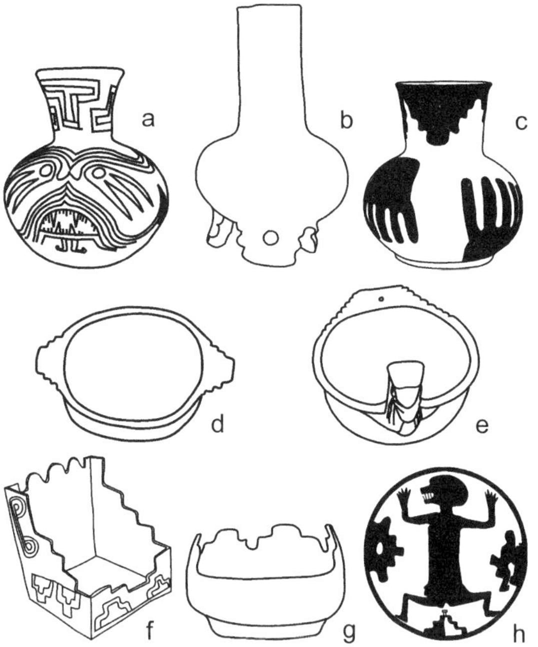

10.8. Mississippian ceramic vessels with terrace motifs: (a) bottle with engraved neck above cat monster, Berry site, Arkansas (from O'Brien 1994:Figure 1.2); (b) bottle with terraced tripod feet, Togo site, Arkansas (from Hathcock 1988:Figure 132); (c) bottle with red and white painted terrace on neck above human hands, Scott site, Arkansas (from Dye 2004: Figure 31); (d) bowl with terraced tabular handles, Nickle site, Arkansas (from Hathcock 1988:Figure 82); (e) cat monster effigy bowl with terraced tail, Bone Bank site, Indiana (from photo by Cheryl Ann Munson, courtesy of National Museum of the American Indian, catalog no. 5/5767); (f) terraced bowl with engraved terrace motifs, Lubbub Creek site, Alabama (from Mann 1983:Figure 41); (g) bowl with terraced orifice, Moundville site, Alabama (from Steponaitis 1983:Figure 83f); (h) red-on-white bowl with infant (female) above and between painted terraces, Rose Mound, Arkansas (from Moore 1910:Plate XII). (Drawings by Della Collins Cook and Cheryl Ann Munson)

eling, incising, and painting also occur at the Lubbub Creek site in Alabama (Figure 10.8f) (Mann 1983:Figures 38, 41, 42) and the Dupree site in Mississippi (Ford 1936:Figure 23h). Related examples are Cahokia area vessels on which modeling was used to create stepped outlines (Holley 1989; Pauketat 1987:9, Figures 9b, 9c, 10b, 10c). Bowls with terraced outlines are considered to be elite display goods in Alabama and are known from mortuary contexts. At Cahokia they were found in domestic garbage in a broken state, but this does not exclude earlier use as display goods.

In the Late Mississippian and protohistoric period in the Mississippi valley, primarily in southeastern Missouri, northeastern Arkansas, and adjacent states, the once-rare terrace motif was used more widely (Figure 10.8a–e). It appears as a painted, incised, or engraved superstructure on the necks of bottles, usually above other symbols—perhaps as a crown over monsters, maces, interlocking scrolls or spirals, ogees, and human trophy emblems, such as dismembered hands and forearms (e.g., Dye 2004:Figure 31; Evers 1880: Plate 17; Hathcock 1988:Figures 63, 67, 142–146, 161a, 239, 241; Lankford 2004:Figures 15, 18; O'Brien 1994:Plates 2f, 6d, Figure 1.2). An unsettling red-on-white painted example is a bowl from the Late Mississippian Rose Mound, Arkansas (Figure 10.8h). The painting depicts what appears to be an emaciated female infant with bared teeth positioned above an opposed red-and-white terrace and flanked by two red ones (Moore 1910:Plate XII).

Additionally, modeling was used during this period to create the terrace motif in abstract form along the edges of tabbed bowls and footed bottles (Figure 10.8b, d) (e.g., Hathcock 1988:Figures 41, 128, 132; O'Brien 1994: Figure 7.8). A cat monster bowl in the Charles Artes collection from the Mississippian Bone Bank site in Indiana has a modeled tail that is stepped (Figure 10.8e) like the Mississippi valley bowls (Munson 2003). Only 50 km to the east, the Angel site has neither cat monsters nor the previously noted engraved serpents represented in ceramics (Black 1967; Hilgeman 2000; Kellar 1967).

Among the ceramic containers, those with modeled terraced orifices in the Moundville region and in the Mississippi valley present the best ceramic analogues to the Angel object, but it is noteworthy that these crown-embellished containers are limited to a small number of sites.

Long- and Short-Nosed God Maskettes

Another group of crowned Mississippian artifacts found in the Midwest and Southeast that exhibit terrace motifs along the edges of ornaments is long-nosed and short-nosed god maskettes made from shell, copper, and even bone (Figure 10.7b–c). These human head maskette earrings are linked to the mythic hero Red Horn, or Morning Star, who wears such ornaments on his ears (Brown and Dye 2007; Diaz-Granados and Duncan 2000; Hall 1989, 1991, 1997:145–153; Interesting Wisconsin Specimens 1956; Lithics Casting Lab 2012; Phillips and Brown 1978; Reilly 2004; Salzer 1987; Salzer and Rajnovich 2000). Several examples of maskette earrings definitely have a terraced crown, but their small size (about 5 cm–8 cm in height) makes them unsuitable analogues for the Angel object. An association of ear ornaments with human skulls or heads may have broader symbolic dimensions. For example, Perino (1971) recovered a small earspool made from human vault bone in a Mississippian burial at the Yokem site in western Illinois, and

Shirley Schermer and Robin Lillie (this volume) present several similar uses of human bone.

Rattles and Masks

The terraced Mississippian artifacts most similar to the Angel object are carved, copper-covered, wooden rattles or masks in the form of human heads with crowns (Figure 10.9a–d). These were found with burials at Etowah in Georgia (Larsen 1957) and Emmons in Illinois (Brown 2004:Figure 33; Conrad 1989, 1991; Morse et al. 1961; Sampson and Esarey 1993). Additionally, there is an agnathous, wooden mask or rattle (Brown 1996: Figure 2-103) and an unterraced but crowned wooden human head mask or rattle from Craig Mound C at Spiro (Brown 1996:533–534, Figure 2-105). Another terraced human head rattle was found at Moundville and described as an exact counterpart of the Etowah rattle (Knight and Steponaitis 2011:228, Figure 24b).

The Etowah and Emmons specimens, because of their terraced crowns, have been compared to long-nosed god maskettes. At the Emmons site, the terraced human head mask or rattle was placed on the upper chest of a 46-year-old male (Brown 2004:Figure 33; Conrad 1991:144–146; Morse et al. 1961:Figure 76). A long-nosed god maskette earring was found previously in a nearby mound (Griffin and Morse 1961). Both the mask/rattle and maskette were copper-covered.

The Spiro site also had four other full-faced, wooden human head masks without crowns; miniature maskettes; and uncrowned, full-faced, wooden heads termed rattles because they were backed with thin wood planks and associated with pebbles (Brown 1996:529–530, 533–534, Figures 2-103, 2-105, Table 2-150). Topknots may stand in for terraced crowns. Examples from Etowah and Spiro have shell teeth, and the Spiro agnathous mask has shell ear ornaments and eyes. The Emmons mask or rattle has whitish, galena-painted weeping eyes. Perhaps shell or pigments were used to block the openings in the Angel object.

Farther afield, uncrowned human skull rattles have been reported many times among the protohistoric Iroquois. They are made from paired parietals of young males and have a form similar to the widely distributed turtle-shell rattles. The single example that was not recovered from refuse deposits comes from a sweat lodge at Moatfield village, Ontario. Curing, feasting, and war preparations have been suggested as contexts for use of these rattles (Williamson 2007). Their construction from the matched parietals of an individual suggests that the identity of the person whose bones these were may have been seen as residing in the artifact.

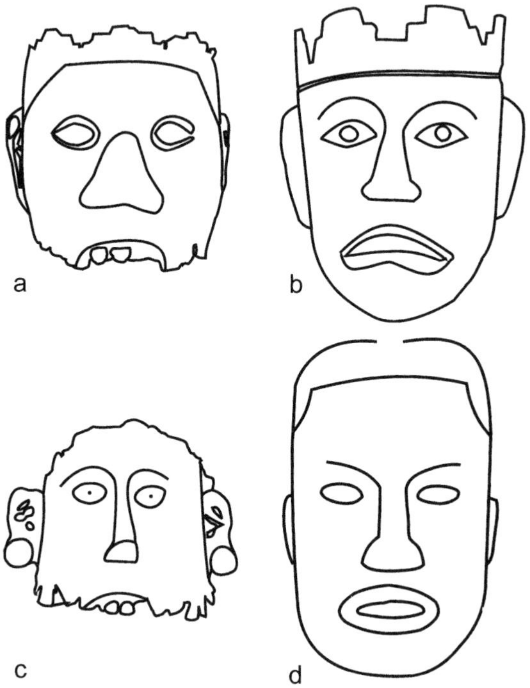

10.9. Wooden rattles and masks: (a) Etowah site, agnathous, copper-covered, wooden rattle (Larsen 1957:Figure 1); (b) Emmons site, full-faced, copper-covered, wooden rattle(?) (Brown 2004:Figure 33); (c) Spiro site, agnathous, wooden mask (or figure or rattle) (Brown 1996:Figure 2-103); (d) Spiro site, full-faced, wooden mask (or figure or rattle) (Brown 1996:Figure 2-105). (Drawings by Della Collins Cook and Cheryl Ann Munson)

The clearly crowned Spiro, Etowah, and Moundville wooden head specimens are agnathous. In contrast, the Emmons artifact and the other four Spiro rattles are full-faced. Brown and Dye (2007) have called attention to severed and agnathous human heads in Southeastern Ceremonial Complex iconography, noting that the theme begins in the thirteenth century and that over time the jawless heads become more common and constitute a distinctive trophy motif.

Are the crowned heads rattles or masks? In general, rattles speak, while masks conceal, disguise, or transform. For example, Blackfoot eagle hunters used a human skull to magically hide themselves (Grinnell 1972). But rattles are not simply noisemakers. Brown and Dye (2007:283) noted, citing Bailey (1995:80), that "Osage gourd rattles were said to symbolically represent the head of a man; the pebbles inside the rattle head were said to be the teeth; and the handle was the forearm."

The Emmons artifact was present as a single piece and so was called a mask, but it may be the preserved front portion of a rattle. The Etowah artifact is most clearly a rattle given its fitted back, top, and bottom pieces. It also contained rounded pebbles for rattling. In addition, the four Spiro wooden human heads lacked sides but were associated with pebbles and thus were initially identified as rattles. The other wooden human head artifacts may also be rattles whose backs and sides were not clad with copper and thus were not preserved; similarly, their "pebbles" may have been composed of dried corn kernels or some other perishable material. The fine polish on prominences on the endocranial surface of the Angel object may be the result of contact with a fine abrasive, such as the phytoliths in corn kernels and cupules or other grass seeds.

All the terraced and unterraced wooden masks or rattles have concave backs. Our conjectural reconstruction of the Angel bone object as a rattle indicates that it would have had a similarly concave back consisting of the interior surface of the frontal squama. Measurements indicate that the Mississippian rattles are good analogues for the Angel object. The reconstructed height of the Angel object is in the range of 131 mm–168 mm. The approximate heights of the rattles are Etowah, agnathous, 106 mm; Emmons, full-faced, 119 mm; Spiro, agnathous, 172 mm; Spiro, reconstructed, full-faced, 110 mm; and Moundville, 103 mm. These measurements are consistent with our estimate of the size of the terraced Angel object.

Human Head Objects in Use

Several artifacts show how a human head rattle may have been used. At Etowah, the Rogan copper plates 1 and 2 also have birdman figures holding a human head or head-shaped object that was part of a dancer's (or impersonator's) paraphernalia (Figure 10.3c) (Brown 2007:Figures 4.1c, 4.1d; King 2004:150, Figure 1; Willoughby 1932:41, Figures 14, 15). These figures are generally thought to be carrying trophy heads, but the angle of the handheld object suggests that use as a rattle is equally probable. An engraved shell gorget from Tennessee (Brown 2007:Figure 4.4a) has a similar theme, as does one from Etowah (Willoughby 1932:Figure 26a). Spiro shell cups further illustrate the use of human head objects held in the hand (Figure 10.3b) (Phillips and Brown 1980:Plates 153, 154).

In a skillful interpretation of a Missouri pictograph, Duncan and Diaz-Granados connected both maskettes and terraced rattles to the adoption of captives by using a Winnebago myth about hero twin boy ancestors. "In one of the wild boy's many adventures, he is decapitated and replaces his own lost head with a rattle. He thus becomes a 'rattle' head" (Duncan and

Diaz-Granados 2000:10). Many ceramic vessels with single or double adornos in the form of human heads have pebbles or fired clay balls inside that create sound (e.g., Evers 1880:Plate 23; Hathcock 1988:Figure 477; Morse 1989:Figure 5e; National Museum of the American Indian 2012). It would be interesting to explore what these vessels contained and in what contexts they were rattled.

The Malden copper plate in Missouri's Wulfing collection (Brown 2004: Figure 23; Howard 1968:Figure 6) shows an object in the form of a small terraced head that is included in the head piece of a birdman (Figure 10.3d). This terraced emblem appears above a beaked nose and diamond-shaped eye. The mandible is not present and the maxilla is represented by another terrace. Other examples of terraced human heads as headdress items are engraved cups from Spiro (Phillips and Brown 1978:Plates 2, 17, 22g). Sampson and Esarey (1993:469, Figure 21) highlighted the association of these human head depictions with headdresses in the high crest style. They argued that the Etowah rattle and the Emmons mask are primarily headdress elements, as indicated by perforations that would provide for their attachment. However, perforations could also have been used to attach the back of the rattle, and the large size of the wooden Etowah and Emmons specimens, as well as the Spiro and Moundville specimens, would indicate a headdress that is far out of proportion to the size of the human head. In the examples mentioned above, the proportion of headdress ornaments is roughly one-third the size of the human head. However, the terraced wooden human head artifacts are similar in size to human heads, and so are much larger than what would be suitable for use as headdress paraphernalia.

Other Human Bone Artifacts at Angel

Three additional, though dissimilar, artifacts from the Angel site are made of human bone and are described below (Figure 10.10). Each was found in midden deposits.

(1) S11D/2372 and 2389 are two fragments of an adult right frontal, parietal, and greater wing of the sphenoid (Black 1967:Figure 327) (Figure 10.10a, b). They were found in adjacent blocks (3L2 and 3L3) in a deposit that had no obvious disturbance (Black 1967:328–329; field records of Glenn A. Black, Indiana University). The field assessment was that two burials had been exposed, and they were assigned burial numbers (numbers 14 and 15 in the block), but refitting proved that these two fragments were a single skull object and not a burial. Domestic refuse characterizes the excavation

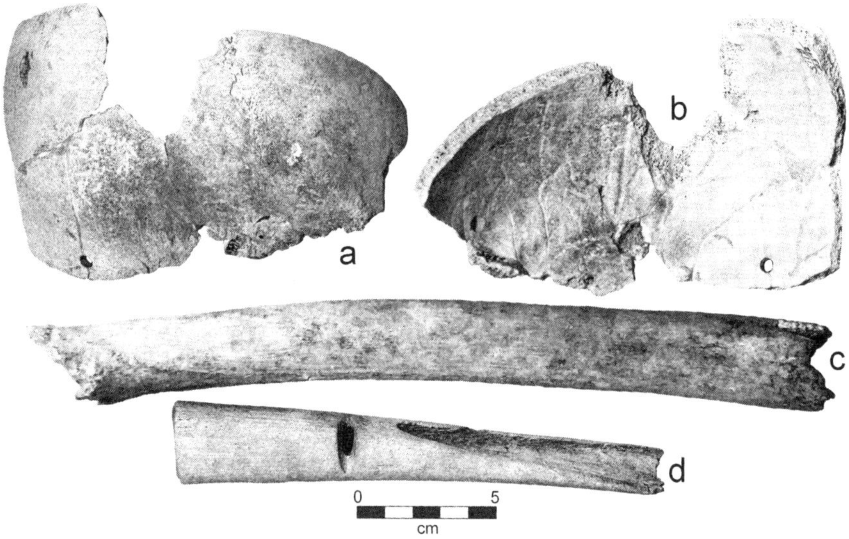

10.10. Other modified human elements from the Angel site: (a) exterior and (b) interior views of two refitted fragments from S11D (the right frontal, parietal, and greater wing of the sphenoid) with defleshing marks, hinge fractures, and drilled perforations suggesting components of a rattle; (c) fragmentary left femur shaft with groove-and-snap treatment, from domestic refuse in X11C; and (d) juvenile left tibia shaft from W11A that was cut, scored, and abraded to produce a spatulate end for a possible flensing tool. (Courtesy of Glenn A. Black Laboratory of Archaeology, Indiana University)

level containing the two fragments, although features of a wall trench house underlie the deposit (Black 1967:Figure 333).

The coronal suture is well consolidated, particularly at pterion, suggesting that this individual was at least 35 years of age at death. The medial margin of the object more or less parallels the midline of the skull about 1 cm lateral to the midline and is perpendicular to the outer surface. The posterior margin is more or less vertical and lies just behind the parietal boss. Both these margins show evidence of scoring of the outer table, snapping, and smoothing of the resulting cross section. The inferior edge shows excavation damage, but was probably prepared in a similar way. The inferior border is more or less transverse, extending from below the frontal boss across the temporal line, below pterion, touching the highest portion of the squamosal suture and removing the parietal notch and posterior-inferior corner of the parietal. There are hinge fractures on the thick portion of the frontal at the base of the zygomatic process and at the posterior edge of the largest frontal fragment, indicating that the object was broken with considerable force when the bone still had fresh fracture characteristics. There are drilled perforations at anterior-inferior and posterior-inferior corners. Fine transverse cut marks above the frontal boss suggest defleshing or scalp removal. The surviving elements of S11D are 91 mm high and 145 mm in anterioposterior length.

This Angel object is dissimilar to the previously noted drilled ornament from the Mississippian St. Thomas site (Hargrave 2005) in having smoothed margins and drilling only from the ectocranial surface. It may compare best with the drilled segments of prehistoric southeastern U.S. parietal objects that Jacobi (2007:323) interpreted as components of "a rattle . . . worn on the legs or arms."

(2) X11C/611 is an adult left femur shaft (Figure 10.10c). Both ends are missing and show a combination of ancient damage and excavation damage. The fragmentary length is 290 mm. There is a shallow, irregular groove medial to the linea aspera that may represent scoring for the purpose of breaking the bone, and there are fine diagonal and transverse cut marks across the linea aspera and at the distal end. The Angel site has abundant evidence of the groove-and-snap technique used in the manufacture of bone tools, but this is the only human long bone displaying this preparation. The location of the worked human femur was grid 0L4, .49 m (1.6 ft) below the surface. The object was found with domestic refuse in a part of the site where basin-shaped pit features occurred (Features 16–18; Black 1967:Figure 89). Several burials are present in the vicinity but not in the grid unit.

(3) W11A/2339 is a highly modified segment of a juvenile left tibia shaft (Figure 10.10d). It has been cut by scoring all the way around and snapping just proximal to the nutrient foramen. There is a beveled opening produced by scraping or grinding from about the midshaft on the anterior crest diagonally to the posterior surface about 3 cm–5 cm from the distal end. The result is a spatula shape with upturned margins consisting of the posterior cortex of the tibia at its distal end. This end was damaged in excavation. Just proximal to the diagonal cut, there is a transverse groove penetrating to the medullary cavity. It was produced by abrading the cortex with a transverse sawing motion until the medullary cavity was reached. The outer surface has been ground slightly throughout. There are numerous fine diagonal striations along the interosseous crest. The tibia was found in grid 5L4 at a depth of .37 m (1.2 ft). This location and depth produced dense domestic refuse deposits that overlie a series of rebuilt wall trench houses (Black 1967:Figure 176).

The length of the W11A specimen is 173 mm; it was longer before the thinned distal portion was broken in excavation. If the end was smooth, it may have served as a shuttle or other weaving tool, a spatula, or a handle for some object. Perforated bone whip handles are known from the historic Plains (Horse Capture and Her Many Horses 2006), and flensing (i.e., flesher) tools of human bone are discussed by Katie Zejdlik (this volume). If the thinned portion widened again toward the distal end, the object would resemble a beamer, but it may be too refined for this purpose and the perforation would be unusual. If the end was pointed or serrated, it may have served as a scratcher, scarifier, or bone pick. Animal bone awls, pins, beamers, a shuttle, and other objects are well represented at Angel (Kellar 1967:448–455). Neitzel (1983:106) illustrated a Natchez three-pronged scratcher made of deer metapodial, and bone scarifiers were reported from the Lawrenz Gun site (Conrad 1991) and from an adult male burial at Emmons (Morse et al. 1961).

While there are no close analogues known to us for the three objects described above, it is worth noting that the choice of human bone as a raw material suggests a special purpose rather than a domestic function.

Discussion

The object with the terraced motif is the most interesting of the four Angel site artifacts made of human bone. There are other associations of rare abstract or nonfigurative motifs with human bone or with representations of human heads in Mississippian iconography. Perhaps the most fascinating example is from Henry County, Tennessee: an adult male, fully articulated primary burial with a herringbone pattern incised on the frontal (Smith 1974). We think it likely that each of these motifs had a specific meaning, and we hope that we have recovered a portion of that meaning for the terraced crown or nimbus. Its uncommon occurrence but wide geographical distribution in the early Mississippian period and its persistence from the thirteenth to the twentieth century, long after the specifics of its symbolism were forgotten, speak to its power.

Based on stylistic elements and size, we propose that X11C/5, the modified human cranial bone object from the Angel site, is probably not a container in the sense of a bowl or cup. Black and Kellar probably thought it was a container because they misunderstood the orientation of the decoration. More likely, it is an additional example of a carved human head rattle with a terraced crown. The abrasion on the interior surface would be consistent with wear from stones, small ceramic spheres, seeds, teeth, or other materials (such as dried corn kernels) used to make a rattling noise. The embedded pigment suggests that this rattle was painted red, making it similar in color to the copper that covered the other carved head rattles. Human head rattles may have also functioned as headdress ornaments, but their large size—nearly the same size as the human face—makes this prospect unlikely. The combined infrequency of Mississippian artifacts made from human bone and of representations of human heads as well as the particular rarity of the terraced- or stepped-crown motif, suggest that this association had an important symbolic valence and was highly ritualized. The Angel site's terraced object thus links the largest Mississippian community in the Ohio valley to representations of Red Horn or Morning Star and to the birdman and thunderbird symbolism of the larger Mississippian world.

Acknowledgments

We thank the Bioanthropology Laboratory, Department of Anthropology, Indiana University; Patricia L. Nietfeld, collections manager of the Smithsonian Institution, NMAI; Sheryl Hartman, Piankeshaw Trails Educational Park; Vincas P. Steponaitis; Vernon J. Knight Jr.; Penelope B. Drooker; and, for permission to study and photograph Figures 10.1 and 10.10, Christopher S. Peebles, former director, and Timothy E. Baumann, former curator, of the Glenn A. Black Laboratory of Archaeology, Indiana University.

11

Modification of Human Bone from Mississippian Caborn-Welborn Phase Sites in Southwestern Indiana and West-Central Kentucky

Cheryl Ann Munson, Della Collins Cook, and Mary Lucas Powell

Artifacts made from human bone are unusual in Mississippian sites, and indeed in most archaeological contexts. Despite the relatively limited excavation of Caborn-Welborn phase sites, three villages have yielded evidence for defleshing and other modification of human bone: Slack Farm (15UN28), Murphy (12PO1), and Caborn (12PO32). The Caborn-Welborn phase is a Late Mississippian occupation centered at the mouth of the Wabash River (Green and Munson 1978; Munson 1998; Munson and Green 1973; Munson and Pollack 1998; Pollack 2004; Pollack and Munson 2003). Radiocarbon dates and occasional European trade goods indicate a time span of approximately A.D. 1400–1650, and perhaps as late as A.D. 1700 (Munson 2003; Pollack 2004). Modified elements include carefully defleshed mandibles, as well as clavicles and long bones with distinct cut marks.

Caborn-Welborn is distinguished from the earlier Angel phase by a dispersed settlement pattern and the absence of both temple mounds and a central town. Continuity with the Angel phase (A.D. 1050–1450) is evident in domestic architecture, plain and fabric-impressed ceramic vessels, and many types of lithic, bone, and shell implements and ornaments. In contrast to the Angel phase, evidence of extraregional trade is extensive in Caborn-Welborn, measured both in quantities of foreign goods (shell, copper, catlinite, chert, ceramic vessels) and in the distance of connections (Minnesota to the Gulf Coast). Mortuary practices are complex and also show some continuity from Angel to Caborn-Welborn (Munson and Cook 2001). In Caborn-Welborn there is evidence of status distinctions as well as diverse burial locations: primary interments in rowed cemeteries, house floors, and village area pits (Munson and Cook 2001; Munson et al. 2001, 2002; Pollack and Munson 1998). Secondary burials and burials of crania occur rarely. The main distinction in mortuary treatments is the occurrence of cemeteries and residential area burials at large Caborn-Welborn villages and small communities, whereas Angel phase burials seem to be restricted to the polity's mound center.

This chapter describes the five Caborn-Welborn examples of modified human bone and discusses their cultural meaning.

Slack Farm Mandible

Unfortunately, the version of Murphy's law that applies to archaeology is at work here. Our most interesting specimen is from the least-controlled archaeological context. The Slack Farm site is a large Caborn-Welborn village in Union County, Kentucky, only 2.7 km from the Murphy site and the mouth of the Wabash River. It was extensively looted in 1987. Data recovery investigations in 1988 in the damaged areas of the site focused on making a legal case against the looters and on documenting the location of still-intact deposits. Excavation was limited to screening the soil disturbed by the looters and mapping the walls and floors of their trenches and holes as well as any exposed burials, features, and stratigraphy. Seven cemetery areas were identified in the village. Analysis of the remains by Powell indicated more than 1,000 individuals of both sexes and all ages were impacted by the looting (Munson et al. 1988; Pollack 2004).

A carefully defleshed and drilled right human mandible (15UN28/5492-1; Figure 11.1a) was recovered at the Slack Farm site from Hole 419, a large looted area that impacted one of the village cemeteries. A minimum of 69 individuals, primarily adults, was identified in an area that showed 30 extended interments in multiple rows (Pollack et al. 1996; David Pollack, personal communication 2009).

The drilled mandible found in this cemetery is that of a robust young adult male. There is excavation damage on all surfaces consistent with a sharp, pointed implement. Fractures through the mandibular symphysis are older than the excavation damage, and the left side may have been separated from the right prior to the looting episode. A drill hole through the right ascending ramus is conical in cross section, tapering from 6 mm on the external surface to 4 mm on the internal surface. The superior margin of the internal opening is rounded and somewhat polished, suggesting that the mandible may have been suspended from a cord for sufficient time to result in wear.

Many fine cut marks are concentrated on the anterior aspect of the condyle, on the lingula, and above the mylohyoid line. These locations are consistent with disarticulation of the temporomandibular joint, cutting of the anterior fibers of the capsule, detachment of the sphenomandibular ligament, removal of the tongue, and scraping away the gingiva. This suggests careful defleshing with a fine, sharp implement and is more suggestive of the use of a cane knife rather than a stone tool (West and Louys 2007).

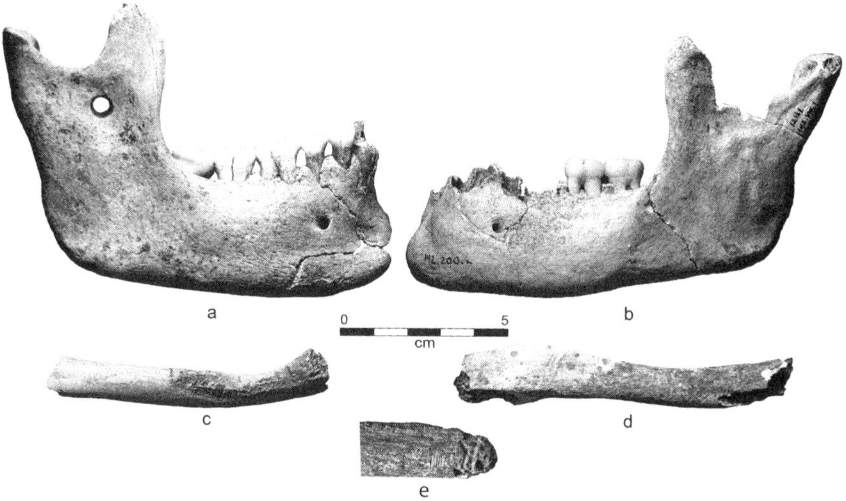

11.1. Modified human bone from Caborn-Welborn phase sites: (a) Slack Farm site, mandible; (b) Murphy site, mandible; (c) Murphy site, clavicle; (d) Caborn site, clavicle; (e) Caborn site, ulna. (Photographs by Cheryl Ann Munson. [a] Courtesy of Museum of Anthropology, University of Kentucky; [b, c] Courtesy of Department of Sociology and Anthropology, University of Southern Indiana; [d, e] Courtesy of Glenn A. Black Laboratory of Archaeology, Indiana University)

Seven teeth are present. No teeth were lost in life in the portion of the mandible that was recovered. Wear is light, and there are no caries. The lateral incisor and canine are fractured, and the fracture surfaces are conchoidal. This fracture pattern resembles damage seen in cadaver skulls in teaching collections. Anatomical or dissection room specimens from teaching collections with intact collagen that have been handled extensively and carelessly show tooth fractures resembling these (Berryman et al. 1991). In contrast, older remains from archaeological contexts show relatively rectilinear fractures that tend to be confined to the enamel. We infer that the Slack Farm mandible was handled roughly for an extended period when it was still relatively fresh. Because this interesting specimen was recovered out of context, we cannot establish whether it was associated with a burial or whether it came from midden deposits.

Murphy Mandible

A second defleshed mandible was found at the Murphy, or Mouth of the Wabash, site in Posey County, Indiana (12PO1/142.200.2; Figure 11.1b). Human bone was not a surprise in the first modern investigations at Murphy. In 1898, Clifford Anderson excavated dozens of burials in rowed cemeteries A, B, and C for Warren K. Moorehead (1906). Munson directed mitigative excavations at the site in 1997–1998 and again in 1999 at two additional cemeteries impacted by the construction of a frame house and by water lines to a well (Havill and Munson 1998a; Munson, Dougherty, and Havill 2001). Human bone exposed on the surface by plowing also has been documented over a large area, with burials clustered in several locales suggesting additional cemeteries (Dougherty and Munson 2001; Havill and Munson 1998b).

The defleshed mandible was recovered from midden deposits at the Frame House Cemetery, which had been disturbed by the house's septic system. In the upper deposits, archaeological excavations revealed that the remains of at least 10 individuals had been completely displaced, but 6 burials in the lower deposits remained partly intact in opposed rows. This mandible was found at the same depth as the uppermost burials, which included adults of both sexes and children.

Construction activities considerably damaged the Murphy mandible. The fracture through the right ascending ramus is older than the other damage. Four bone fragments and five teeth were recovered. The Murphy mandible was not drilled in the same region of the ascending ramus as the Slack Farm mandible. However, we cannot rule out drill holes in the missing right gonial region nor suspension without drill holes from the missing right condyle. The mandible is from an adult female with fully erupted third molars. The right anterior premolar was lost in life. The texture of the alveoli suggests that the first molars may have been carious, and it is possible that one or both were lost shortly before death. The left second molar was fractured through the pulp canal in life, since the fracture margins show wear. The right lateral incisor is heavily worn, resulting in pulp exposure and a small apical abscess. There is healed trauma to the inferior border of the mental region. Fine cut marks are present on the inferior border at the anterior limit of the masseter muscle insertion, on the inferior border of the mandible, on the coronoid processes, and along the mylohyoid line. Again, careful defleshing is indicated, including severing of the masseter and temporalis muscles and removal of the tongue.

It is possible that the worked mandible was associated with one of the burials that were disturbed by the septic system, but it is equally possible that a broken, defleshed mandible was deposited with the refuse that comprised the midden. Sherds, debitage, rock, daub, faunal bone, and charcoal were recovered from this midden. A mostly in situ burial in the lower part of the midden deposit was accompanied by a jar with combined decorations typical of Campbell Punctate and Campbell Appliqué (O'Brien and Fox 1994:40–44; Phillips 1970:61–62). Soot on the exterior of this vessel has been radiocarbon dated to cal A.D. 1445–1650 (BETA 119794) (Munson 2003: Table I.1).

Murphy Clavicle

A right clavicle fragment, also from the Murphy site, represents a small adult, probably female (12PO1/142.15.2; Figure 11.1c). There are five deep cut marks on the ventral edge in the region of the conoid ligament. The cut marks might relate to cutting the deltoid muscle in order to open the shoulder joint or to separate the humerus from the shoulder girdle. The lateral edge of this fragment is weathered or chewed, while the medial edge terminates in recent breakage.

This modified clavicle fragment was found with typical village refuse plus a small fragment of human cranium (unmodified) in the fill of a pit that was intrusive into an earlier filled-in house basin (Munson 1998). Corn kernels on the floor of this structure are radiocarbon dated to cal A.D. 1405–1480 (BETA 119391) (Munson 2003:Table I.1), a terminus post quem for this disarticulated clavicle.

Caborn Clavicle

An incomplete right human clavicle (12PO32/7109/982; Figure 11.1d) of a small adult, possibly female, was recovered during test excavations that sampled features and a buried midden deposit at the Caborn site in Posey County, Indiana (Munson, Jones, and Ruby 1989). The clavicle was found in the uppermost sealed midden deposits that filled a swale at the edge of the habitation area. The lower part of the midden is radiocarbon dated to cal A.D. 1300–1430, also terminus post quem.

The clavicle has fine, parallel cut marks on the superior aspect in the region of the conoid tubercle. There is a diagonal scraping mark on the inferior aspect near the medial convexity. Again, the cut marks might relate to cutting the deltoid muscle in order to open the shoulder joint.

Caborn Ulna

An incomplete right ulna (12PO32/7109/2464; Figure 11.1e) was found within 2 m of the clavicle in the same upper midden deposit. The shaft was recovered in two pieces. This bone is very robust, likely from a large adult male. Broken ends and a midshaft break are transverse and stepped, suggesting that these fractures occurred long after death.

The distal end shows numerous fine, parallel striations in the region of the pronator quadratus attachment. Striations are oblique on the anterior, or palmar, side and transverse on the posterior, or dorsal, side. Distal to these marks, the end of the ulna segment is battered but preserves portions of two deep transverse grooves that may represent score-and-snap modification. These grooves are in the portion of the distal shaft that has no muscle attachments. There are no defleshing marks along the portions of the shaft that underlie the forearm muscle origins. We can suggest no simple scenario—bead or bone tube production, hand removal, defleshing—that would explain these multiple modifications. Together, they are strikingly unlike the patterned modification of the tibia shaft segment that Zejdlik (this volume) has described at Aztalan.

Discussion

Given the small number of excavated burials and human remains from the Caborn-Welborn phase that have been subjected to careful analysis, we have compiled a remarkable list of bone modifications. All modifications were made on bones of adults. The drilled Slack Farm mandible is clearly some type of object, given its careful preparation, but the question arises whether the other examples are parts of disturbed secondary burials or are objects made of bone.

Caborn-Welborn Mortuary Data and Frequency of Bone Modification

Mortuary data from other Caborn-Welborn villages provide context for interpreting the functions of modified human bone. Nine sites have identified human remains. Table 11.1 summarizes the available data on the number of burials found and the range of treatments identified.

Our review of these human remains shows that defleshing and secondary burial are present but very rare in Caborn-Welborn. The only analyzed bundle interment (Mann site)[1] was the one burial associated with defleshing cut marks. Therefore, the modified mandibles, clavicles, and ulna that lack this treatment are not likely to have been associated with secondary inhumation, but are probably bone objects. But what kind of objects?

Modified Bones as Objects

A wider comparison to other analyses of alterations of human bone may be helpful in assessing the Caborn-Welborn specimens. White (1992) presented a complex catalog of alterations that suggest butchering for consumption as food. This is an unlikely interpretation in our case for two reasons. First, cut marks on the Caborn-Welborn specimens are primarily fine rather than coarse and are limited in location to the attachments of the toughest connective tissues. They correspond in location to cut marks that have been reported elsewhere as evidence for defleshing (Olsen and Shipman 1994; Raemsch 1993). Second, there is no evidence of percussion for marrow extraction (White 1992). These observations suggest that defleshing for burial preparation or artisanal activities, rather than butchering, fits the Caborn-Welborn phase evidence.

Skull Elements

The Slack Farm and Murphy mandibles are skull objects. Although they were not found with modified crania, they may have had associated crania. It is helpful to review both modified crania and mandibles in the Eastern Woodlands in order to assess the Caborn-Welborn specimens.

One example of a cranial bowl from the Mulberry Creek site in the Pickwick Basin of Alabama (Jacobi 2007) has opposed drilled holes for suspension. A particularly interesting child's cranium bowl or cup was recovered from a Fort Ancient burial in Franklin County, Indiana (Lilly 1937:60, 220; Quick 1881; Setzler 1930:467–481, 500, 515). Fletcher (1882) interpreted the closely spaced drilled perforations in this skull cup as mending holes, analogous to those frequently seen in ceramics because they are adjacent to a crack, but it seems equally plausible that this small object was a distinctly concave gorget.

Skulls that are decorated may also be considered objects. The Chucalissa site in western Tennessee has a burial accompanied by defleshed skulls, two with cut marks that suggest scalping and one decorated with red paint (Jacobi 2003). A burial at the Harris site in the Guntersville Basin in northern Mississippi was interred with three painted skulls. A unique human skull decorated by engraving rather than painting has a herringbone design on the frontal of an intact, fully articulated burial from the Mississippian Thompson Village site in western Tennessee (Smith 1974), making this cranium both an object and part of an individual. Another non-bowl human skull object, which may be part of a rattle, is from the nearby early Mississippian Angel site in Indiana (Black 1967; Cook and Munson, this volume). Reports of other Mississippian objects made from human mandibles have not been identified.

Oneota sites have several examples of defleshing cut marks on mandibles, or fragments thereof, which have been interpreted as trophies or possible trophies. These include a mandible and a cranium of two individuals in a pit in the Sanford Archaeological District near La Crosse (west-central Wisconsin) (Holtz-Leith 2006); mandibles and crania at Diamond Bluff (west-central Wisconsin) (Owsley et al. 1977) and Armstrong (northwestern Wisconsin)

Table 11.1. Burial Data for Nine Caborn-Welborn Phase Sites

Site	Site Type	Investigations of Burials	Extended Burials in Rows	Bundle Burials	Stone Slabs	Skeletal Modification	Comments	References
Slack Farm (15UN28)	large village	1,000+ burials disturbed by looters in large village; documentation of 304 partly intact extended burials; no evidence of secondary burials or stone slabs	present in multiple cemeteries	–	–	–	time-constrained field and laboratory study; looted bluff top burial mounds area; associated stone slabs; recorded orientation for 291 burials	Munson et al. 1988; Pollack 2004; Pollack et al. 1996
Murphy (12PO1)	large village	170+ burials in 3 separate cemeteries excavated 1898 for Moorehead; extended burials based on Anderson's village sketch map and letters	opposed rows in cemetery B, unknown in cemeteries A and C; scattered burials in residential area	2 of crania (without mandibles)		–	R. S. Peabody Museum, Andover, Massachusetts, curates a small series of disarticulated elements, primarily arms; Smith sonian Institution curates 1 cranium (adult male) (262137) and 1 mandible (elderly male) examined by Cook; no cut marks	Moorehead 1906
		portions of 30 partly in situ extended burials and 17 disturbed, completely disarticulated individuals excavated during data recovery investigations	opposed rows in cemetery B and a 4th cemetery	absent	absent	observed cranial and postcranial healed trauma, including scalping	1 additional cemetery identified and Moorehead's cemetery B locale confirmed; no indication of defleshing or processing of cranial or postcranial elements	Havill and Munson 1998b; Munson, Dougherty, and Havill 2001, 2002

		surface surveys across the site identified portions of at least 66 individuals from plow-disturbed burials	–	–	present in at least one cemetery	–	2 additional cemeteries identified, plus scattered burials throughout the village area	Dougherty and Munson 2001; Havill and Munson 1998a; Munson and Spencer 2009
Caborn (12PO32)	small village	surface survey identified 29 spatially discrete clusters of plow-disturbed, flood-washed human bone	–	–	–	–	burials occur throughout the village area; 1 burial minimally exposed during test excavations but not investigated; no data on secondary burials or cut marks	Munson, Jones, and Eisterhold 1989; Munson, Jones, and Ruby 1989
Bone Bank (12PO4)	large village	burials first excavated by Charles Alexandre Lesueur in 1828; his drawings and notes suggest multiple rowed cemeteries	probable	–	–	–	a single skull from Lesueur's work is curated at Musée de l'Homme, Paris; hundreds of burials are reported to have been washed away by bank erosion	Elliot and Johansen 1999:Figure 30; Munson 2003

Continued on the next page

Site	Site Type	Investigations of Burials	Extended Burials in Rows	Bundle Burials	Stone Slabs	Skeletal Modification	Comments	References
Mann (12PO2)	hamlet or small village	rescue excavations mapped and recovered fragmentary remains of 9 adults and adolescents and 17 children and infants from extended and bundle burials; elements recovered from plowed contexts indicate at least 3 additional adults were buried in the cemetery; 1 of 2 bundle burials was analyzable for modification	opposed rows, 2 on west, 1 on east	2; 1 bundle burial was analyzable for modification	absent	defleshing cut marks on cranium in bundle burial; another cranium has 2 deep cut marks	rescue excavation by Lacer in 1964; bundle burials placed on knees of extended burials; deep cut marks suggest scalping	Lacer 1980; Munson and Spencer 2009; Ruby 1997; Spencer 2007; Spencer et al. 2007
Leonard (12PO38)	hamlet	excavation of 25 burials; 8 collected for study	present	–	–	none on 8 crania	Indiana State University field school excavation and curation; osteological analysis by Susan Spencer	Henn 1971; Munson and Spencer 2009; Spencer et al. 2009
Mulligan (15HE625)	hamlet or small village	dozens of burials excavated by several nonprofessionals; hundreds of artifacts but only 4 crania collected	present	–	–	none on 4 crania	no evidence of skeletal trauma or defleshing on 4 adult crania	Munson and Spencer 2009

Hovey Lake (12PO10)	large village	8 in situ and partly in situ burials and 11 disarticulated individuals in residential context; plow-disturbed burials in both residential and outlying areas	not observed	not observed	present in at least 1 cemetery	no cut marks on 1 complete adult	residential areas and house contexts excavated in 1978–1979; removal of most elements of adult and older juvenile burials after interment in house floor	Munson and Cook 2001; Munson et al. 2008
		reports of looting in 1980 of 15 cemeteries outside the palisaded residential area; testing during 1996–2007 seasons identified but did not excavate 7 prehistoric (possibly Native American) burials in other residential areas and in central plaza	reports of multiple cemeteries outside the residential area with burials in opposed rows; scattered burials in residential area and plaza	–	–	–	fragmentary remains of disturbed burials too small to observe modification	Munson et al. 2008; Munson and Spencer 2009
Galt (11G20)	small village	about 25 burials in cemetery with opposed rows	2 rows, perpendicular, not opposed	not observed	not observed	–	10 adults and 1 juvenile documented; poor preservation precluded observation of cut marks or other modifications	Cobb 1999
Ries-Hasting (12PO590)	hamlet	scattered burials	–	–	not observed	–	testing revealed 1 disturbed burial; surveys identified fragments of 8 disturbed individuals	Munson laboratory inventory (2013)

Note: Cells containing a dash indicate that no information is available.

(Savage 1978); and a mandible and a complete skull from a pit at Blood Run (northwestern Iowa) (Schermer 1987b:62, 65). A mandible with numerous cut marks found in midden deposits at the Wever site (southeastern Iowa) is most similar to the Murphy specimen (Hollinger 2005:64, Figure 5; Hollinger and Vradenburg 2004).

Multiple Oneota sites have engraved or incised crania (Hollinger 2005; Hedman, Lillie and Schermer, this volume). Hollinger (2005:248) interpreted the Oneota cranial objects that have engraved designs and evidence of scalping as human trophies of war. He further suggested that these, along with engraved red pipestone tablets, are markers for the Classic Oneota horizon (Hollinger 2005:252–253). No engraved human crania are known from Caborn-Welborn villages, but similar engraved birdman and thunderbird motifs occur on stone tablets and catlinite pipes (Munson 1997:Figure 4; Munson, Jones, LaBudde, and Turner 2004:26).

Skulls described as possible trophies are rare at Mississippian sites (Jacobi 2007; Ross-Stallings 2007), although the Murphy site included two burials of groups of skulls without mandibles (Moorehead 1906). A context that includes cranium-and-mandible burials is the Crenshaw site, a Caddo cemetery in southwestern Arkansas (Powell 1977). The word "trophy" is loaded with unexamined meanings and is sometimes used casually by archaeologists and anthropologists. The interpretation of defleshed crania as trophies may need rethinking. Are these crania those of strangers, friends, or family? Does perimortem trauma or postmortem damage support the notion that these represent war captives or battlefield spoils?

Fine cut marks or groups of marks from sawing or scraping suggest the careful removal of flesh. Multiple fine cut marks on a frontal and an ulna from Edwards I—a Plains Caddo tradition site—are interpreted as evidence for mortuary defleshing (Owsley et al. 1994). Missing mandibles in bundle burials (Agogino and Galloway 1963), burials of crania without mandibles, and cut mandibles have all been observed in protohistoric Plains sites (O'Shea 1984). Ancestor worship and similar interpretations may be more appropriate than trophy terminology in some cases.

Middle Woodland and Late Woodland sites have yielded many more examples of ornately worked human bone than have Mississippian and Oneota sites, and the analysis of Woodland trophy skulls, masks, bowls, and pendants is more advanced. Mark Seeman's (1988) observation that Middle Woodland trophy skulls are those of young adult males of "draft age" with good teeth lends support to the interpretation of the Slack Farm mandible as a trophy, but not the Murphy mandible. Using Seeman's (1988) criteria, the Slack Farm mandible is unlike Middle Woodland human mandible ornaments that are trimmed, highly polished, and more modified. The Murphy site mandible is female and has several dental pathologies, and thus also does not fit the Middle Woodland trophy model in any regard.

Postcranial Elements

The two Caborn-Welborn clavicles and the one worked ulna present an abbreviated set of modified postcranial elements. Cut marks on postcranial elements are less commonly reported, but they occur widely in the late prehistoric period from the Plains to the Midwest to the Southeast. A Plains Caddo defleshed ulna is an example (Owsley et al. 1994). Investigations of disturbed contexts at the Blood Run Oneota site recovered a human femur with cut and puncture marks (Schermer 1987b:6). A femur at the Madisonville site (southwestern Ohio) has been tapered (Drooker 1998:Plate 860). At the Younge site (southeastern Michigan), long bones and a manubrium of one burial were drilled (Greenman 1967). In Lohmann phase contexts at Cahokia, cut marks are found on a femur, fibula, and radius from Submound 51 (Hargrave and Cook, this volume), and on four clavicles and one ulna from the Halliday site (Hargrave and Hedman 2002). At Wickliffe Mounds (western Kentucky), cut marks were observed in analyses of no less than 200 individuals, but none were reported as associated with particular elements (Matternes 2000; Wesler 2001; Hugh Matternes, personal communication 2000). Jacobi (2007:Table 11.3) reported the inclusion of additional arms in burials at two Guntersville Basin sites, which may represent trophies, but did not analyze bone modifications. The Caborn ulna is most similar to examples from Late Woodland sites in Michigan that have been interpreted as showing careful defleshing (Raemsch 1993; Redmond 1982), except that the Caborn ulna shows many more cut marks at the distal end and lacks longitudinal marks on the shaft.

Tools made from human postcranial elements are uncommon. An awl made from a human radius is reported from a historic spring site on Lake Poygan, Wisconsin (Munson, Cook, and Martin 2001), and there are a few other examples reported in the present volume. We are more inclined to less utilitarian interpretations. For example, the Caborn ulna corresponds well to defleshing as a component in producing the still-articulated forearm trophy segments that are prominent in southeastern Mississippian iconography (Dye 2007). The groove-and-snap evidence could also be interpreted as a stage in the manufacture of an ulna tube. A Virginia late prehistoric sucking tube or smoke-blowing tube manufactured from a human humerus shaft identifies the man with whom it was buried as a shaman or curer (Holliman 1970).

Further attention to soft tissue as a potential focus in bone modification is needed. Mensforth (2007) reported a trophy arm lying across the torso of a burial from an Archaic site in Kentucky. The arm was detached by cutting through the clavicle, and one might be tempted to view the Caborn site clavicle as evidence of removal of the arm at the shoulder for similar purposes. If so, the operation was not carried to completion. One might imagine that a person used to performing this operation on deer might be surprised to find the clavicle, because ungulates lack a clavicle, and the forelimb is easy to remove by cutting the scapula free of the ribcage. However, the Caborn-Welborn phase has many connections to the broader Mississippian world, including Southeastern Ceremonial Complex motifs and Southern Cult ceramic effigy vessels.

In particular, female human-effigy bottles—the "old grandmother" vessels—suggest that some Mississippians were quite aware of the clavicle as a peculiarity of human anatomy.[2] Compare, for example, the Caborn-Welborn female effigy bottles from Murphy (Moorehead 1906:Figures 20–21), two of Lesueur's 1828 illustrations of Bone Bank effigies (Bonnemains 1984:Plates 164, 168; Elliott and Johansen 1999:Plates 28, 44), and a third illustrated by Hathcock (1988:Figure 544), with examples from the Mississippi valley (e.g., Hathcock 1983:Figures 314, 315, 1988:Figures 498, 499, 501, 504, 506, 507, 508, 526, 527, 531, 532, 536, 538, 539, 540, 541, 542, 543, 545, 547, 548, 549, 551, 556, 557, 561, 563, 567, 568; Holmes 1886:Figures 452, 454, 455, 1903:Figures 26c, 26d). The disarticulated cut clavicles from Murphy and Caborn could represent dismemberment of the arms of either relatives or enemies, but their deposition in refuse contexts points toward the separated clavicles being refuse and their status as lower than that of curated trophies.

Drilled Bones

Drilled holes may suggest suspension, rearticulation, or binding of bones to other objects. The Angel site yielded an articulated parietal and frontal segment with two perforations (Black 1967; Cook and Munson, this volume). Williams (1975) and Jacobi (2007) reported other drilled cranial objects that may be comparable. The perforations in those objects are very similar in size and shape to the drill hole in the Slack Farm mandible. A similar calotte with four perforations is reported from Pinson Mounds in Tennessee; it is interpreted as a rattle (Jacobi 2003). At Cahokia, a fragmentary parietal with a drilled hole was found at the Stirling phase site 11MS54 (Hargrave 2005). Iroquois made rattles from paired human parietals (Williamson 2007), and the protohistoric Senecas suspended a human skull by its zygomatics (Sublett and Wray 1970).

Suspension is the most interesting feature of the Slack Farm mandible, but the absence of drill holes does not mean that the other modified bones were not suspended. For example, Henschen (1966:Plate 20) illustrated a young man in Borneo wearing a trophy skull with the mandible tied in place at the condyles and the symphysis, a modeled nose ornament, and a suspension cord passed through the zygomatic arches.

Hrdlička reported many examples of drilled human bones from his pre-Koniag horizon on Kodiak Island. He inferred that this was "drilling of skulls or bones for suspension as charms or trophies" (Hrdlička 1941:14). One of his examples is a mandible that closely resembles the Slack Farm artifact. Drilling of the mandible incidental to the production of drilled teeth is reported for Adena (Webb and Baby 1957) and may have been quite widespread since drilled teeth have been recovered for many groups. The location of the Slack Farm drill holes does not correspond to tooth drilling. Whole trophy skulls with perforations are reported from the Plains (Owsley et al. 1994) and from Michigan (Collins 1943; Hinsdale and Greenman 1936). Drilled perforations in skulls for removal of plaques or rondelles for manufacture of gorgets is particularly common in Late Woodland sites from the region surrounding Lake Erie and continues into late prehistoric Iroquoian contexts (Redmond 1982).

Experimental evidence suggests that many months of suspension would be required to produce the rounding observed on the upper margins of the perforations in the Slack Farm mandible. Suspension might suggest that these items were included in medicine bundles, but there is little information supporting this interpretation. In a careful study of Pawnee bundles in the collections of the Field Museum and the American Museum of Natural History, Ray DeMallie (personal communication 2000) found that just one contained human bone: the skull of a former keeper of the bundle. Voegelin (1944) reported that spirit bundles kept by mourners among the tribes of the Great Lakes contained hair of the deceased. Alternatively, the absence of evidence for suspension in the Murphy mandible may suggest stationary display or inclusion in some container or wrapping, as opposed to an item suspended from a person, pole, or building (cf. Owsley et al. 1977).

Going somewhat further afield, drilled holes may suggest that the Slack Farm mandible was bound to other skeletal elements. The absence of drilled holes does not preclude binding or suspension, and the following examples may represent far more extensive artisanal use, which might be invisible in the archaeological record. Mesoamerican representations of skulls and mandibles worn as masks (Coggins and Shane 1984; Matos Moctezuma 1988; Schele and Miller 1986) echo Mississippian iconography, and the drilled mandible from Slack Farm might well have been worn—alone or in combination with cranial elements—as a mask. The drilled vault segment from the Mississippian Angel site (Cook and Munson, this volume) might represent a plausible element in such a composite mask. Its drill holes and fine cut marks are remarkably similar to those on the Caborn-Welborn phase material, and the anterior drill hole is associated with a hinged fracture that suggests wear and tear while the bone was still flexible. Drilled and copper-covered deer mandibles were recovered from a mound at the Mississippian Mitchell site north of Cahokia (Howland 1877) and are curated at the National Museum of the American Indian. These items are connected at the symphysis and may have been "pendants or mask elements (MAI 10/3333, 3334)" (Winters 1974:38, 42), perhaps worn in the mouth by a deer impersonator. Composite masks using bear, wolf, or cougar bones have been recovered from several Middle Woodland contexts in the Midwest (Berres et al. 2004; Webb and Baby 1957). Finally, perforated bones articulated as a skeleton puppet are reported from northern Mexico (Ravesloot 1988). Redmond (1982) argues that the extensive drilling of long bones and skulls in Great Lakes Late Woodland sites may have been done in order to rearticulate skeletons for display during feasts associated with secondary burial.

Ethnographic aspects of all these reports suggest that the use of human bones for artifactual purposes is seldom solely utilitarian. Any of these scenarios may well fit the Caborn-Welborn phase mandibles. Further, all these reports show that modification of human bone is so culturally and geographically widespread in the later prehistory of North America that drawing any specific connections for the Caborn-Welborn examples would be a mistake.

Summary

The Caborn-Welborn modified human bone presents two probable uses. The mandibles appear to be modified for some type of ritual display and are thus more similar to Oneota cranium and mandible "trophies" than to Mississippian examples, which are often from grave contexts. The modified clavicles and ulna may also have been associated indirectly with display. The clavicles would not likely have been displayed themselves, but were likely the byproduct of removing trophy arms. The ulna, on the other hand, could have been a part of a person that was actually displayed. The disposal of the modified clavicles and broken ulna in refuse contexts suggests that the body parts were taken from enemies rather than being the prepared remains of family that were memorialized.

Review of the ethnohistoric literature indicates that the display of scalps, heads, and other dismembered body parts was a common occurrence in the historic Southeast and Midwest (Dye 2007; Hollinger 2005). In addition, iconographic representations of human body parts are evident archaeologically on Mississippian ceramic vessels and shell objects. Mississippian sites in the Ohio valley have produced only a limited number of culturally modified human bones, and the same is true of Mississippian, Oneota, and other late prehistoric sites elsewhere in the Midwest and beyond. Close analysis of Caborn-Welborn phase materials and their contexts bridges the gap between the bony evidence and the ethnographic and iconographic representations. Thus, display rather than use as containers, rattles, tools, or ornaments was the likely cultural meaning of Caborn-Welborn modified human bone. Preparing parts of enemies for exhibition is likely; venerating parts of ancestors is less plausible.

Acknowledgments

Portions of the data in this chapter were presented at the annual meetings of the Indiana Academy of Science in 2001, the Bioarchaeology and Forensic Anthropology Association in 2002, and the Kentucky Heritage Council Archaeology Conference in 2002. We wish to acknowledge multiple institutions for their support of our field and laboratory investigations: for Slack Farm, the National Park Service, the Kentucky Heritage Council, the University of Kentucky, and the Glenn A. Black Laboratory of Archaeology, Indiana University; for Murphy, the Department of Anthropology, Indiana University, the National Park Service's Historic Preservation Fund, and the Indiana Division of Historic Preservation and Archaeology; and for Caborn, the Indiana Historical Society, the Glenn A. Black Laboratory of Archaeology, the Department of Sociology and Anthropology, University of Southern Indiana, and the Department of Anthropology, Indiana University. Permission to study and photograph elements in Figure 11.1 was granted by several institutions: Figure 11a, by the Museum of Anthropology, University of Kentucky; Figures 11.1b and c, by the Department of Sociology and Anthropology, University of Southern Indiana; and Figures 11.1d and e, by the Glenn A. Black Laboratory of Archaeology, Indiana University. We thank Rexford C. Garniewicz, Terrance J. Martin, Timothy R. Pauketat, and Thomas E. Emerson for their assistance in this project, and Patrick J. Munson for his comments on butchering and deer anatomy.

Notes

1. Charles Lacer of Evansville, Indiana, carried out the rescue excavations of the Caborn-Welborn cemetery at the Mann site, after he discovered multiple burials be-

ing plowed out in the spring of 1964. We are indebted to him for his efforts in the excavation and curation of the collection.

2. One of the Caborn-Welborn "old grandmother" effigy bottles with prominent clavicles is displayed at the National Museum of the American Indian, Our Peoples gallery, section 1491. See catalog number 5/5712, http://www.nmai.si.edu/searchcollections/item.aspx?irn=60238&catids=2&catnum=5/5712&src=1-5.

III

LATE PREHISTORIC PERIOD

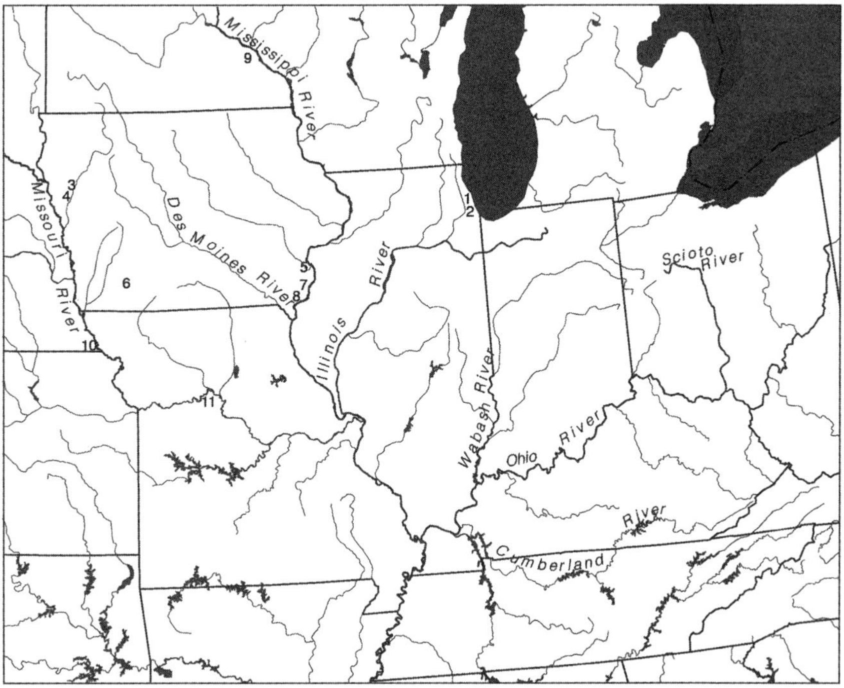

Late prehistoric sites. *Illinois*: (1) Anker (chapter 12); (2) Hoxie farm (chapter 12). *Iowa*: (3) Anthon site (chapter 14); (4) Dixon site (chapter 14); (5) McKinney site (chapter 14); (6) Nodaway River findspot (chapter 14); (7) Schmeiser site (chapter 14); (8) Wever site (chapter 14). *Minnesota*: (9) Red Wing locality (chapter 13). *Nebraska*: (10) Leary site (chapter 14). *Missouri*: (11) Utz site (chapter 14). (Courtesy of Illinois State Archaeological Survey, University of Illinois)

12

Human Bone as Ritual Object?

Modified Human Bone from the Hoxie Farm and Anker Sites, Cook County, Illinois

Kristin M. Hedman

The use of human bone in the manufacture of objects, in ritual activities, and as symbols of personal, political, and spiritual relationships occurs in virtually every culture and time period (Baby 1956, 1961; Chacon and Dye, ed. 2007; Cybulski 1978; Hackenschmidt 2005; Hrdlička 1941; Mensforth 2007; Pereira 2005). Across the midwestern United States, culturally modified human remains have been documented from a number of late prehistoric sites (Table 12.1) and are often associated with Classic Oneota (A.D. 1300–1700), Caborn-Welborn (A.D. 1400–1700), and Caddoan (A.D. 1250–1750) occupations (Brose et al. 2001; Pollack 2004). The two main categories of human bone modification identified at these sites are (1) the cut marks attributed to scalping, defleshing, or disarticulation of remains after death and (2) the manufacture of objects for utilitarian and/or ritual use from human remains. Examples of manufactured objects include polished and incised human bone fragments; cranial and dental elements perforated or grooved for suspension; calvaria used as vessels or bowls; gorgets, masks, and rattles constructed from cranial bone; and, less commonly, the modification of human long bones for use as beads, tubes, awls, rasps, handles, and pipestems.

This chapter focuses on examples of culturally modified human bone from two late prehistoric sites in northeastern Illinois, Hoxie Farm (11CK4) and Anker (11CK21). Located approximately 3.2 km from one another and likely overlapping temporally for a portion of their occupation history, Hoxie Farm and Anker share many similarities in site organization, material culture, subsistence practices, and mortuary treatment. The types of human bone modification and the contexts in which they were found, however, differ significantly between these two sites. I explore these differences and their possible social and cultural implications and significance.

Table 12.1. Oneota Sites with Modified Human Bone

Site	Location	Type*	Element Description	Context	References
Hoxie Farm	Illinois	I	human parietal fragment (adult?) incised with geometric crosshatched design	pit feature with domestic debris, left tibia also present	this chapter
		S	cut marks on isolated parietal (adult)	looter-disturbed context, no other human bone identified	this chapter
		S	cut mark across anterior aspect of sagittal suture (adult female)	Burial 1 (Bluhm's excavations)	this chapter
Anker	Illinois	O	"pipestem of human bone" (human tibia)	associated with Burial 7B11, associated with white stone disk pipe, placement unknown	Bluhm and Liss 1961:97–98, 128; Brown and O'Brien 1990:90; this chapter
		O	"rasp of human long bone" (human femur)	associated with Burial 7B11, placement unknown	Bluhm and Liss 1961:97–98,128; this chapter
		O	"worked bone" (human femur)	associated with "mass of animal jaws and bones above pelvis" of Burial 2XF	Bluhm and Liss 1961:96; this chapter
		O	"notched bone—long bone cut at both ends" (human humerus)	associated with Burial 2XA, found along left side of ribs	Bluhm and Liss 1961:96–97, 128; this chapter
		O	"fragment of human skull covered with copper" (temporal of human infant stained with copper)	associated with cluster of artifacts between legs of Burial 2X	Bluhm and Liss 1961:97; Brown and O'Brien 1990:90; this chapter
Norris Farms	Illinois	S, D	scalping, decapitation, and violent death evidenced for multiple individuals	primary and secondary burial contexts	Santure et al. 1990
Adams County	Iowa	S	cranium incised with forked-eye, bird-man, and other classic Oneota designs, deeper cuts score skull for possible partition into smaller sections	found eroded on a sandbar of the Nodaway River; original context and temporal or cultural affiliation unknown	Schermer 2009; Lillie and Schermer, this volume

Dawson	Iowa	S	cut marks consistent with scalping on left temporal bone	unit JJ, level 4; isolated element from nonburial context	Moffat et al. 1990:408–410, referenced in Lillie 2002c
Wildcat	Iowa	D	cut marks consistent with disarticulation on mandibular ramus	domestic pit feature, isolated mandible fragment from nonburial context	Moffat et al. 1990:401, referenced in Lillie 2002c
Dixon	Iowa	D, S, O	cranium with cut marks consistent with defleshing and disarticulation of the mandible, also removal of portion of right parietal with patterned notching and polishing of cut margins (adult male); small right parietal fragments recovered from this feature	feature context, habitation area	Fishel 1999:115; Lillie and Schermer, this volume
		I	human cranial (frontal) fragment incised with diamond-shaped or crosshatched design, four-sided star, and anthropomorphic birdman figure (private collection)	eroding from cutbank	Lillie 1999; Nansel 1989, referenced in Fishel 1999; Schermer et al. 2008; Lillie and Schermer, this volume
Lane Farm Mound Group (Grant village)	Iowa	O	perforated human cranial fragment with worked edge	identified as "Burial C, Mound 14"	McKusick 1973:47; Schermer and Lillie, this volume
McKinney	Iowa	I or S	2 incised parietal fragments	plow zone	Fokken 1979
		I or S	1 burned and polished parietal fragment (adult) with 6 incised lines	from unit 120	Lillie 1996c
		I or S	burned occipital fragment (young adult) with 34 cut marks made after burning and fragmentation, also with area of abrasion	from unit 123	Lillie 1996c

Continued on the next page

Site	Location	Type*	Element Description	Context	References
		I, O	several cranial fragments with deliberate incising, polish, and smoothing of edges; one highly polished fragment incised with crosshatch pattern after bone was burned	from plow zone, roasting pit, other nonmortuary pit feature contexts	Schermer et al. 2008; Lillie and Schermer, this volume
Phipps	Iowa	V	bowl made from human cranium	Mill Creek	Fugle 1962, referenced in Henning 1970:120
Schmeiser	Iowa	I or S, V?	polished parietal fragment with incised lines in a parallel pattern and abrasion mark (not clear if modified as fragment or when whole), possibly used as bowl, cut marks do not cut into exposed edges of bone and likely extended onto now-absent bone, cut marks as illustrated look similar to scalping or defleshing marks	plow zone and midden contexts	Lillie and Hollinger 2002; Lillie and Schermer, this volume
Wever	Iowa	I, V?	polish and burning on 2 cranial fragments, 1 also exhibits cut marks and rounded edges	recovered from pit feature	Hollinger and Vradenburg 1994; Lillie 2002c; Lillie and Schermer, this volume
Blood Run	Iowa	S	mandible with cut marks (defleshing)	recovered from pit feature	Schermer 1987a:52
		S	skull with cut marks (defleshing)	recovered from pit feature	Schermer 1987a:54
		O	human femur shaft fragment with 3 deep, wide cut marks, each with circular puncture about 1.5 mm from cut mark	recovered from mound context (Feature 11)	Schermer 1987a:55

Armstrong	Wisconsin	S, O	cranial fragment with modified (cut) suture edge	pit feature associated with house structure	Savage 1978:124–128, in Hurley 1978
		O	skull base with red ochre staining	house basin	Savage 1978:124–128, in Hurley 1978
		I, O	burned mandible with incised lines	pit feature associated with house structure	Savage 1978:124–128, in Hurley 1978
Tremaine	Wisconsin	V	bowl made from human cranium	nonmortuary context	Hollinger, personal communication 2002; referenced also in Vradenburg 1993:149.
		S	2 individuals with cut marks consistent with scalping	scattered remains	O'Gorman 1995
		S	2 individuals with evidence of scalping, 1 individual with embedded projectile points	burials	O'Gorman 1995
Guthrey	Missouri	O	human canine, root tip grooved for suspension	refuse area	Henning 1970:83
Utz	Missouri	V, I	burned bowl made from human cranium (adult), portions of parietals and occipital present, exterior surface covered with fine scratches, incised line runs parallel to cut and polished edge of occipital	trench 21, nonburial feature	Henning 1970:120
		I	cranial fragment engraved with crescent and star surrounded by circular lines	refuse pit	Hollinger 2005:247; Lillie and Schermer, this volume

Continued on the next page

Site	Location	Type*	Element Description	Context	References
		O	human femur shaft (19.5 cm) incised with anthropomorphic figure and other motifs	surface of field near Utz site	Betancourt 1965:262, 272
Edwards I	Oklahoma	S	human frontal (adult female) and ulna with scattered cut marks	fortification ditch	Owsley et al. 1994
		O	human femur (adult female) with 31 deep cuts across linear aspera	fortification ditch	Owsley et al. 1994
		O	human femur (adult female) with 7 V-shaped grooves on anterior suface, polish also evident	fortification ditch	Owsley et al. 1994
Leary	Nebraska	I	cranial fragment engraved with possible "thunderer" and "lightning bolts"	surface of site	Hollinger 2005:194; Lillie and Schermer, this volume
OT (Tremaine complex)	Wisconsin	O	"trophy skulls"	mortuary and nonmortuary contexts	Bray 1961, referenced in Henning 1970:120; Vradenburg 1993:149

Note: *I = incised, decorative, or symbolic lines, often with polish or burning; D = disarticulation, dismemberment; S = scalping or defleshing; V = vessel or bowl made from human cranium; O = other forms of bone modification.

Hoxie Farm Site

The Hoxie Farm site (11CK4) is a large and intensively occupied site located adjacent to Thorn Creek in Cook County, Illinois. Material culture and radiocarbon dates place the Hoxie Farm occupation from the late fourteenth through the sixteenth century, corresponding to the Late Fisher (ca. A.D. 1100–1400) and Early Huber (ca. A.D. 1500–1650) phases of the Upper Mississippian period in this area (Emerson and Hedman 2007; Herold et al. 1990; Jackson and Emerson 2013; Jackson and Hedman 2009). Although this site has been heavily looted over the years, archaeological investigations conducted by Chicago's Field Museum of Natural History in 1953 (Herold et al. 1990) and the Illinois Transportation Archaeological Research Program (ITARP) at the University of Illinois, Urbana-Champaign, from 2000 to 2003 identified and excavated more than 2,500 features, including several structures and over 50 burial features (Hedman and Jackson 2009; Herold et al. 1990). Two roughly contemporaneous areas of occupation were identified by ITARP: a Fisher phase fortified village (Jackson and Emerson 2013) and the larger Fisher/Early Huber phase main occupation area. The majority of the burials and isolated human elements, including the modified bone presented here, were associated with the main occupation area (Hedman and Jackson 2009).

Human remains were encountered in a number of different contexts at Hoxie Farm. Burials occurred in the occupation area of the site; no discrete mortuary area was identified. Mortuary treatment included primary extended interments and a small number of secondary burials (Fricker et al. 2003). Artifacts were found in small numbers in association with over half of the documented burials and included lithic and bone tools, copper artifacts and copper staining, red ochre inclusions, animal bone, at least one pipe, and several ceramic vessels (Emerson and Hedman 2007; Hedman and Jackson 2009; Herold et al. 1990). One older male was interred with several unusual items. These included a stone pipe incised with a bird design, several projectile points arranged in a tight cluster (suggesting they may have been a quiver of arrows), and three animal skulls (two young beaver, one bobcat) placed at the shoulders and upper chest. Red ochre had been applied to the animal skulls, and copper caps or inserts covered the eye sockets. Elements of the forepaws were also present, which suggests these may have been components of bags or perhaps a sash (Foster 1994; Zedeño 2008). A similarly decorated otter skull was found with a burial excavated at this site in 1953 (Herold et al. 1990). Skull fragments from a small animal were found on the chest of at least one other burial during ITARP excavations, also suggesting the presence of a bag, bundle, or sash.

A number of isolated and fragmentary human elements were also recovered during the excavation of domestic pit features, post molds, and midden fill, as well as from both prehistorically disturbed and more recent looter-disturbed contexts at the site. A small number of these fragments show evidence of burning. These isolated elements may reflect modern or prehistoric disturbances of burials; a mortuary program that involved the secondary processing of remains in the habitation area; cultural practices that included the curation, display, and ritual use of human remains, including possible trophy taking; and/or noncultural disturbance by burrowing animals and roots (Hedman and Jackson 2009; see also Birch 2010).

Anker Site

The Anker site (11CK21) is located along the Little Calumet River in Cook County, Illinois, approximately 3.2 km from Hoxie Farm. Archaeological information about this site is derived largely from information provided by local collectors and professional salvage excavations directed by Elaine Bluhm and the University of Illinois in the late 1950s prior to construction of a housing development (Bluhm and Liss 1961; Brown and O'Brien 1990; Jackson 2010). Material culture and radiocarbon dates place Anker in the late fifteenth through early seventeenth centuries, or the Late Fisher to Early Huber phases of the Upper Mississippian period (Bluhm and Liss 1961; Jackson 2010). The absence of any European artifacts in the Anker assemblage suggests a pre-seventeenth-century occupation (Jackson 2010; Mazrim and Esarey 2007).

Two burial areas were identified at this site, each associated with a ceremonial longhouse structure, and while an estimated 60 burials were excavated at the Anker site, most by collectors, the description of "fragments of recently disturbed skeletons" (Bluhm and Liss 1961:92) suggests that additional burials had also been disturbed (Jackson 2010). Most isolated or scattered human bone at Anker could be attributed to modern looter disturbance and construction activities. The number of burials, the apparent clustering of burials into distinct areas each associated with special-use structures, and the number and variety of exotic artifacts included with burials is very different from the pattern at Hoxie Farm. At both sites, primary extended single interments were most common, although secondary bundle burials, often containing the remains of multiple individuals, were also present. The types of artifact placed with burials at Anker (e.g., vessels, projectile points, pipes, copper, ochre) are similar to those found with burials at Hoxie Farm; however, artifacts occur in greater numbers and in association with more individuals at Anker. Furthermore, the often exotic or "unique" nature of the materials found in association with the burials at Anker reflects far-reaching trade relations and has led researchers to suggest that Anker was an important ceremonial site (Bluhm and Liss 1961).

Artifacts found in association with Anker burials included shell-tempered vessels, copper items (including snakes, beads, rings, bangles, and sheet copper), red ochre, shell spoons and hoes, ground stone tools and triangular projectile points, marine shell beads and shell gorgets, a single mask fragment, and three maskette gorgets with weeping eye motifs (Bluhm and Liss 1961; Jackson 2010). Sixteen pipes were recovered from burial contexts: four elbow, four stone disk, one modified disk, one vase-shaped, one rectangular block, one truncated cone, one bear effigy, two human-face effigy, and one celt-shaped incised with a bison and a heart-line (Bluhm and Liss 1961:Figures 64, 65).

At least six burials had clusters of animal bone and other artifacts placed on or near the body, which are thought to represent medicine bags or bundles (Bluhm and Liss 1961). Several of these clusters included animal skulls with copper caps or inserts over the eye sockets and red ochre application to the skull. Bones of several animal species are represented in these clusters, most commonly the jaws and teeth of otter, mink, raccoon, loon, beaver, wolf, dog, bobcat—and human.

Modified Human Bone from the Hoxie Farm Site

Peri- or postmortem cut marks were identified on human cranial fragments from one burial and five isolated feature contexts at Hoxie Farm (Hedman 2003, 2008; Hedman and LeFagre 2002). Distinct cut marks crossing the sagittal suture of an adult female (Bluhm's Burial 1) suggest possible scalping, although no other clear evidence of trauma is present. Cut marks on isolated parietal fragments from pit Features 144 and 767 also suggest scalping or defleshing cuts; however, the small size of the bone fragments prevents an accurate interpretation of their significance. Several parietal fragments exhibiting unusually fine, shallow cut marks, very different from those typically associated with scalping or dismemberment (Hamperl and Laughlin 1959; Raemsch 1993), were recovered in flotation samples from Feature 329 and the adjacent Feature 322. The precise patterned incisions clearly reflect the intentional cultural modification of human cranial bone.

Features 329 and 322

Feature 329 was a large, elongated, flat-bottomed Fisher phase pit feature located in the northern portion of the Hoxie Farm site in an area of high feature density. In addition to the cranial fragments described above, Feature 329 contained a human tibia shaft of an adolescent or adult, as well as multiple elements of an infant. Although human remains were present in the feature fill, the quantity of nonhuman bone and other cultural material recovered suggests that this was primarily a domestic pit feature, possibly used secondarily for the interment of an infant. Feature 322 was a small oval pit that was superimposed on Feature 329. The degree to which features in this area of the site overlay one another makes it difficult to assess the original context of the human remains recovered from these features.

Several cranial fragments exhibiting unusually fine cut marks were recovered in flotation samples from Feature 329 and mend with incised cranial fragments recovered from Feature 322. Once reconstructed, the element was identified as a left human parietal fragment measuring approximately 7 cm x 10 cm. The thickness of the bone suggests it was from an adolescent or gracile adult.

The surfaces of the parietal fragment are in fair condition, although cortical flaking and erosion have obliterated some of the surface morphology. After reconstruction, a diluted solution of polyvinyl acetate (PVA) was applied to the outer surface of this element to prevent further exfoliation of the cortex and to permit casting of the element. Unfortunately, while protecting the surface from further erosion, it also created a somewhat shiny or glossy exterior. The external surface of this bone did exhibit a slight patina prior to the application of PVA that is attributed to use or handling. Although determining the orientation of this skull fragment is difficult due to the obliteration of, or damage to, nearly all anatomical landmarks, the design appears to lie just above the temporal ridge and roughly parallel to the sagittal suture. The edges of the design are interrupted by old breaks, but the design likely would have continued onto bone that was not recovered. The posterior portion of the design is obliterated by erosion of the bone surface.

The incised design consists of three parallel bands of paired triangles that run from the anterior end (nearest the coronal suture, or the front of the skull) toward the back of the skull, where they intersect with and possibly extend beneath a perpendicular curved line (Figure 12.1). The uppermost band measures approximately .7 cm in width and 5.5 cm in length and contains portions of four paired triangles. The center band measures approximately 1.3 cm in width and 5.5 cm in length and contains at least three paired triangles, each filled with fine crosshatching. The lowermost band extends .7 cm in width from the broken edge of the bone fragment and approximately 3 cm in length and contains portions of at least two paired triangles, each filled with fine crosshatching.

It is impossible to tell whether the cranium was complete or fragmented

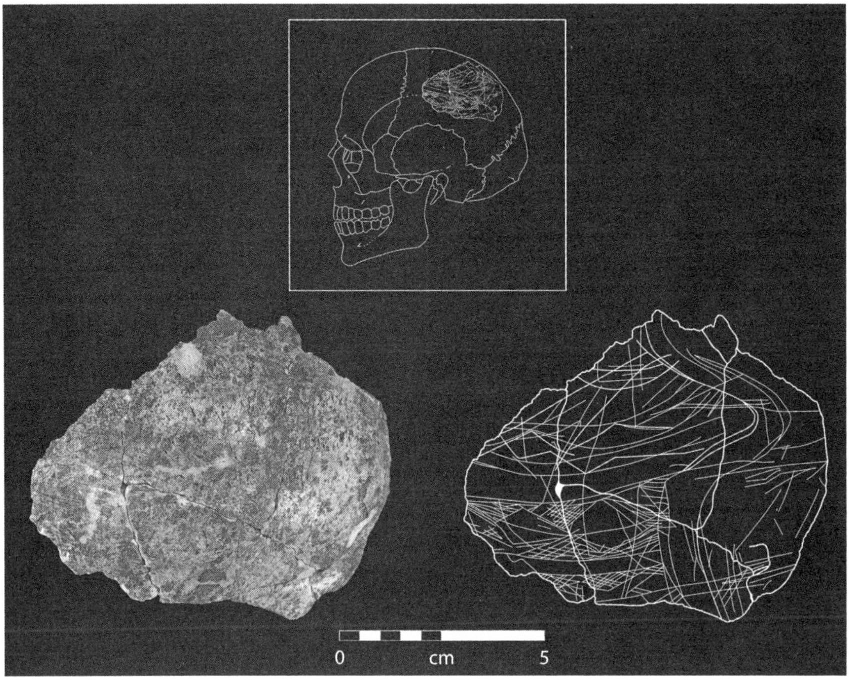

12.1. Incised design on a human parietal fragment from Hoxie Farm. (Courtesy of Illinois State Archaeological Survey, University of Illinois)

when the design was incised. The lack of appreciable flaking of the surface of the bone suggests that the cranial fragment retained fresh bone characteristics at the time it was modified. The level of detail and precision in the execution of these lines indicates that the cranium was defleshed at the time it was incised; however, no scalping or defleshing cuts can be identified with certainty. The design elements are similar to those used in the depiction of serpents and thunderers, both important in late prehistoric cosmology (Benn 1989). The feature context and fragmentary nature of the remains provide little evidence of where the skull fragment originated and who or what it represents.

Modified Human Bone from the Anker Site

Among the array of associated mortuary artifacts at Anker, four modified human long bones and one copper-covered human cranial fragment were recovered from primary burial features (Bluhm and Liss 1961:96–98, 128–129). The modified long bones are identified as a notched bone tube, a worked bone tube, a rasp, and a pipestem (Bluhm and Liss 1961:96–98, 128–129;

Hedman 2008). The manufacturing techniques applied to all are similar. The ends of the bones were grooved and snapped to remove the articular ends; then, the cut ends were polished or smoothed. Abrasive cleaning of the diaphysis is evidenced by fine scratches. The long bones are all hollow to a degree; however, there is no evidence that they were intentionally reamed out. Cancellous bone remains in the medullary canal in varying amounts.

The available information suggests that these were found with primary adult burials and that most were included in clusters of bone and other material interpreted as remnants of bags or bundles. Some of the modified bone artifacts described below were not initially recognized as human bone, suggesting that modified human bone may be more prevalent at Anker (and other sites) than these numbers suggest. Much of the Anker site material remains in private collections. Several elements described below were generously made available to me for documentation.

Burial 2XA

Burial 2XA, the extended primary burial of a probable adult, was exposed and largely destroyed during the laying of a sewer line; only the upper portion of the body remained at the time of excavation. Artifacts found in association with 2XA include two rim sherds, a shell-tempered jar with a notched rim and loop handles placed to the right of the head, and pieces of red ochre inside the vessel; a marine shell gorget, tubular marine shell beads, mussel shell pendants, and a mussel shell hoe also near the skull; a celt-shaped pipe incised with a bison and an arrow heart-line beneath the left side of the skull; and two marine shell beads on the chest. A bone tube, described as a "long bone cut at both ends with three notches along sides," was found near the left side of the body along with two raccoon canines and a wooden earplug covered with sheet copper (Bluhm and Liss 1961:96–97, 128).

The modified "long bone" described above was recently identified as the shaft segment of a human left humerus measuring approximately 12 cm in length (Figure 12.2). Bone size and cortical thickness suggest it was from an adult. The ends of the element appear to have been scored and snapped, then smoothed by abrasion. Four irregularly spaced, V-shaped beveled grooves occur on the shaft. These grooves are roughly 2 cm in length and roughly 2 mm in width, placed perpendicular to the length of the shaft and across flat planes demarcated by points of muscle attachment; they are not aligned along a single surface as on a rasp. A 2 mm–3 mm lip of bone on the distal end may have served to haft or tie an object to the shaft (inset in Figure 12.2). Polish, fine striations, and a very small area of red ochre staining on this lip are visible under magnification.

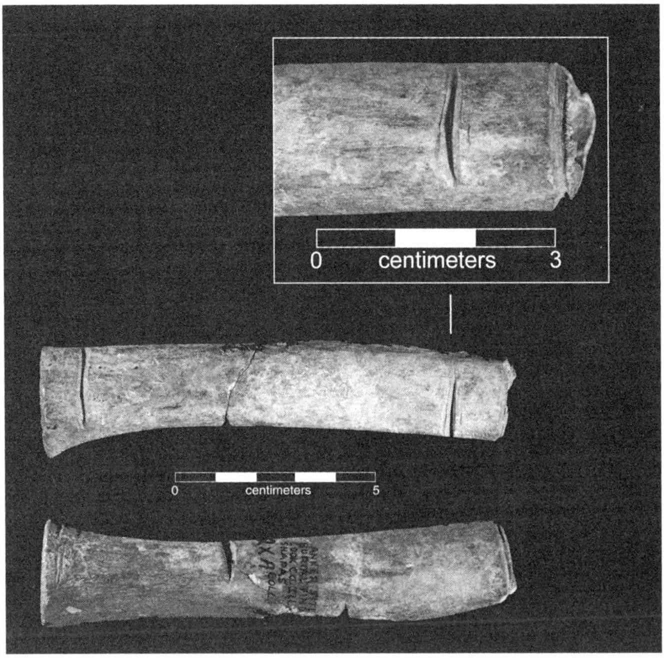

12.2. Burial 2XA, humerus with grooves and lipped end; (*inset*) close-up of distal end of modified humerus with evidence of possible hafting. (Courtesy of Illinois State Archaeological Survey, University of Illinois)

Burial 2XF

Burial 2XF was an extended burial of an adult. A "mass of animal jaws and bones" (including wolf and bobcat) was placed over the pelvis of this individual (Bluhm and Liss 1961:96). The clustering of these items suggests that they represent the contents of a bag or bundle. In this mass of bone was a bone tube identified as a modified left human femur shaft segment (Figure 12.3a). Other artifacts found in association with 2XF include a copper ear ornament and a small copper wire coil to the right of the skull; a copper snake to the left of the skull; and a large calcite crystal and piece of chert on the chest (Bluhm and Liss 1961:96).

The femur segment is approximately 16 cm long. The size and cortical thickness suggest that it was from an adolescent or gracile adult. Both ends of this modified shaft have been scored, snapped, and abraded smooth. Fine striations running roughly parallel to the length of the shaft and similar striations encircling either end likely reflect abrasion by fine sand or reeds in order to remove adherent tissue and periosteum from the bone surface

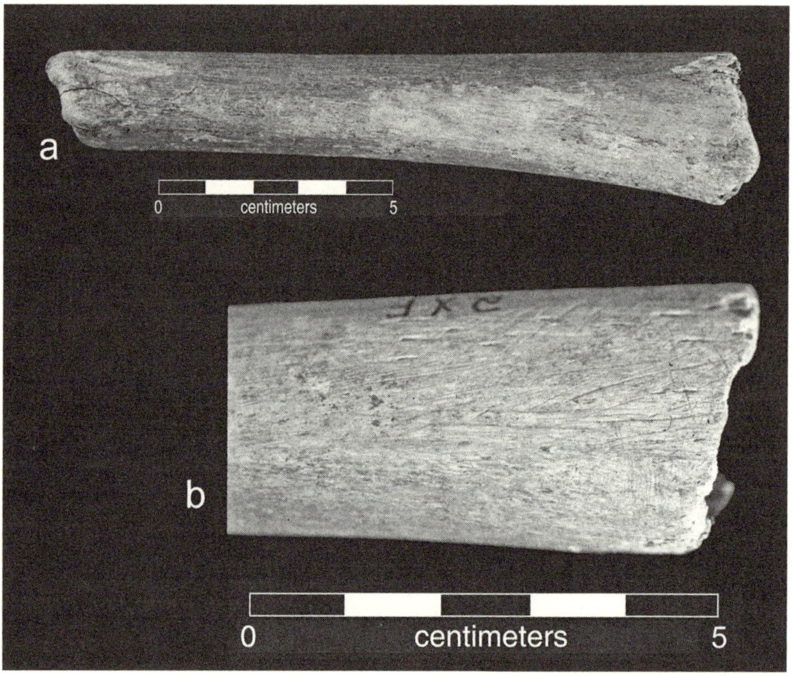

12.3. Burial 2XF: (a) modified left human femur; (b) close-up of modified left human femur showing striations along the outer surface. (Courtesy of Illinois State Archaeological Survey, University of Illinois)

(Figure 12.3b). A faint polish or patina on the shaft indicates use or handling. A "notch" is present on the lateral aspect of the proximal end; it is not clear whether this notch was intentional and functional, whether it was incidental to the cutting and snapping of the shaft, or whether it is the result of use-wear. The surfaces of this notch show abrasions and polish, indicating that the object was used for some period after the notch was made and does not reflect postdepositional damage.

Burial 7B11

Two examples of modified human long bones were found in association with Burial 7B11. These are described by Bluhm and Liss (1961:97–98) as "a rasp of human long bone" and a white stone disk pipe "with a pipestem of human bone." No plan maps are available for Burial 7B11, thus little can be said about the placement of these items or the location of the burial itself. Other materials found in association with 7B11 include 41 triangular projec-

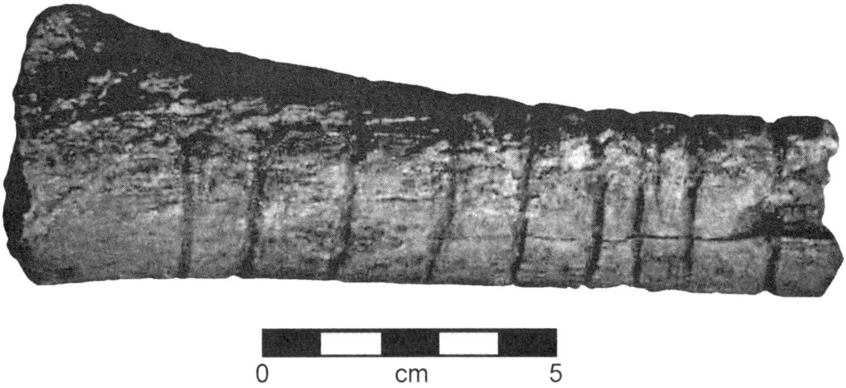

12.4. Burial 7B11, modified human femur interpreted as a rasp. (Courtesy of Illinois State Archaeological Survey, University of Illinois)

tile points arranged along the arms, an antler handle, two sandstone abraders, and a human-face effigy pipe (Bluhm and Liss 1961:97–98, 125, Figure 65).

The rasp was not available for study, but photographs of this object indicate that it is a human femur segment approximately 14 cm long (Figure 12.4). Age and sex could not be estimated from the photograph beyond noting that the femur was not that of a young child, but more likely an adolescent or adult. Grooves cut at regular intervals appear to encircle the shaft and are consistent with bone rasps from Mesoamerican contexts (Pereira 2005; see also Koelikamp 1974).

The pipestem is a 16 cm segment of a left human tibia (Figure 12.5a). Bone size and cortical thickness indicate that the bone was from a robust adult, probably male. The surface is marked by equally spaced, shallow depressions that encircle the shaft. Unlike the grooves on the rasp described above, the depressed ridges on the tibia are neither cut nor abraded, but appear to be the result of compression and use (Figure 12.5b). A photograph in McKusick's *Men of Ancient Iowa* (1964:Figure 8.8) shows a small Oneota "bone ceremonial object decorated with copper rings," which produced a similar effect (Figure 12.6). Like the example illustrated by McKusick, the depressions on the Anker tibia shaft are uniform in width and spacing—as if individual rings had been placed around the shaft rather than a continuous spiral binding. No staining is evident on the bone surface to indicate what material (e.g., metal, plant fiber, animal sinew) might have caused the depressions. Although weathered and eroded to some degree, the bone surface shows significant patina indicative of handling.

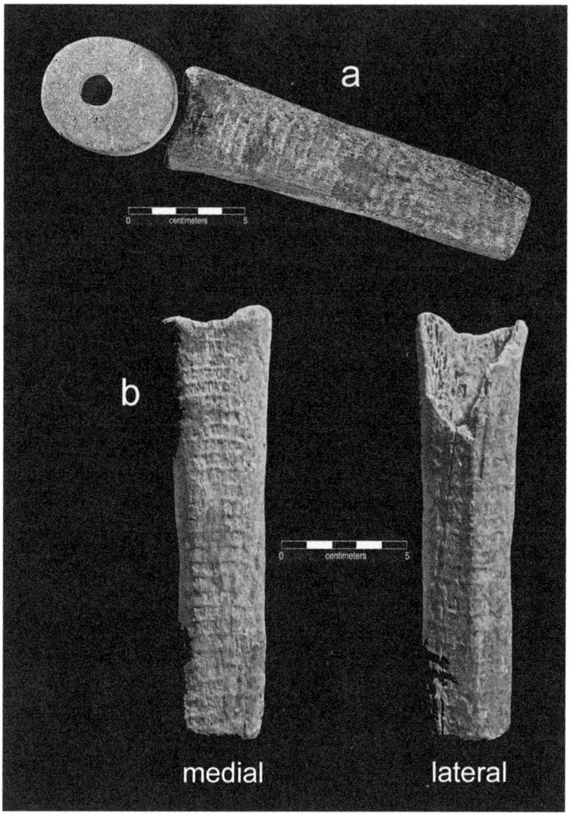

12.5. Burial 7B11: (a) modified left human tibia with limestone pipe bowl as discovered in situ during excavation; (b) close-up of depressions along the surface of the modified tibia. (Courtesy of Illinois State Archaeological Survey, University of Illinois)

Burial 2X

The final example of modified human bone described for Anker is a "fragment of human skull covered with copper" found in association with Burial 2X. Burial 2X had been impacted by excavation for a sewer line, and only the lower portions of the femora and the lower legs remained of what was likely the extended burial of an adult. Several artifacts were found clustered between the legs of Burial 2X. In addition to the copper-covered skull fragment, these include a drilled wolf mandible, four bone disks (no species identification provided), one antler projectile point, an antler flaker, a modified

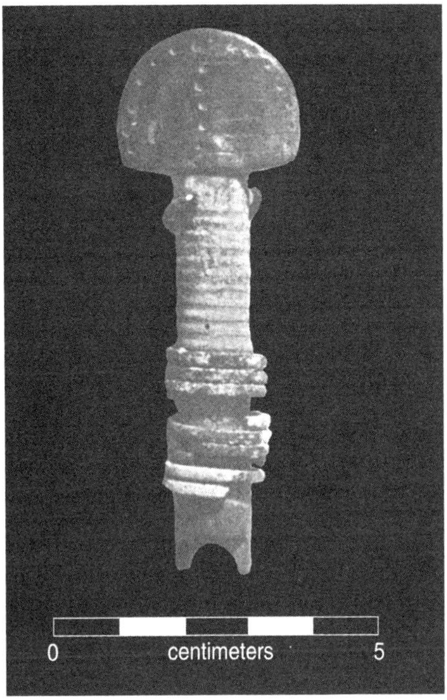

12.6. Bone ceremonial object. (McKusick 1964:Figure 8.8A)

scapula (nonhuman), a tubular shell bead, a mussel shell spoon, three beaver teeth, and three dog or wolf canines (Bluhm and Liss 1961:97).

Although most material from Burial 2X remains in private collections and unavailable for study, a portion of a left temporal from an infant aged 6–30 months was identified, which had been commingled with curated faunal material from Burial 2X. It exhibits green copper staining suggesting it might well be the human skull fragment described above. No further modification to this element was noted. The absence of additional infant remains in this assemblage, combined with its reported inclusion in a cluster of animal bone, supports the interpretation of this stained cranial fragment as culturally modified human bone. The disturbed context of Burial 2X does, however, leave open the possibility that the infant cranial fragment is displaced from a disturbed burial or represents a poorly preserved infant interred with Burial 2X.

Discussion

As addressed throughout this volume, many motives have been attributed to the retention and modification of human remains. They may be kept as trophies of war or relics of venerated ancestors. They may be a source of power to the possessor, whether an individual or the community. Several lines of evidence have been used to address the question of how these items may have functioned in society and the role they may have played.

A standard biological or osteological analysis of modified human remains provides identification of the particular skeletal elements. It may be possible to estimate the age and sex of the individual from whom the skeletal remains were derived and to identify evidence of disease, injury, or mortuary processing. Morphological or chemical evidence might also be useful in determining the cultural affinity or place of origin of an individual or element. Demographic and morphometric data can be utilized to determine if modified remains are derived from within a specific population or from an outside group—whether they are more likely to represent the remains of a venerated elder or member of the society, a memento mori of a loved one, or a body part taken in conflict as a trophy or retribution (see Johnston, this volume).

Artifact analysis looks at the material type used in the manufacture of an object as well as taphonomic evidence for how that material was modified and used. This approach can provide information on how soon after death an element was modified, identify evidence of dismemberment or trauma indicating a possible trophy origin, or identify evidence of defleshing or scraping away of soft tissue prior to modification. The characteristics of cut marks, striations, abrasions, perforations, punctures, grinding, staining, or pigment application can provide evidence for the mode of manufacture and the sequence of steps in bone modification. The degree of polish or patina on the bone surface may provide evidence of the handling and use of an object.

Archaeologists tend to draw heavily on ethnographic and historic sources in their interpretations. "They scour historical and ethnographic sources to find an analogy that will magically unlock the meaning behind the image or the structure" (Howey and O'Shea 2006:262). The shape of an object and its similarity in form or context to other, perhaps more familiar objects from archaeological or ethnographic contexts can suggest possible function. The context in which a modified human bone was found may provide clues to less tangible concepts such as use, ownership, and symbolism. If an object or pattern cannot be easily attributed to factors such as subsistence, warfare, or trade, for example, it is often deemed a "ritual" object—intangible, elusive, and unknowable. However, ethnographic evidence can provide valuable clues to interpreting the meaning and significance of more esoteric objects.

Hoxie Farm Parietal

The Hoxie Farm parietal fragment was derived from an adolescent or gracile adult. The bone is relatively thin with no marked musculature evident. While one cut mark suggestive of possible scalping has been noted, no scalping or defleshing marks were identified with certainty, nor were striations observed to suggest it was cleaned with abrasives prior to incising. The lack of these modifications may be due to the postdepositional surface erosion and weathering present on this element. Decomposition of soft tissues would have made cleaning easier, and some decomposition may have occurred prior to final cleaning and modification. The sharp, fine lines and lack of cortical flaking or fracture during incising suggest that the bone still retained the elastic qualities of fresh bone when it was modified (Owsley et al. 1994). Since bone can retain these characteristics for several months after death, depending on conditions, it seems likely that the modification occurred sometime during the first year or so following death.

The Hoxie Farm parietal fragment might well represent cranial remains taken in war (i.e., a trophy). The presence of a fortification surrounding a portion of the Hoxie Farm site; the skeletal evidence for scalping and violent death in the Hoxie Farm mortuary population; and the presence of fragmentary, burned, cut, and scattered human bone in the habitation areas all suggest that Hoxie Farm inhabitants engaged in conflict and were at least the occasional victims of scalping. Removal and modification of the head was not evidenced in the mortuary treatment at Hoxie Farm. The lack of evidence for intentional removal or retention of skulls (or other elements) from primary or secondary burials at this site suggests that the modified cranial fragment was not intentionally derived from a member of the Hoxie Farm burial population.

This modified fragment may have been part of a larger object, which is suggested by the interruption of the design at the broken edges. The Nodaway cranium, recovered from a sandbar in Adams County, Iowa (see Lillie and Schermer, this volume), makes a convincing analogy for the Hoxie Farm parietal and other isolated, incised cranial fragments at Oneota sites. The Nodaway cranium was incised with symbols that had meaning across a wide geographical area, including motifs of the Southeastern Ceremonial Complex and geometric and crosshatched designs similar to those on the Hoxie Farm parietal. It was then scored into parts. Whether these scored segments were ultimately to be separated and distributed is not known, but it seems probable.

There is little evidence to suggest that the Hoxie Farm fragment was manufactured for decorative use. There are no suspension holes on the portion remaining. While a slight patina is present, there is no significant polish or wear, and the design is seemingly crude, with overlapping lines and images, suggesting that little emphasis was placed on creating a finely crafted representational image. The act of incising or creating the design may have been as important or more important than the completed object.

The designs found on the Hoxie Farm parietal are similar to those found on human and nonhuman bone, stone, ceramic, and shell objects at many Oneota sites (Figure 12.7, Table 12.1; see also Betancourt 1965; Bray 1963; Fishel 1999; Hedman and LeFagre 2002; Henning 1970; Lillie and Schermer, this volume). Most descriptions of these artifacts emphasize the symbolic iconography rather than how the object functioned in the society (Knight 2006). The most common design elements are geometric patterns, mythical beings, and human and animal figures. These motifs represent "elements of sacred myths and ritual" that could be "recombined and reused in fresh forms to meet the needs of new situations" (Hall 1997:108). The importance of the object may have been based largely on the act of creating the design motif(s) and the role the object served rather than on the particular material (or individual) used to create it. The material upon which the design was rendered likely enhanced or changed the meaning, the power, or the story of the motif or sequence of motifs. The material (in this case, a human cranium), the individual from which it came, the context in which it was obtained (e.g., trophy of war, mortuary processing of friend or relative), and the particular design or sequence of designs likely combined to create the symbolic or ritual power of both the image and the object.

The Hoxie Farm parietal fragments, like other incised objects described above (see also Lillie and Schermer, this volume), occur exclusively in nonmortuary contexts, as do the majority of incised cranial fragments presented in Table 12.1. The disposal of modified human bone in midden or domestic pit contexts suggests a communal function or finite use of the object. The disposal, discarding, or placement of these objects in a midden or pit feature rather than in a burial feature suggests that these modified elements were viewed not as individuals (or parts thereof) or personal possessions, but as objects with a finite functional life. Their discard or placement in midden and feature contexts may reflect an end to their functional life or, conversely, may represent the transfer of the power or purpose of the object from the individual to the earth, where it may have continued to serve (or impact) the broader community. A correlate might be the smashing of vessels or figurines, marking a dedication or termination event (Stross 1998) or a sym-

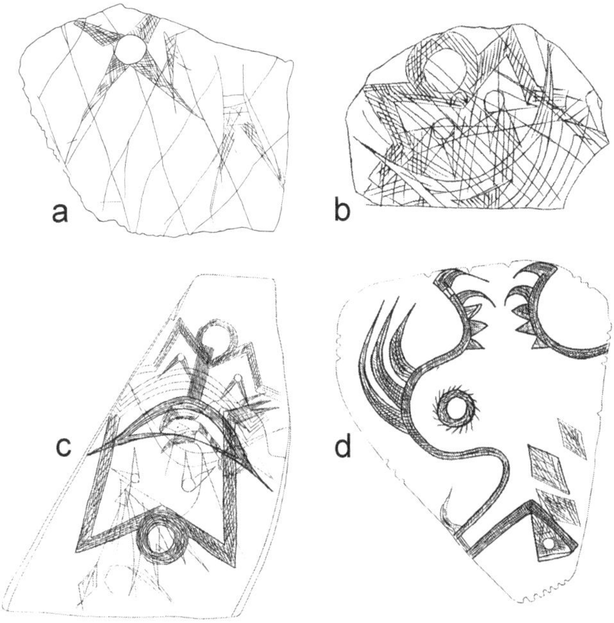

12.7. Incised catlinite tablets from midwestern Oneota sites: (a) modified superior frontal bone from the Dixon site (13WD8) (drawing by Liz Niec); (b) Millard tablet from the Utz site, Missouri (from Bray 1963:10); (c) Utz tablet from the Utz site, Missouri (from Bray 1963:6–7); (d) Stiles tablet from the Bastian site, Iowa (from Bray 1963:18). (Bray figures courtesy of Missouri Archaeological Society, Missouri State University)

bolic transference of power from the individual to the community (Luby and Gruber 1999).

Anker Modified Bone

The modified long bones from Anker differ in several key aspects from the incised cranial fragments described from Hoxie Farm and are similar in others. The cutting, polishing, and compression characteristics indicate that, like the Hoxie Farm example, the long bones from Anker were manufactured from fresh bone. A score-and-snap technique was used to remove proximal and distal portions of the long bones, and striations along the shafts indicate that bone surfaces were abraded with sand or grasses to remove adherent tissues. The absence of defleshing cuts along areas of diaphyseal muscle attachment suggests that some decomposition of soft tissues had occurred prior to modification. It must be noted that only midshaft segments are represented; the articular ends and their associated areas of muscle attachment, where evidence for disarticulation would be found, are not present.

The elements were taken primarily from adults or adolescents, and differences in the sizes of the elements suggest that both sexes are represented. There is insufficient evidence to determine if the elements or the objects derived from them were obtained through trade, as trophies of war, or as part of the mortuary treatment of group members. Bundle burials are present at Anker, so it is possible that elements were selected from curated remains prior to final burial. It is also possible that they represent trophies or elements taken from individuals outside the community. Although information is limited, there is no archaeological or osteological evidence for interpersonal violence at Anker.

Modified human bone at Anker was identified exclusively in primary mortuary contexts in direct association with a fairly small number of the documented burials. If the copper-covered cranial fragment described for Burial 2X is included, modified human bone has been identified with four burials at Anker, or about 10 percent of the available sample. All appear to have been associated with burials of adults. They may have been possessions of the individuals with whom they were found, used during life, or symbolize group membership or the individual's position in the society. They may have been placed with the individual after death to offer power or protection or to serve the deceased in the afterlife.

In at least two cases, modified human bone was included in clusters of animal bone and other items interpreted as medicine bundles or bags. These bundles were found in association with only six individuals at Anker, all adults, suggesting that bundles, like modified bone objects, may have been restricted to certain individuals or indicative of a particular position or role in the society.

Ceremonial or medicine bundles are well documented for historic Algonquian and Siouan groups; often made from the pelt of particular animals (e.g., otter or mink), they symbolized an individual's membership in religious societies and their role in the community (Foster 1994; Harrington 1914). These bundles contained items of spiritual importance to the possessor, such as pebbles, crystals, animal bone, locks of hair, and other items. They were carried during life and were often interred with the individual at death (Foster 1994; Harrington 1914).

Bundles are far more than a collection of objects; they are repositories of knowledge about specific rituals shared among initiated individuals, and although they share a number of significant characteristics, each bundle is unique and powerful, with a life history, personality, and position in society (Zedeño 2008). Each object chosen for inclusion has specific properties, and the combination of the individual materials creates a new object, the bundle, that is specifically tailored to that individual or situation (Foster 1994). Bundles were, and still are, associated with tribes across the Plains, Prairie, and western Great Lakes. Each clan within a tribal group may have its own pipe and several different types of bags, each associated with specific rituals and uses (e.g., war bundles, pipe bundles, medicine bundles).

The use of human bone in the manufacture of ritual or sacred objects, rather than the use of readily available nonhuman bone and antler, and the inclusion of these objects in bundles was clearly intentional. Human bone was not used simply because it was available. Human bone, perhaps even the particular element or the particular individual from whom it was taken, was undoubtedly ritually or symbolically significant (Zedeño 2008). Bone is often linked to the spiritual world both as a symbol of death and as a means of communicating with spirits in ritual contexts (Turpin 1996).

The objects manufactured from human bone at Anker all have performative characteristics. Their forms suggest pipestems, rasps, rattles, handles, staffs, or hollow bone tubes described ethnographically as staffs, soul catchers, or sucking tubes—objects that have been associated historically with ritual, witchcraft, healing, and religious practices and practitioners (Walker 1998; see also Baby 1961; Gilliland 1975; Hester 1969a; Koelikamp 1974; Mensforth 2007; Owsley et al. 1994; Willoughby and Hooton 1922).

Pipes, smoking, and tobacco have played a crucial role in Native American cosmology, spirituality, and ritual across the continent from early prehistoric times to the present (Rafferty 2004). Smoking is most often depicted as a formalized ritual behavior that occurred at both community and individual levels. The tobacco and hallucinogens inhaled or ingested could produce altered states of consciousness. Trance, or symbolic death, and other altered states are an integral component of many shamanistic belief systems (Turpin 1996). Smoking is often a ritualized act related to cosmology, social regulation, spiritual purification, and mortuary rituals (Rafferty 2004:7–9). The pipes themselves, which often depict animal symbolism, may have totemic properties, and the placement of pipes in special function features, such as mounds, burials, and artifact caches, speaks to their importance. In addition to the stone platform pipe and its pipestem made from a human tibia, and the rasp made from human bone, Anker Burial 7B11 included a human-effigy pipe (Bluhm and Liss 1961). The various "human" representations interred with Burial 7B11 are distinctive and striking.

The use of human bone in the manufacture of musical instruments—crania resonators, femora rasps, bone rattles and flutes—is well documented (Pereira 2005; Turpin 1996). Like smoke, the music produced by rasps and other instruments was a means of communicating with spiritual realms. In the Mesoamerican context, the Tarahumara word for sorcerer is "the one who rasps" since that person projected evil magic through notched rasping sticks. Spanish accounts indicate that rasps produced a very sad music and were generally performed at the funerals of rulers or to commemorate fallen warriors or sacrificial victims (Turpin 1996:267). Others have noted bone's phallic significance and the use of rasps in both erotic festivals and at funerals, contexts primarily concerned with life and rebirth (Turpin 1996:267).

Bone tubes are more ambiguous and might have functioned as staffs or handles for rattles or other objects. Rattles constructed of sticks, bone, or antler handles with noise-making objects attached were used in healing and religious contexts (Foster 1994:188). Hollow bone tubes, most typically bone from birds or animal, are often described in healing treatments, used for extracting disease or for exorcisms. Cybulski (1978:27) described a human humerus as a possible "soul receiver," which he defined as a hollowed-out bone shaft (human or animal, especially bear or caribou) with open ends, while others have described long bones as containing the "soul of animation" (Birch 2010; Williamson 2007).

Modified human long bones are uncommon at late prehistoric sites in this region. Only a few examples of similarly modified elements were found in the literature. In southwestern Oklahoma, two modified human femora were recovered from a fortification ditch associated with the protohistoric Wheeler phase (A.D. 1450–1750) occupation of the Edwards I site (Owsley et al. 1994). These elements are grooved, with one femur portion showing polish on the grooved surfaces. Bone tubes, some decorated by carving or pigments, are known from several sites in Texas (Hester 1969a). Most were recovered with burials, and several were associated with tubular stone pipes, including "two large tubular stone pipes, one of which had a mouthpiece fashioned from a human ulna" (Pearce 1938:221). Numerous other segments of hollow bone were present and were interpreted as spare mouthpieces for such pipes. The age and culture of these sites, however, is not well established (Hester 1969a).

Multiple Narratives of Modified Human Bone

Objects are integral to human action and have always been the center of archaeological research (Gosden and Marshall 1999). Cultural objects are often seen and interpreted mainly as functional items, vital to the social process but rarely informing it (MacGregor 1999). The biographical approach to artifact analysis allows us to explore how social interactions involving people and objects create meaning, and how these meanings change and are renegotiated through the life of an object (Gosden and Marshall 1999:169).

Viewing objects far removed from contemporary Euro-American society will, according to Stevens (2007:197), "always disappoint if we expect this experience to provide us with a complex history. . . . [Cultural objects] represent so much more on a cultural, political, and historic level than a museum label can ever explain." Objects must be understood within the context in which they were created, exchanged, used, and ultimately taken out of circulation. Some objects are "inscribed" with meaning: they become socially powerful at the time of their production, their meaning and significance either inherent at the time of manufacture or through the act of creating them, although it can change through time. Other objects are "lived," or everyday, objects that acquire meaning through social action—who used them, how they were used, and how and when their use-life ended (Joy 2009:545). Their form and how they were experienced, their appearance, the smell, touch, sound, and taste associated with their use, all combine to illuminate function (MacGregor 1999).

A small, incised bone fragment would have been visible to the individual holding it and to those in close proximity. Functioning more as a talisman or symbol of personal magic, its power lay in the act of creating it more than in the final object. In contrast, bone tubes, rasps, and smoking pipes would have been visible or audible at a distance, their effect experienced (e.g., seen, smelled, or heard) by others; the objects themselves were likely emblematic of the role of the individuals using or possessing them. For these, power was inherent in the object itself and in its use in performative contexts.

Conclusions

The way a culture treats the dead, how bodies are handled, where they are placed, the materials that are placed with them all together shed light on social, political, and spiritual aspects of past societies (Gowland and Knusel 2006; Parker Pearson 1993). The examples of modified human bone identified at Hoxie Farm and Anker, and the contexts in which they occurred, provide a window into cultural continuity and change at a figurative and actual crossroads in late prehistory. The incised human bone at Hoxie Farm is similar in form, context, and potential function to incised bone, stone, and ceramic objects from contemporaneous sites elsewhere in the Midwest (Lillie and Schermer, this volume). This suggests a degree of shared beliefs and cultural practices. The bone tubes, pipestem, and associated bundles interred with individuals at Anker are markedly different from what was recorded at Hoxie Farm and imply a change in religious beliefs and mortuary practice, or perhaps a change in the ethnic composition of the population at Anker.

At first glance, Hoxie Farm and Anker share much in terms of location, temporal associations, and culture. However, as Betts (2007) noted, similarities in material culture may mask substantial underlying differences in life experience, language, and ethnic identity. The social landscape of the Upper Midwest was complex and rapidly changing in the late prehistoric period. Population movement and the threat of violence occurred in many regions during this time (Birch 2010; Milner et al. 1991; Owsley et al. 2007; Santure et al. 1990). Cultural material at Anker reflects wide-ranging trade relations and suggests that Anker was a ceremonial center attracting people from beyond the immediate area. Although there was no direct European contact in this region until the mid-1600s, far-reaching trade relations between Anker and groups to the south and east would have foreshadowed changes to come (Betts 2006, 2007; Dobyns 1992; Green 1993; Ramenofsky 1987). Population coalescence in the face of disease, social change, and environmental decline may well have characterized Anker (Birch 2010; Hickerson 1997).

Religious beliefs and practices tend to be conservative in nature and are often retained as a marker of ethnic identity after other trappings of ethnicity (e.g., dress, material culture) change. The cultural diversity associated with a ceremonial center such as Anker may account for the apparently sudden appearance of new religious paraphernalia in this area. The increased visibility of religious or spiritual paraphernalia and specialists could well have been a response to new and frightening environmental stressors (Wallace 1956).

The meaning and significance of modified human bone from Hoxie Farm and Anker remains elusive, but these objects hold stories that deserve examination. Descriptions and ethnographic analogies provide some points of discussion. Engaging in dialogue with Native American descendant groups might further illuminate the role and significance of these objects, both as prehistoric artifacts and as cultural elements with meaning for contemporary lives.

Acknowledgments

I would like to thank Tom Emerson, ISAS director; ISAS production staff Mike Lewis, Linda Alexander, and Mike Farkas; my colleagues Eve Hargrave, Shirley Schermer, Robin Lillie, Doug Jackson, Cheryl Munson, Della Cook, Dale Hutchinson, Dale Henning, Eric Hollinger, Mary Hynes, and Julie Bukowski; and Wayne Pitard, director, Spurlock Museum.

13
Grooved Teeth from Red Wing Locality Sites and the Loss or Gain of Identity

Kathleen T. Blue

Postmortem cultural modification of human bone is a fairly common practice at precontact sites in the Upper Midwest, defined here as Minnesota, Wisconsin, northern Iowa, and eastern portions of North and South Dakota. However, the manipulation of human teeth into cultural objects appears confined to the Red Wing locality of southeastern Minnesota and southwestern Wisconsin in the period A.D. 1050–1300 (Blue 2006). Although there is a dearth of known precontact human remains from the Red Wing locality, 21 teeth from multiple sites exhibit a specific and similar form of cultural modification. This modification is related to the suspension of the teeth for the assumed purposes of adornment, status marker, or symbol of affiliation.

Although the phenomenon is uncommon in Minnesota, the use of human teeth as personal adornment dates back at least 40,000 years (White 2007; White et al. 2003). This chapter details the evidence and contexts of teeth from the Red Wing sites and explores the use of teeth as a medium for self-expression and cultural membership. More particularly, I address the transformative aspects of self-identity as seen in the usage of teeth as cultural objects; the disintegration of the body as the loss of the individual; and the incorporation of disparate skeletal elements, specifically human teeth, as one component in the forging of a collective identity at the familial or societal level.

The Use of Teeth as Ornaments

Drawing on inferences from the Red Wing locality data set and from the archaeological and ethnographic literature, this chapter will attempt to elucidate the overarching question, what does it mean? By this, I refer to the use of human body parts for cultural purposes and, specifically, to the use of human teeth as adornment or emblems. Several lines of inquiry present themselves. Why teeth? Which teeth? Why these particular teeth? And what does the incorporation of human dental elements into another's persona accomplish for either the group they belong to, or for that person's position in the society?

Perhaps the earliest example of teeth as cultural objects is seen at Arcy-sur-Cure in central France, where researchers have discovered dozens of animal teeth that were grooved for suspension (Zilhão 2007; Zilhão and d'Errico 1999). These teeth may date to 45,000 years ago and are, according to Zilhão, the work of Neanderthals. Assuming the temporal affiliation is correct, the teeth represent one of the only known uses of symbols by Neanderthals. The use of *human* teeth as ornaments is seen only slightly later in the Aurignacian (40,000–28,000 years ago) at multiple sites in France (White 2007; White et al. 2003). By the end of the Paleolithic, shell and tooth ornaments are ubiquitous and possibly reflect "significant transformations in human society . . . including individual and group identities, as well as the beginnings of defined gender and economic roles" (Edgar 1999:3). Tooth and species choices were not random; ivory or bone facsimiles of teeth were also produced (White 1993).

Oxford University's Pitt Rivers Museum collections contain more than 275,000 items, roughly 600 of which are cultural objects composed of human remains, both bone and teeth (Pitt Rivers Museum 2009). The museum's collections come from all parts of the world, including Asia, Europe, Oceania, Africa, North America, Australia, and South America. A review of just some of the literature finds references to human teeth as ornaments from at least four Upper Paleolithic sites in France, among the Incas, and among modern groups in the Amazon basin, Fiji, New Zealand, Hawaii, and Borneo (Beck 2009; Best 1934; Skinner 1916; Tsintjilonis 2000; White et al. 2003). So common was the use of human teeth as personal adornment that in the 1800s Sachse of Austria and other firms made a lucrative living out of exporting ceramic teeth to Asia, Australia, and Africa (Beck 2009; Pitt Rivers Museum 2009) for use presumably in adornment. In North America, grooved or perforated teeth have been reported from Archaic, Hopewellian, and Mississippian contexts (Cobb, this volume; Jacobi 2007; Lillie 1996b; Nawrocki and Emanovsky, this volume; Schermer and Lillie, this volume).

Grooved teeth have not been found at any other sites in Minnesota outside the Red Wing locality, and other references to teeth as ornaments in the Upper Midwest are sparse, although there is a perforated human tooth from an unspecified archaeological site in Iowa (Cobb, this volume; Lillie 1996b; Schermer and Lillie, this volume). But elsewhere the use of human teeth for decorative purposes is widespread throughout both time and space. There are several possible reasons for this. A review of the ethnographic record as well as a web-based search brings up numerous references to teeth as the "ornaments of the face" (Blackwell 2004; Guerini 1909). Teeth perhaps gain our attention since they are part of what we see when we listen to another person speak. Additionally, they are used as a means of nonverbal communication. In humans, a grin is generally considered nonthreatening and a sign of goodwill, and in other primates a grin is often a form of appeasement, while baring of the teeth is a threat display (Goodall 1986; Hall 1963).

While teeth function to break down food items into smaller and more manageable pieces, thus aiding digestion (Hillson 1996), it is apparent that they are so much more. Cultural references to our "pearly whites" (the term is first used around 1895 [Dictionary.com 2013]) are numerous, and many human groups worldwide, both now and in the past, equate good teeth with both health and beauty. Teeth act as ornament displays in animals, signaling "genetic quality, developmental history and current disease state to potential rivals and prospective sexual partners" (Hendrie and Brewer 2012). In the case of human females, Hendrie and Brewer (2012) found that the appearance of the teeth also conveyed residual reproductive value—that is, the possible number of years of remaining reproductive ability.

Prehistorically, teeth were colored, sharpened, reshaped, and inlaid, all in the interests of aesthetics or status (Goose 1963; Guerini 1909). Today in the United States, teeth whitening, straightening, and other cosmetic surgery, including the addition of bling in the form of implants or a grill, attest to our obsession with our teeth (Ceatus Media Group 2009). Given their role in conceptions of self-identity, it is perhaps not surprising that this interest in teeth should carry over into their incorporation, after death, in a new role as an ornament or object in the creation of another individual's self-identity.

The form of teeth lends itself to their function as ornaments. Teeth are made of enamel, the hardest substance in the human body. Teeth are also naturally white and, in life, stand in contrast to our pink gums and red lips, as well as the generally darker tones of human skin, regardless of ethnicity. In the Cartesian duality often encountered when probing into human processes of assigning meaning, "white" for many peoples equates with pure, clean, or good, while for others it is the opposite: white is the color of death or evil. Regardless of which way a group may view the color white, it is often replete with powerful imagery and symbolic connotations that may play a role in the use of teeth as cultural objects. In addition to their color, the small size and portable nature of teeth also make them desirable as ornaments, as does their simple form, particularly in the single-rooted types. Their division into two parts: the crown, which acts as the ornament itself, and the root, which provides a handy surface for attachment via grooving or drilling without impacting the aesthetic of the crown, also facilitates their use in ornamentation.

Like hair and fingernails, teeth can be "cast off." They are an entity unto themselves, distinct from the rest of the body. Unlike bone and other bodily tissues, such as skin, teeth are easily separated from the body with minimal pain. As children, we lose all of our deciduous teeth; teeth are also lost through injury or disease, or are removed for medical or cultural reasons. All individuals, regardless of background, have some familiarity with teeth as objects separate from their bodily origin.

However, despite this disconnect from their point of origin in the human body, in many societies teeth are considered to be imbued with their owner's essence. Teeth, as well as hair and nail parings, are thought by some to contain some portion of their original owner's life force or to be a distillation of their spirit (Frazer 1922; Gonzalez-Whippler 1991; Tanner 1968). Accordingly, they can be used to subtract from, or cause harm to, the entity from which they arose. If they can be subtracted, they can also be added, imparting prestige, favor, knowledge, or power to their new "owner." Furthermore, teeth are, if you think about it, readily available.

All, or at least some, of the above likely figured into the use of teeth as cultural objects at the Red Wing locality. Given the use of teeth worldwide for this purpose, it is interesting to ponder why teeth are commonly used in this manner at precontact Red Wing sites but only rarely occur elsewhere in the Upper Midwest.

The Red Wing Locality

The Red Wing locality is situated along the northern reaches of the Mississippi River approximately 40 mi southeast of St. Paul and just north of the river's expansion into a broad body of water known as Lake Pepin. The Red Wing locality, as defined by archaeologists, includes sites in both Minnesota and Wisconsin. These sites are located on high terraces overlooking the Mississippi River and on the adjoining deltas of the Cannon and Trimbelle rivers (Figure 13.1). Over 2,000 mounds, eight large villages, and many smaller sites have been identified in this 58 mi^2 area. The majority of the mounds and habitation areas of the Red Wing locality date to between A.D. 1050 and A.D. 1300 (Dobbs 1993). Artifacts from these sites can generally be classified as Silvernale (a Middle Mississippian–like culture) or Oneota (a more local tradition that appears to bracket the Mississippian-like items in time, occurring both earlier and later than the so-called Mississippian component). Some Red Wing locality sites include only Silvernale or Oneota assemblages while other sites exhibit both types. The Silvernale culture appears to have been influenced by Middle Mississippian groups to the south, with styles and

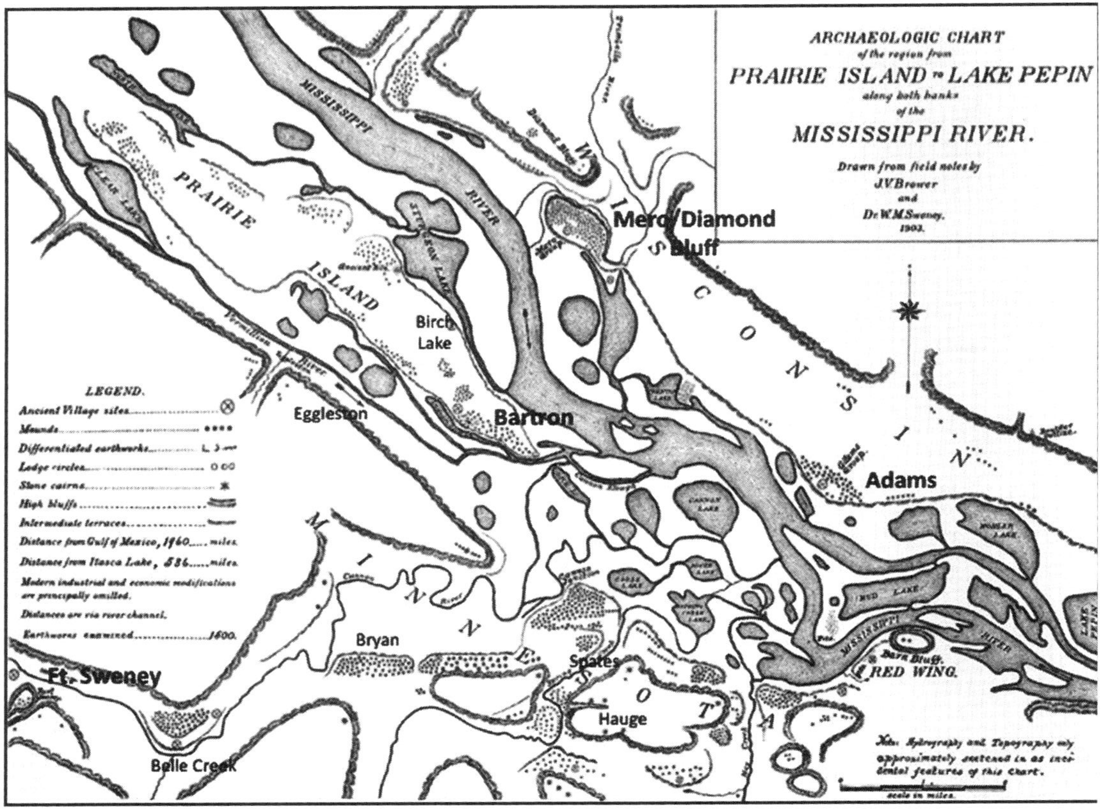

13.1. Major Red Wing locality sites. Those in bold type have yielded teeth modified for suspension. (Map modified from Brower and Sweney 1903)

Table 13.1. Red Wing Locality Sites

Site	Type	Number of Teeth	Excavator/Source
Fort Sweney (Minnesota)	mound burial	11	Jensen, Science Museum, Minnesota, 1960–1962 (Jensen 1960)
Mero/Diamond Bluff (Wisconsin)	habitation	7	Alex, University of Wisconsin, Milwaukee, 1974 (Alex 1974)
Bartron (Minnesota)	habitation	2	Wilford, University of Minnesota, 1948 (Gibbon 1979)
Adams (Wisconsin)	habitation	1	Dobbs, Institute for Minnesota Archaeology, 1984–1985 (Nelson 1999)

motifs more similar to Apple River Mississippian from northwestern Illinois than to those of Cahokia (Ronald Schirmer, personal communication 2012).

Red Wing locality sites have yielded human remains from several different interment and disposal contexts. Although large mortuary complexes consisting of numerous mounds and sizable villages characterize Red Wing locality sites, no large cemeteries are known from the area. Most of the over 2,000 mounds are no longer in existence, but those that were investigated by earlier archaeologists yielded only a few remains. The known human remains come from mounds and habitation areas and include both primary and secondary interments. Much of the human skeletal material consists of single elements found in nonmortuary contexts, such as refuse pits.

Postmortem skeletal modifications are fairly common and occur at six of the eleven sites with human remains. Cut marks are present on bone from two sites, while burning occurs at three of the sites. Approximately half of the bones from Mero/Diamond Bluff refuse pits are charred. This pattern is similar to many of the other mortuary sites in Minnesota, where secondary burial with cut marks related to defleshing is frequent; burning, given that it occurred in a habitation area, may be unintentional. Two examples of modified human remains from the Red Wing locality do not fit the characteristics of modification related strictly to mortuary processing or accidental burning. A cranial disk, or rondelle, was recovered from a burned house feature at the Bryan site (21GD04) along with the so-called trophy skull from which it was derived. Also present was another charred "trophy" skull (Blue 1997a). Teeth grooved for suspension were found at four other Red Wing locality sites (Table 13.1). These are fairly novel modifications in the context of the Upper Midwest. Rondelles are known from a small number of sites in Iowa, and the only other tooth modified for suspension is perforated, rather than grooved. This unprovenienced tooth is also from Iowa (Lillie 1996b; Schermer and Lillie, this volume).

Red Wing Sites Yielding Modified Teeth

Fort Sweney

Fort Sweney (21GD86) is located on a high promontory above the south bank of the Cannon River a little distance from its confluence with the Mississippi River. The site is composed of 7 mounds and another 30 embankments, pits, and other earthworks (Blue 1997b; Peterson 1986). When investigated by Edward Schmidt at the beginning of the twentieth century, Schmidt (1909) thought the location and earthworks were indicative of a fortress, hence the name of the site, but later archaeological investigations have not supported this (Borden 1963). Unlike most of the other Red Wing sites, Fort Sweney has no associated habitation area.

Five of the mounds at Fort Sweney were excavated in 1960–1962 by the Science Museum of Minnesota (Borden 1963; Peterson 1986). Five individuals were recovered during these excavations; all were primary burials (Blue 1997b). Four of the known remains were ostensibly recovered from Mound 1 while the fifth was discovered in Mound 3. Field notes are missing for the 1961–1962 excavations, but various newspapers reported the excavation of between two and six burials. A report in *American Antiquity* stated that eight individuals were recovered, but the remains were too fragmentary to assess sex or age (Borden 1963). Peterson (1986) also indicated that the Science Museum of Minnesota excavated five of the six known burial mounds and recovered eight burials. As noted above, only five individuals could be identified from the remains present at the time of my analysis. The most compelling of the burials is perhaps Mound 1, Burial 1: a young child found lying supine on a bed of Oneota dolomite pebbles and accompanied by 11 human teeth grooved for suspension (Woodbury 1961), likely the remains of a necklace (Figure 13.2). The child was 4.5–5.5 years of age and evinced a number of markers of stress, including growth retardation, Harris lines, cribra orbitalia, and endocranial lesions (Blue 1997b).

Duplication of elements, differential wear, and degree of root completion indicate that the teeth were from at least three individuals. O'Connell's (1995) analysis of the teeth prior to reburial noted that the root tip was incomplete in one of the teeth, a lower first premolar, indicating the individual

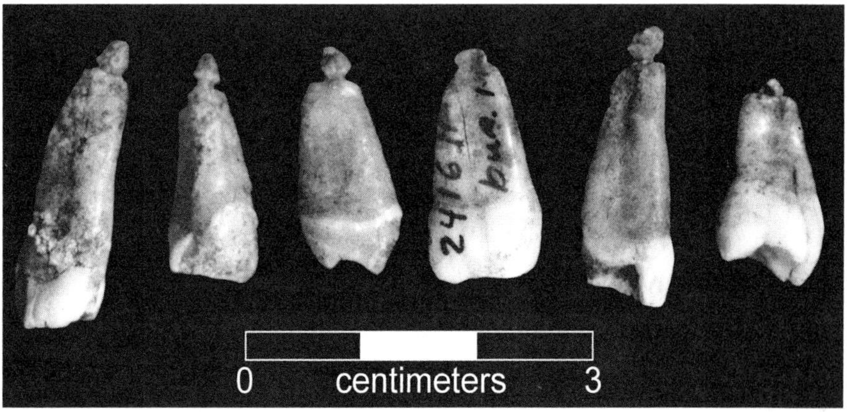

13.2. Teeth F–K from Fort Sweney (21GD86), showing typical Red Wing locality modification. (Photo by Kathleen Blue)

was less than 12–13 years of age, while the rest of the teeth show heavy wear and are likely to be from two older adults. A majority of the teeth are maxillary, and most are from the right side (Table 13.2). Most common were upper premolars, followed by incisors and then canines. Only one molar is present, and it has only a single root preserved. The tooth appears to have been modified after it was broken.

Mero/Diamond Bluff

The site with the next largest number of grooved teeth is Mero/Diamond Bluff (47PI02), located on a glacial outwash terrace overlooking the delta of the Trimbelle River in Pierce County, Wisconsin. Excavations and analyses of the site have been carried out by a number of researchers (Goldstein 1995; Masluk 1997; Maxwell 1950; Rodell 1991). Mero/Diamond Bluff is a mound and habitation site with over 300 mounds and a 15-acre village. The human remains from the site are from both mortuary (mounds) and nonmortuary (village) contexts. The mound burials (minimum number of individuals = 11), which include both primary and secondary inhumations, exhibit no modification.

Material from the habitation area includes approximately 85 isolated fragments currently housed at the Science Museum of Minnesota. An additional 200 fragments were unearthed during Alex's excavation (Alex 1974; Masluk 1997) and are curated by the University of Wisconsin, Milwaukee. Some of these fragments were recovered from "refuse pits," while others are merely described as being from the habitation area. Over 50 percent of the bone fragments from this area evince burning—possibly unintentional, given their

Table 13.2. Modified Teeth by Site

Fort Sweney	Mero/Diamond Bluff	Bartron	Adams
R I^1	upper R C	R I^1	L P^2
R I^2	R I^2	R M^3	
upper R C	L I^2		
R P_1	upper R C		
R P_2	R P^1		
R P^1	L P_1		
L P^1	R M_3		
L M_1 or M_2, mesial half			
L P^1 or P^2, crown missing			
R I^1			
upper R C			

context. Nine percent show some sign of cultural modification, including cut marks and grinding on bones and the grooving of seven teeth for suspension (see Table 13.1). As at Fort Sweney, multiple individuals are represented by the modified teeth. Also similar to the Fort Sweney example, the most commonly modified teeth are single-rooted, anterior maxillary teeth (see Table 13.2). The Mero teeth, however, differ from the Fort Sweney material in that they lack specific context and are also not associated with a specific individual. It is not known if the teeth were at any time associated with each other or were possibly awaiting incorporation into a future object.

Bartron

The Bartron site (21GD02) is located at the southern end of Prairie Island, a low-lying island situated between the Mississippi and Vermilion river deltas. Bartron is a small village site located on slightly higher land away from the water's edge. There were roughly 300 mounds on Prairie Island when it was mapped by Theodore Lewis in 1885 (Winchell 1911), some of which lay in close proximity to the Bartron site. Two teeth, both grooved for suspension, were found by Lloyd Wilford during his 1948 excavations at the site (Gibbon 1979:Plate 17.2): an adult right upper-central incisor and a right upper-third molar (see Table 13.2). The teeth are from separate excavation units (C and D) and were both found in the first level. The central incisor shows two distinct hypoplastic bands, suggesting the possibility of episodes of childhood stress. Both teeth are worn and could represent a single individual. However, different techniques used in the modification of the teeth most likely preclude this possibility. The incisor's root is grooved circumferentially while the root of the molar bears grooves, or notches, only on its lingual and buccal aspects.

Adams

The Adams site (47PI12) is a village and mortuary complex of at least 97 mounds in Pierce County, Wisconsin. Located on a terrace on the east side of the Mississippi, it is approximately six mi south of the Mero/Diamond Bluff site and has been extensively cultivated. The osteological analysis of material collected during 1984–1985 field seasons by the Institute for Minnesota Archaeology was carried out by Gretchen Nelson (1999). A small amount of human skeletal material was recovered, including three isolated bone fragments and five teeth. At least three individuals are represented based on age and the repetition of elements. A single tooth grooved for suspension was recovered from the top level of an arbitrary excavation unit in the village area (see Table 13.2). There is no further contextual information. Like the modified teeth from Fort Sweney and Mero, the grooved tooth recovered from the Adams site is a single-rooted, anterior permanent tooth from an adult individual.

Cultural Context of Red Wing Locality Teeth

Although all four sites had associated mortuary components, only Fort Sweney represents a clear mortuary context and thus preserves the modified teeth in their presumed cultural milieu, that is, as objects of personal adornment for the purposes of aesthetics, affiliation, or status marking. The description of the position of the 11 teeth from Fort Sweney implies they were likely suspended as part of a necklace or as decorations around the neck opening of an item of clothing. Of particular note is the fact that they are adorning a young child. In contrast, all the remaining grooved teeth were recovered from habitation areas and in nonmortuary contexts, including some described as refuse pits. Perhaps these teeth were accidently lost or were purposely discarded, either as a ritual act or merely as objects no longer important to their possessor.

The Manufacture of Teeth into Cultural Objects

The modified teeth from Red Wing locality sites show similar modification: one or more grooves have been cut into the roots within millimeters of the root's apex. The teeth, however, exhibit two different modes of manufacture. While some of the roots have been notched on opposing sides (e.g., on the buccal and lingual surfaces), others exhibit a groove around the entire circumference of the root. Specifics of manufacture were collected from three of the sites: Fort Sweney, Bartron, and Adams.

The teeth from Fort Sweney exhibit both styles of manufacture. Teeth A–F are notched on the buccal and lingual aspects of their roots, while Teeth G–K are grooved completely around the tooth root (O'Connell 1995). The single tooth from Adams is described as having a circular groove, .83 mm in width, which extends around the entire root with a visible starting and stopping point (Nelson 1999). The two teeth from Bartron differ from each other in their manufacturing techniques. The root of the incisor is grooved circumferentially similar to the Adams tooth and to the Fort Sweney G–K teeth. The molar resembles the Fort Sweney A–F teeth, being grooved on its buccal and lingual sides only. Interestingly, all recorded notching occurs buccolingually rather than mesiodistally. This orientation may be related to a preference for the labial/lingual side of the tooth crown to be visible when suspended.

The two types of manufacture, and the presence of both types at a single site, suggest that more than one individual in Red Wing society was involved in the manufacture of human teeth into ornaments. Pereira (2005) analyzed culturally modified bone from Zacapú, Mexico, and found similar styles in overall bone modification at Zacapú but also noted subtle stylistic differences, suggesting more than one manufacturer. The same seems to be true for the Red Wing locality sites. The comparable placement of the modification on the root and the use of only two different techniques (circumferential and buccolingual notching) suggest that there is some cultural or physical constraint on tooth modification techniques in the Red Wing locality. It may be that strong traditions hold sway and limit the amount of cultural variation. On the other hand, physical limitations may be at work. The innate qualities of the teeth or their intended usage may have varied. Perhaps perforation, another common method for the suspension of teeth, was not possible due to the size or fragile nature of the teeth.

Choice of Tooth Type

Drawing on the Red Wing data, a pattern emerges in which only the permanent dentition was used in the production of tooth ornaments, and anterior teeth were preferred over posterior teeth (18 vs. 3). Teeth from the right side were twice as likely to be used (14 vs. 7) than those from the left. The most frequently used teeth were premolars (8), followed by incisors (6), canines (4), and molars (3). Maxillary teeth were far more commonly used than mandibular teeth (16 vs. 5), and all molars used were single-rooted.

Chi-squares were performed for the following categories: left vs. right;

Table 13.3. Chi-Squares for Left vs. Right, Maxillary vs. Mandibular, Anterior vs. Posterior, and Tooth Type

Left vs. Right

	Observed	Expected	(O-E)	$(O-E)^2$	$(O-E)^2$ / E
left	7	10.5	3.5	12.25	1.166
right	14	10.5	3.5	12.25	1.166
					2.33

Maxillary vs. Mandibular

	Observed	Expected	(O-E)	$(O-E)^2$	$(O-E)^2$ / E
maxillary	16	10.5	5.5	30.25	2.88
mandibular	5	10.5	5.5	30.25	2.88
					5.76*

Anterior vs. Posterior

	Observed	Expected	(O-E)	$(O-E)^2$	$(O-E)^2$ / E
anterior	18	10.5	7.5	56.25	5.36
posterior	3	10.5	7.5	56.25	5.36
					10.72**

Tooth Type

	Observed	Expected	(O-E)	$(O-E)^2$	$(O-E)^2$ / E
incisor	6	5.25	.75	.5625	.11
canine	4	5.25	1.25	1.5625	.30
premolar	8	5.25	2.75	7.5625	1.44
molar	3	5.25	2.25	5.0625	.96
					2.81

Note: *p = .05
**p = .01

maxillary vs. mandibular; anterior vs. posterior; and tooth type (Table 13.3). The anterior vs. posterior and maxillary vs. mandibular categories were found to be significant; that is, preferences for both anterior teeth and maxillary teeth exceeded that expected by chance alone.

All of the teeth from Red Wing, as well as all other similarly modified teeth that could be located in the literature (Bishop Museum 2010 [1892]; Ifantidis 2006; Jacobi 2007; Pitt Rivers Museum 2009; Skinner 1916; Webb and DeJarnette 1942, among others), are from the permanent dentition. This preference for permanent teeth may reflect functional or practical considerations (such as their larger size and the fact that they generally occur in greater numbers in the mouth compared to the smaller, less numerous deciduous teeth); in addition, the roots of permanent teeth are also more apt to be long enough for modification compared to the roots of deciduous teeth, which often are significantly resorbed on all but the youngest dentition. The preference for permanent (i.e., adult) dentition likely also reflects the way children are perceived in these societies. Deciduous teeth are understandably associated with children, and children in many societies lack status and are not considered full members of the group before their transition into adults. In societies where ancestor worship is prominent, death in childhood prohibits individuals from attaining an ancestor position since they will produce no descendants. Teeth themselves often figure into this determination of status. Among the Igbos of Nigeria, children who die before they have cut their first teeth are not accorded burial in the communal cemetery but are instead thrown away or placed in the bush (Basden 2009), while in the Buntao society of Southeast Asia infants without erupted teeth receive different mortuary treatment than individuals with teeth, who are deemed adults (Tsintjilonis 2000).

At Red Wing and generally speaking elsewhere, there appears to be a predilection for anterior teeth (Bishop Museum 2010 [1892]; Pitt Rivers Museum 2009; Skinner 1916). A few exceptions to this pattern are noted, however, including a single perforated molar from Dispilio, a Neolithic site in Greece (Ifantidis 2006); the incorporation of human molars into the design of a historic Hawaiian sash currently housed in the Bishop Museum, Hawaii; and a fairly even division among all four tooth classes (incisors, canines, premolars, and molars) in the 150 or so teeth associated with the "dentist" or "bone picker" burial at the Bluff Creek site in Alabama (Jacobi 2007; Webb and DeJarnette 1942). Several likely reasons for choosing the anterior teeth present themselves. Possibly, anterior teeth are more favored because they are the teeth that can be easily seen. Modifications to the teeth in living individuals (ablation, sharpening, semiprecious stone insets, among others) are all performed on anterior teeth since they are the ones visible. It is also true that their form more closely resembles shells and other preferred ornaments than do molar teeth. Another possibility is their similarity to the nonhuman teeth often used for ornamentation by different human societies—the incisors of elk or deer or the canines of bears or wolves (Carr and Case 2005; Issenman 1997). Most likely, it is the presence of a single root that is the deciding factor in their usage as cultural objects. Single roots make anterior teeth easier to remove; they also play a role in the propensity of anterior teeth to simply fall out of their crypts after death. Molars, which commonly have more than one root, are the most infrequently used teeth in Red Wing, and those that are present have single roots: two are single-rooted third molars while the third example, which originally possessed more than one root, was likely broken before being fashioned into an ornament. In its current state, this molar exhibits a single root.

There also appears to be a strong preference for maxillary teeth at Red Wing. The reasons for this are not known, but perhaps they are preferred because of their larger overall size or the fact that in living people maxillary teeth are more visible than mandibular teeth. Another possibility is that the mandible of deceased individuals is considered to be a separate cultural object. This conjecture is supported by the discovery in refuse pits at Mero/Diamond Bluff of three charred mandible fragments and four nearly complete mandibles bearing cut marks. Additionally, there are reports of five nested mandibles uncovered elsewhere at Mero/Diamond Bluff, although the veracity of this story cannot be confirmed and the present location of these remains is not known (Clark Dobbs, personal communication 2006). At Bryan (21GD04), another Red Wing locality site, a complete mandible with two puncture-type perforations was recovered from a refuse pit (Blue 1997a). If these reports are accurate, they lend credence to the idea that mandibles were defined as cultural objects in their own right. This is not surprising, given the significance that mandibles appear to have had for both Hopewellian and Mississippian peoples. Both groups frequently used human mandibles as ritual objects and as items of adornment (see chapters in this volume by Cobb; Johnston; Munson, Cook, and Powell; Nawrocki and Emanovsky; Schermer and Lillie).

Another noted characteristic of the grooved teeth from the Red Wing locality was their overall poor condition. While the teeth show little post-deposition damage, the majority of them were worn, several showed signs of antemortem breakage, and one exhibited hypoplastic bands. These conditions occurred during the life of the original possessor(s) of the teeth. Obviously, the teeth were not chosen for their pristine condition. Was it just happenstance that these were the available teeth? Or do they instead represent the teeth of relatives (or enemies)? Is it the tooth or the individual it came from that is most important?

Conclusions

The grooved teeth from the Red Wing locality do not exist in a vacuum. They are merely one facet of the elaborate mortuary treatment present at Red Wing sites in the period A.D. 1050–1300. This treatment includes disaggregation of the body, burning, cut marks, drilling, grooving, puncturing, and the creation of trophy skulls. The Red Wing locality itself is part of a larger scenario seen throughout precontact Minnesota, which stressed secondary burial and the defleshing and disarticulation of at least some of the deceased.

When we contemplate the grooved teeth from Red Wing, we see two processes at work. The first concerns the fragmentation of the body and the subsequent loss of identity. Mortuary studies stress that death is a process that transforms a deceased's status from that of "actor" to "object" (Parker Pearson 1999). The human body plays a significant role in the construction of self-identity. In addition to an individual "being defined as a single person by the boundaries of the body" (Sofaer 2006:22), the body affects our self-image and acts as a medium for transforming our image during life (e.g., tattoos, piercings, weight loss or gain, body building, among others). The physical body can be altered for the purposes of status or affiliation, as is seen in artificial cranial modification (Blom 2005). At death, the body begins a journey from a social persona to a purely biological entity. The increasing fragmentation of the body after death results in a loss of individual identity. This process can be speeded up by deliberate defleshing and disarticulation, as well as by the incorporation of the resultant fragments into building blocks, so to speak, of another individual's social persona.

In many instances, this newly constructed social persona is not purely the work of the individual incorporating the teeth but is an ongoing mediation between the individual and the group. Therefore, the disembodied teeth represent the loss of individual identity, but simultaneously represent the acquisition of group identity. Hegmon (1992) noted that the stylistic information that is highly visible is most often used to indicate group or ethnic boundaries. Personal adornment has its beginnings in the Paleolithic. Teeth, first those of other animals but followed quickly by those human in origin, are some of the first materials to be used for this purpose. Several researchers, including White (1993), have tied the phenomenon of adornment to the use of clothing and other manipulations of the body to address, convey, and comment on major social categories, such as sex, age, and status. These categories are associated with the very beginnings of society and social communication.

A number of archaeologists have commented on various forms of stylistic communication (Hegmon 1992:References). Wiessner (1983) identified two types of stylistic communication: emblemic, which has a distinct referent and is used to convey ethnic or boundary information; and assertive, which speaks more to individual identity and expression. These are similar to distinctions put forth by Macdonald (1990), which he labels "protocol" and "panache": protocol deals with group identity while panache is more individualistic. The modified teeth from Red Wing seem to more closely align with emblemic or protocol types of stylistic expression, given their widespread appearance throughout the Red Wing locality sites and their absence outside of this region. They appear to function as cues to social identities, perhaps as devices that indicate to participants what categories of people are present and "overcommunicate" their affiliation for the purpose of behavioral expectations (Schortman 1989).

The grooved teeth from the Red Wing locality have two possible sources: they are either the disaggregated remains of kin or the remnants of outsiders. As I have argued elsewhere (Blue 2006), our present knowledge more fully supports the idea that specialized long-term mortuary treatment is reserved for members of the group. The inclusion of the grooved teeth from Fort Sweney in a young child's grave gives credibility to this supposition, given the unlikelihood that the child acquired the teeth as a result of battle—a common scenario for the acquisition of enemy body parts in societies elsewhere in the world (Best 1934; Chacon and Dye, ed. 2007; Harrison 2006). It seems much more likely that the teeth at Fort Sweney instead signify a group or lineage demarcation specific to the child with whom they were interred. Ample evidence of the incorporation of a family or group member's body parts into the society's rituals by which membership is affirmed can be found in the anthropological literature (see, e.g., Barley 1995; Knudson et al. 2009). However, regardless of their original provenience, Parker Pearson (1999:52) suggested that "the disaggregation of the body may be an ideological imperative by which the individual is denied and the collective asserted; the physical body acts as a metaphor of social organization." Grooved teeth at Red Wing, by their very nature, act as a symbol of group identity. This is especially true if the incorporated teeth represent the remains of kinfolk.

During the late precontact period in Red Wing, identity was in large part created and maintained by the construction of the mounds and the associated mortuary rituals carried out as part of the overarching burial program. The use of human teeth as cultural objects is but one element in that larger picture. The manufacture and possession of these teeth may have functioned on several levels, serving to delineate clans or lineages within the larger group, while simultaneously acting as emblems of the group at large.

Acknowledgments

I wish to thank the Minnesota Indian Affairs Council and Barbara O'Connell, professor emerita, Hamline University, for allowing access to the skeletal material. I would also like to thank Ron Schirmer for his help and the Red Wing Publication Project for financial support. Additionally, I am grateful to the anonymous reviewers of the book for their helpful comments and to the editors, Eve Hargrave, Kris Hedman, Robin Lillie, and Shirley Schermer, for their input and hard work.

14

Design Motifs and Other Modifications of Human Bone from Iowa Late Prehistoric Oneota Sites

Robin M. Lillie and Shirley J. Schermer

Archaeological evidence of the late prehistoric Oneota tradition can be found throughout the Upper Midwest (Green 1995; Hollinger 2005). In Iowa, Oneota sites date from around A.D. 1150 to 1700, with villages primarily concentrated in the northeastern, northwestern, southeastern, and central parts of the state (Alex 2000). Archaeological and osteological studies from Oneota sites in Iowa add to the growing body of evidence that demonstrates the diversity of Oneota treatment of human remains (Schermer and Lillie 2007). Oneota cemeteries were often separate from village areas (e.g., Bray 1961; Orr 1934; Schermer et al. 1998), with burials occasionally intruding into Woodland mounds (e.g., Lillie 2002a; Orr 1934, 1937; Schermer et al. 1998). Primary and secondary interments have been found within villages (e.g., Gradwohl 1973; Lillie 1996a; McKusick 1973; Schermer et al. 1995), with incomplete skeletons and isolated skeletal elements frequently recovered from cache pits (e.g., Hodges 1994; Hollinger and Vradenburg 1994; Lillie 1990; Moffat et al. 1990) and village middens (e.g., Lillie 2002b; Moffat et al. 1990).

Each of these contexts has yielded culturally modified human bone. Alterations include burning, cut marks, the application of red ochre, engraving or incising, and polishing. Intentionally placed cuts, incised designs, deliberate polishing, or some combination of these elements suggest the purposeful transformation of human bones, imbuing them with deeper cultural meaning.

Examples of Purposeful Bone Modifications

"Incising" or "engraving" on bone is defined here as cut marks that result from deliberate decorative embellishment rather than defleshing, disarticulation, or scalping. All of the Iowa examples of incising on human bone occur on cranial elements, and the described examples come from domestic contexts in late prehistoric Oneota villages. Several fragments display polishing

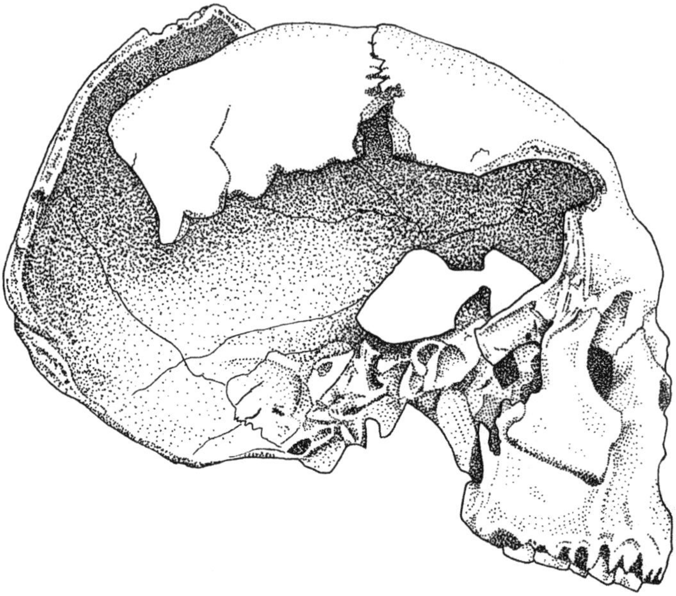

14.1. Right lateral view of modified cranium found eroding from a cache pit at the Dixon site (13WD8). The right parietal and frontal modification of the inferior edge produced notches that were smoothed, perhaps from wear. The bone inferior to the notched edge was not recovered. (Drawing by Liz Niec, courtesy of University of Iowa Office of the State Archaeologist)

or smoothed edges in addition to deliberate incising. "Polishing" here refers to abrasion, patina, or smoothing resulting from intentional modification or from handling or wear. Although most examples consist of fragments, one nearly complete cranium from the Dixon site displays deliberate cutting, serration, and polishing.

Dixon

The Dixon village (13WD8) is situated along the Little Sioux River in western Iowa and dates to A.D. 1300–1440, identified as the Correctionville phase (Fishel 1999:134). The site has yielded two distinctive examples of culturally modified cranial remains.

A cranium collected from the bottom of an eroding cache pit (Figure 14.1) represents an adult male, approximately 25–35 years of age at time of death (Lillie 1999). Although portions of the ectocranial surface were eroded, numerous fine cut marks are present on the frontal bone, left parietal, left temporal, occipital, right zygoma, and both maxillae. The location and orientation of some of these cut marks suggest, minimally, defleshing and

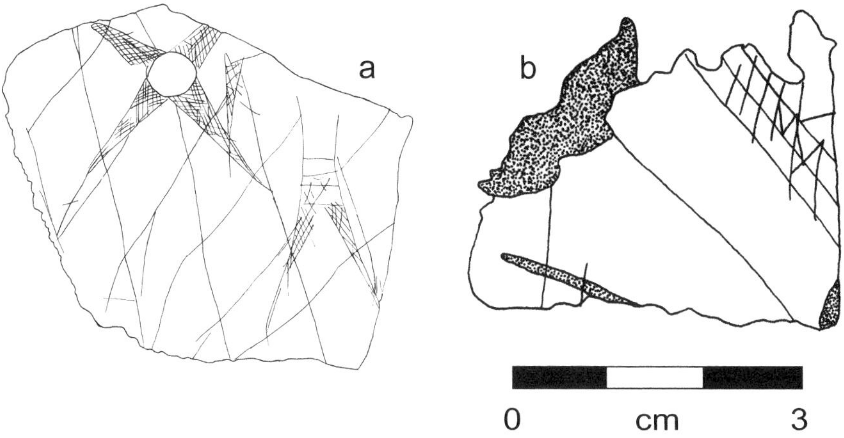

14.2. (a) Modified superior frontal bone from the Dixon site (13WD8); (b) burned, polished, and incised fragment from the McKinney site (13LA1). Note the similarity in the crosshatching between the McKinney fragment and the Dixon details. (Drawing by Liz Niec, courtesy of University of Iowa Office of the State Archaeologist)

disarticulation of the mandible. The right parietal and the right lateral portion of the frontal bone exhibit further cultural modification. The bone was cut approximately 7 cm inferior to the sagittal suture. The modified margin is 8.1 cm in length, affecting the anterior two-thirds of the parietal and extending onto the frontal bone. Along the posterior half of this modified margin, cuts approximately 1.2 cm apart form three downward-pointing V or U shapes, creating a notched border. The notching continued anteriorly, as at least one more point had broken off postdepositionally. The edges of the cut margin are smoothed and rounded. Notching as seen in this cranium is an unusual type of bone modification for Oneota sites and others in the Midwest.

A finely incised frontal fragment, now in a private collection, reportedly was recovered from a cutbank at the Dixon site (Fishel 1999; Schermer and Owsley 1989–1990b) (Figure 14.2a). The ectocranial surface is covered with a widely spaced diamond-shaped or crosshatched design. A circle with four triangular-shaped projections resembles a star or sun, perhaps representing the four cardinal directions. Each of the four projections is filled with fine, closely spaced crosshatching. An adjacent motif appears to be the body, tail, and wing tips of a bird-like figure, possibly the lower portion of an anthropomorphic figure.

Schmeiser

The Schmeiser village (13DM101) is located in southeastern Iowa on a low terrace in the broad Mississippi River floodplain (Straffin 1972a, 1972b; Tiffany 1979, 1982). Schmeiser is the typesite for the Oneota Burlington phase. Most dates from Burlington phase sites fall in the early 1300s (Alex 2000:193).

Two parietal fragments, likely from different individuals, were recovered from the plow zone and midden during excavations conducted in the early 1970s. One fragment was unmodified. The second fragment consists of the parietal just posterior to the coronal suture and superior to the squamosal suture, measures 47 mm x 51 mm, and ranges from 4 mm to 8 mm in thickness. Twelve finely incised lines are observed on the ectocranial surface, varying in length from 1.66 mm to 43.89 mm (Lillie and Hollinger 2002:43). Most of the lines run roughly parallel to one another, with two lines transecting them. Some of the cuts extend to the fragment margin, suggesting that the incisions may have continued onto adjacent, now absent, bone. The entire ectocranial surface has been polished. The inferior edge displays evidence of rounding and polishing resulting from handling or wear. Hollinger (2005:67) speculated that this fragment derived from a larger cranial portion used as a bowl.

Wever

About 28 km south-southwest of Schmeiser is the Wever village (13LE110). The site dates to A.D. 1250–1350 and also is included in the Burlington phase (Hollinger 2005:47).

Excavations at the site revealed probable burials in the village (defined on the basis of feature stain shape and size and the presence of human bone or teeth on exposed feature surfaces that were unexcavated), one flexed burial in a cache pit, and one case of partially articulated elements encountered in a cache pit (Hollinger 2005; Hollinger and Vradenburg 1994). A number of isolated human elements and bone fragments were recovered from the site surface, village midden, and cache pits.

One incomplete cranium recovered from a cache pit possibly represents a young to middle-aged adult female. The cranium shows incised cuts on the ectocranial surface, polishing ectocranially and endocranially, and small areas of burning. One edge of the left parietal displays evidence of rounding and polishing resulting from handling or wear. Hollinger (2005:61–62) suggested possible use of this cranial portion as a tool, dish, or bowl.

McKinney

The McKinney village (13LA1) is located on a bluff overlooking the Mississippi River in southeastern Iowa, approximately 16 km upstream from the Schmeiser site (Fokken 1979; Hollinger 2005; Hollinger et al. 1999; Lillie 1996c, 2002c; Slattery 1979; Slattery et al. 1975; Tiffany 1988; Young 1981a, 1981b). The site dates to A.D. 1400–1650 (Hollinger 2005:53). A number of burials have been found at the site among storage and refuse pits and in large post structures that probably represent houses.

One partially excavated refuse feature contained an articulated forearm missing the hand (Hollinger 2005:103). Several cranial fragments, all apparently from adult individuals, exhibit artificial polishing, smoothing, deliberate incising, or some combination of these modifications. Two parietal fragments, recovered from the plow zone above a hearth, exhibit polishing both ectocranially and endocranially. One, identified as a right parietal, has seven roughly parallel, incised lines approximately 45 mm in length extending from bregma toward the temporal bone (Fokken 1979:1). Just posterior to the parallel cut marks is an eighth incised line that curves slightly, transecting two of the parallel lines. A shorter cut mark extends from the curved line to the coronal suture just anterior to the posteriormost of the seven parallel lines. Although the fragment was not available for our examination, the published drawing (Fokken 1979:2) indicates that several of the incised lines continued onto now-missing bone.

Several isolated pieces of human bone—a vertebra, a metatarsal, and cranial fragments—were found in what Hollinger (2005:101) termed a large communal roasting pit. A burned occipital fragment from the area of the occipital protuberance measures 39 mm by 31 mm, and contains 34 incised lines ranging in length from about 3 mm to 24 mm (Lillie 2002c). Incising occurred after the fragment was burned since the marks clearly cut through the burned outer surface. Several of the incised lines extend to the edge of the broken medial margin, suggesting that they likely continued onto the adjacent bone. The fragment shows evidence of having been burned again after it was broken. The longest mark is also significantly wider and deeper than the other cuts, indicating repeated cutting or sawing. A small area of abrasion, about 8 mm x 8 mm, is noted in the superior-lateral portion of the fragment. Another small, highly polished parietal fragment found in the plow zone (Figure 14.2b) measures 18 mm x 13 mm, and exhibits 17 cuts forming a crosshatch pattern (Lillie 1996c). The lines range in length from 4 mm to 11 mm. This bone also had been burned prior to the polishing and incising. The crosshatched marks extend to the coronal suture and may have extended onto the frontal bone.

An unsided parietal fragment, probably from an adult, was recovered from a bell-shaped pit that likely had been used for storage and then refilled with refuse (Lillie 2002c). The fragment is from the inferior margin, including a portion of the squamosal suture, and measures 21 mm anteroposteriorly and 16 mm superioinferiorly. The bone is burned heavily and blackened on the inferior two-thirds, with polishing on the burned portion of the endocranial surface. Breakage along the superior margin occurred after the fragment was burned. The fragment displays six cut marks ranging in length from 3 mm to 11 mm. Five are oriented in an anteroposterior direction with the sixth angling slightly toward the superior margin.

Cultural Meaning of Incised and Polished Bone

The majority of cut marks and burning observed in material from late prehistoric Iowa sites appears to be associated with defleshing, disarticulation, other processing, and/or ritual. However, the examples presented here show evidence of deliberate cutting or incising, polishing, and burning, which suggests purposeful transformation into objects with deeper cultural meaning.

Hollinger (2005) divided the Oneota tradition into four horizons: Emergent (pre-A.D. 1150), Developmental (A.D. 1150–1400), Classic (A.D. 1400–1650), and Historic (A.D. 1650–1800). The Schmeiser and Wever sites are generally contemporaneous with the Dixon site, and all are from the Developmental horizon, while occupations at the McKinney site are part of the later Classic horizon.

Incising on human cranial remains has been described for several late prehistoric and Oneota sites across the Upper Midwest and Great Plains (e.g., Hedman, this volume). The Schmeiser and Wever sites are contemporaneous with sites belonging to the Bold Counselor phase in west-central Illinois, which contain evidence for violence and trophy taking. To date, there has been sparse osteological evidence of violence in Iowa Oneota sites, although cut marks on cranial fragments and remains have been attributed to scalping and violence (e.g., Hollinger 2005; Moffat et al. 1990). The small size of many of these fragments makes it difficult, if not impossible, to differentiate between cut marks that may have resulted from scalping, disarticulation, or some other form of cultural manipulation. One documented example of injury possibly resulting from violence comes from the early Oneota Anthon site (13WD10) in western Iowa. Burials disturbed during construction included the remains of an adult female with a complete projectile point embedded in the arch of one of nine recovered thoracic vertebrae. The individual had survived long enough for some degree of healing to occur and for the adjacent rib to fuse to the arch (Anderson 1971:11).

The Dixon site is contemporaneous with the Leary site in extreme southeastern Nebraska and with the earliest occupations at the Utz site in Missouri. The incising and polishing of human bone has been reported for both Leary and Utz. Similarities in pottery styles suggest contact among inhabitants of these villages and Correctionville phase villages in northwestern Iowa, including Dixon (Henning 1970). Hollinger (2005:194) illustrated a human calvarium from the Leary site with cut marks, polish, and an incised image he refers to as a "thunderer" (similar to images described elsewhere as a birdman or thunderbird). The Leary illustration was provided by an anonymous collector who reportedly found the bone on the surface of that site; we were unable to directly view the modified bone. Two culturally modified crania from Utz also were illustrated by Hollinger (2005:247). Both have worked edges that he describes as bowl lips. One of the crania, consisting of an incomplete left parietal, has an encircled four-projection "star" design with linear fill and a separate crescent design to one side. Although there are some stylistic similarities, this motif differs from the Dixon fragment's crosshatch-filled projections emanating from a central circle (see Figure 14.2a). Henning (1970:120) also described a burned portion of a "skull bowl" from Utz consisting of an occipital and both parietals. He noted a cut and polished edge on the occipital, a cut parallel to the polished edge, and "fine scratches" covering the exterior surface. Bray (1991:85, 88) described and illustrated three other incised human cranial fragments from Utz. While most purposely incised human bone from Oneota contexts is cranial, Betancourt (1965:262) illustrated an unusual example of a modified human femur shaft incised with an anthropomorphic figure and other motifs.

Cut marks are reported from a number of other Oneota sites in the Midwest, and more examples of deliberate modifications likely exist. Written descriptions of cut marks are not always clear enough to permit the reader to distinguish between cut marks indicative of scalping or defleshing from those with a more "decorative" or symbolic purpose. Also, researchers routinely attribute cut marks on small fragments to scalping rather than considering other causative actions.

One recently discovered example of intentional, possibly decorative incising may provide insight into the manufacture of these incised fragments. A cranium of a young adult female found on a sandbar in the Nodaway River in Adams County, southwestern Iowa, is of uncertain cultural affiliation (Schermer 2009). While the original context of the cranium is unknown, it is assumed to have eroded from a site upstream. Although found on a river sandbar, the cranium was not sun bleached nor characterized by abnormal weight due to mineralization, suggesting fairly recent erosion from a nearby site. So far, efforts to locate that site have been unsuccessful. The preponderance of the osteological evidence suggests that the racial affiliation is prehistoric American Indian. The cranium is missing the maxillae, palatine bones, zygomatic arches, and nasal bones. Postdepositional damage includes a fracture on the right parietal starting at the sagittal suture and extending to the inferior

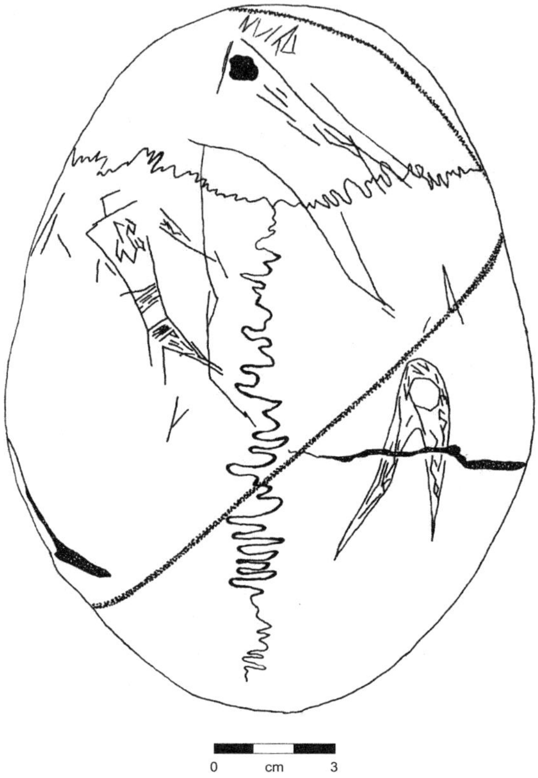

14.3. Superior view of the Nodaway River cranium, illustrating two of the incised images, a birdman and a forked eye. (Drawing by Liz Niec, courtesy of University of Iowa Office of the State Archaeologist)

border. The occipital base was intentionally removed, creating a nearly symmetrical excised area with smooth and slightly polished margins, possibly as a result of use-wear. Two deep, wide, grooved cuts cross the frontal and parietals. The first groove, 182 mm in length, starts on the left parietal, crosses the sagittal suture, and intersects with the second cut. This second groove, 178 mm long, starts above the left orbit, angles superiorly across the frontal bone, and crosses at the right coronal suture onto the right parietal. Numerous fine incised cuts across the ectocranial surface form a "forked eye," a "birdman," and other classic Oneota motifs (Figure 14.3). The entire cranium has weathered to a light brown, and all the cuts—both the wide, deep cuts and the small, fine cuts—have weathered to the same color and patina. Large areas of bone cortex have exfoliated.

Several of the designs on this cranium are similar to Oneota iconography found on pottery, catlinite tablets, and petroglyphs. An anthropomorphic birdman/thunderbird is located on the left parietal. The line-filled wings/arms flare out from the body; the line-filled tail/legs are bifurcated and end in points. Two bands of horizontal lines are located on the main body. The head, although slightly damaged, is complete enough to tell that it was a simple square without a beak. Eric Hollinger (personal communication 2009) noted the unusually shaped heart-line, which is a mace-like form with three points. He likened it to a similar heart-line on a thunderbird on a hematite tablet from Utz. A line intersecting one leg and one arm/wing extends onto the frontal, terminating at a long, vertical, curved line. Several elements of this motif are similar to the birdman/thunderbird images on the Dixon cranial fragment, on a potsherd from the McKinney site (Hollinger 2005:105), and on the New Albin tablet (Bray 1963:34). Although an incised "thunderer" was present on a human calvarium from Leary (Hollinger 2005:194), the two images share only a few common elements. A range of variations in stylized representations and specific attributes in birdman/thunderbird/thunderer images is illustrated in Benn (1989:247) and Hollinger (2005:274). Benn also discussed the Oneota ceramic motif of nested chevrons as stylized representations of the thunderbird's wing.

A forked eye located on the right parietal of the Nodaway cranium consists of a circle surrounded by a line-filled zone that projects beyond the circle to form two points, or "forks." Similar forked eyes are seen on catlinite tablets and pottery (e.g., Betancourt 1965; Bray 1963; Hollinger 2005). A second, incomplete birdman/thunderbird is incised posterior and inferior to the forked eye. Also posterior to the forked eye, and on the same section of cranium, are three pointed, line-filled projections emanating from an unclearly defined center. A fourth projection, which would complete an image similar to the four-pointed star seen at Dixon, and some common elements with the example described from Utz may be present but cannot be completely defined. Scattered throughout the cranial vault are partial motifs or images as well as small areas of seemingly random shallow cuts that may have had meaning to the inscriber or may indicate the start of unfinished motifs. Variations in the depth of the cuts of some motifs suggest multiple episodes of incising.

The Nodaway River drainage and surrounding drainages flow into nearby northwestern Missouri, emptying into the Missouri River near St. Joseph. The upper reaches of the Nodaway, the Platte, and the Grand rivers in Iowa are only miles apart (in adjacent counties). While there are no recorded Oneota sites in this part of Iowa, there may be a possible relationship to Oneota sites in southeastern Nebraska, northeastern Kansas, and Missouri. Historically, the Iowa tribe camped at various times along the Nodaway River, and the

Otoe and Kansa peoples had villages along the Missouri near the mouth of the Nodaway (Blaine 1995:83, 134, 175, 210, 237).

The Nodaway River cranium may shed light on the production of smaller fragments. The deep, saw-mark-like, grooved cuts appear to divide the cranium into three sections. These cuts, similar in appearance to scoring seen on some catlinite tablets (Dale Henning, personal communication 2009), likely required a different tool than that used to make the finer marks. Each of the three sections contains specific design elements. Assuming that the deep scoring would serve to ultimately divide the cranium into separate pieces, we cannot determine why the process of division was interrupted. This could be the only documented example of how the smaller culturally modified cranial fragments may have been created. If smaller segments were curated or somehow utilized over a period of time, they may have become even more fragmented and worn along some edges, resulting in pieces containing only portions of the original design. Some of the small fragments with cut marks previously attributed to possible defleshing or scalping may actually have broken from larger, deliberately modified pieces of bone.

Many of the described incised lines reflect motifs found on Oneota pottery, catlinite tablets, and rock art, possibly a manifestation of the power or importance of these particular images in the Oneota belief system. The choice of these motifs may suggest particular uses or meanings for the incised bone. The most distinct motifs on the examples described are the four-pointed star, forked eye, and birdman or thunderbird. The four-pointed star and other astronomical images seen on the cranial fragments from the Dixon and Utz sites and on the Nodaway River cranium may reflect an aspect of a group's cosmology. Death was associated with night and stars in several historic Plains groups (Fletcher and La Flesche 1992; Hall 1997).

Birds played a significant role in the life of prehistoric peoples, and some may have seen them as sacred animals. A great variety of birds have been identified in the faunal assemblages from late prehistoric archaeological sites throughout the midwestern region. They were used for food, feathers, artifacts, ornamentation, ceremonial paraphernalia, medicine bundles, and symbolic designs. Ethnographic accounts have documented the important role that raptors (especially hawks, eagles, and falcons) played in the ceremonial life of many Plains and midwestern Indian groups (e.g., Blaine 1995; Hall 1997; Radin 1990; Skinner 1926). The eye of a falcon appears as a "forked-eye" design to the viewer (Benn 1989:249). Possibly, this motif symbolized the raptor's defining characteristics of excellent vision and hunting skills and helped transmit these abilities to human beings.

In Oneota iconography, a bird image is sometimes morphed into a part-bird, part-human motif, hence the use of the term "birdman." Benn (1989: 245) described the birdman image as a blend of cosmological and human themes where birds are anthropomorphized by rendering wings as arms and tail feathers as legs. Although Benn (1989) and Hollinger (2005), among others, have associated the thunderbird or thunderer with warfare, others have proposed a different or more expanded role. Radin (1990) described a dualistic cosmological theme for the Winnebagos (Ho-Chunks), which is expressed in their concept of an upper world and a lower world; the need to maintain balance in both nature and social order; and the need for the renewal of order in a chaotic world. The Thunderbird clan, the largest and most important clan in the upper world, was paired with the Warrior clan, which conducted wars for the tribe. "Thunderbirds are powerful spirits who are approachable by humans as guardians and helpmates. Lightning flashes from their eyes, and thunder is caused by the flapping of their wings" (Birmingham and Eisenberg 2000:117). A Meskwaki world origin story depicts Thunderer as a benevolent, earth-shaping spirit (Green 1996:7; Michelson 1930:120–121).

Conclusion

The small, highly polished cranial fragments bearing decorative incising and the modified crania seem to imply a cultural practice other than or beyond simply violence or warfare-related trophy taking. Possibly, such modification and subsequent use of human bone fulfilled a necessary rite or ritual, served a symbolic role reflecting ideology, or was a remembrance of a person or event. Cranial fragments with worn edges and polishing provide evidence of handling that can be interpreted as curation or ritual use, possibly short term since the objects were ultimately discarded. Some of the fragments exhibit a sequence of modifications (such as incising followed by burning followed by wear and polishing) that could suggest changes in the function of the object over time. A critical factor underlying the ultimate disposal of such remains may have been returning them to the earth once the object had served its purpose. This explanation may account for the seemingly casual discarding of modified bone in middens or cache pits. Just as we do not know how the Oneota viewed these objects, we do not know how the Oneota viewed the pits and middens in which they are found. It may be culturally biased to presume they were defined as "garbage pits," as locations for unwanted items. Possibly, the culturally decorated or modified bone was purposely placed in villages, especially in locations shared by a select group of individuals (cache pit) or, potentially, all residents (midden). Alternatively, the final disposition may not have been a critical factor once the remains had served their purpose.

Oneota peoples across the midcontinent likely would have recognized the meaning and significance of the widely used motifs described in this chapter. All of the above examples of incised human bone except one are cranial remains, which in itself could be significant. Cranial bone may have been purposely selected as symbolic of the identity, "soul," or power of the deceased, whether sourced from a specific member of the community or from an outsider or adversary. Use of the cranium as a medium may have enhanced or increased the significance or strength of the iconographic images, subsequently aiding in the transmission of powers or abilities to human beings.

While the meaning or purpose of culturally modified cranial fragments remains elusive, the Nodaway sandbar cranium reveals much about the process of their origin, manufacture, and use-life. That scattered pieces of cranial bone in a site could have been derived from a single cranium may imply a shared meaning for Oneota groups—either all members of a village or a select few, such as the family of the deceased, or a broader regional shared symbolism or ideology. If a cranium or skull was the starting point of modification, this could mean that the individual from whom it came may have been more significant than isolated cranial fragments would suggest. Portions of a single skull could be shared among members of a kin or social group, with the village as a whole, or with other communities. The ultimate disposal of these fragments also indicates that their usefulness was finite; whether veneration, symbolism, or ritual, it came to an end when they were returned to the earth somewhere in the village. The symbols or figures chosen for incising carried meaning for the Oneota people as part of their mythology or ideology, part of their shared identity. The disposal may thus have reflected a "release" of that meaning.

These examples have documented the complexity and difficulty of interpreting the treatment of human bone by the Oneota people. The dead were not simply interred nor left to decompose naturally; trophies were not taken from enemies as singular events. Rather, something about human bone and, in these cases, something about cranial remains held meaning beyond the death of the individual from whom they were obtained.

IV

PERSPECTIVES

15
The Meaning of Scalping in Native North America

Linea Sundstrom

The unique contribution of osteoarchaeology lies in its ability to move beyond a strictly biological approach to the human body toward a broader anthropological perspective. In recent decades many anthropological theorists have called for greater integration of the human body into culture studies—in other words, researchers should treat the human body as a necessary part of the analysis, rather than as a hidden, unexamined presence (Lock 1993). In western philosophical traditions, dichotomies are drawn between nature and culture, the physical and the mental, self and other, but in nonwestern traditions people may have very different ways of thinking about physicality, corporality, disease, and autonomy. Much of western scholarship is predicated on the dualistic notion that the body is a physical object that can be dissociated from person, being, or mind (Lock 1993:135). In contrast, advocates of an "embodied" anthropology point out that all human experience is mediated through the body—that of the subject and that of the anthropologist—in ways that need to be brought to the forefront. Personhood cannot be separated from the body and the physical and sensual experiences of the individual. The body is not a given, but a subject of inquiry in its own right.

Body, Body Parts, and Cultural Practices

All cultures map abstract ideas onto the body. In some European traditions, the head, heart, liver, spleen, and intestines are associated with concepts of intelligence, compassion, courage, anger, and fortitude. The heart is widely used as a metaphor for emotion and courage. In the ancient and medieval worlds, the left (sinister) was associated with evil and uncertainty, the right with righteousness and order. Such views are culture-bound, not universal. Not all cultures include the notion that a soul resides in the body until, but not after, death. If a soul or self potentially remains with the dead body, then the very notion of "death" and "body" (as separate from being) can be seen as culturally specific. Under the Native American Graves Protection and Repatriation Act, such divergent perspectives have come into sharp and sometimes irreconcilable focus. For example, many Native American cultures include the concept of some nonphysical essence of the person remaining in the bones and/or hair after death. This essence may allow the deceased person to be restored to life—for example, if the bones go through a sweat-lodge ceremony—or may exert influence over the lives of surviving relatives.

The idea of human bones harboring some potential to come back to life or to influence others' lives occurs in western religious traditions as well. For example, Roman Catholic doctrine holds that relics (e.g., saints' bones) retain some of the spiritual potency of the deceased. Under such belief systems, but not in the physical sciences, "dead" bones require careful treatment and maintenance. To disturb them is thus not merely disrespectful but actually dangerous in awakening their dormant power.

Because we all have bodies, stepping back from our own cultural constructs may prove particularly challenging. We can imagine vividly the distress accompanying practices such as genital cutting or the amputation of fingertips. The idea of having one's corpse cut up and fed to vultures may horrify a westerner, just as the idea of one's corpse being locked into a box and deeply buried may be equally troubling from a nonwestern perspective. A modern American may accept the idea of orthodontia as normal and healthy, while expressing disgust at historic Chinese foot-binding. But both practices involve pain, expense, and physical limitation in service to a body ideal. Both reflect the extent to which the body is culturally malleable and symbolic of such external factors as familial wealth and a desire that children uphold the family's social status. The complex and often unarticulated ethnographies of the body mean that an anthropology of the body must be contextualized from both sides: that of the subject of the study and that of the researcher (Turner 1991).

As the foregoing chapters demonstrate, ancient Native American societies treated human bone in ways that hint at long, complex traditions regarding power, protection, and identity. The specifics of these traditions are elusive because those who practiced them are long gone and more recent expressions of their beliefs were disrupted or suppressed during European colonization of the Americas. The misunderstandings inherent in sudden contact between very different cultures further painted some body practices as odd, barbaric, or violent. Unfamiliar practices became fodder for the discourse by which invading nations legitimized the subjugation of indigenous populations.

One such practice—scalping—has perhaps been more persistently misunderstood and more often pressed into the service of dispossession of American Indian nations than any other. Unlike other practices treated in the preceding chapters, the indigenous meaning of scalping is available via ethnographic and historic records. A careful reading of old accounts—one that separates the statements by indigenous people from the western-biased language in which they were recorded—can provide a glimpse of the profound religious belief(s) encoded in the practice of scalping.

Recent and old publications alike equate scalp taking with the acquisition of war trophies (Clark 1885:326; Denig 1930:492; Jacobi 2007:301; Lewis 1942:59; Mensforth 2007; Welch and Stekler 1994).[1] In this view, scalping was done to prove that a warrior killed an enemy, to humiliate the enemy, and to disable the dead enemy in some way. Such interpretations rely on the accounts of white fur traders and military men—in other words, those most likely to be on the receiving end of the practice. But the interpretation of scalping as the acquisition of war trophies—something brought back from battle as a tangible symbol of victory—finds little support in the accounts of American Indians and the anthropologists who recorded their customs (e.g., Curtis 1909:36; Dorsey 1902; Dorsey 1885; Hall 1997; Smith 1937; Wallis 1947:31). Fear of American Indians, a mission of conquest and subjugation against them, a lack of even the most rudimentary knowledge of comparative religion, and the imposition of European attitudes onto Native American practices—and, later, the call for dramatic and unambiguous Hollywood story lines—incubated a simplistic and biased view of scalping that lingers today.

It is telling that scalping is frequently mentioned in the same breath as torture or cannibalism (e.g., Goodrich 1997; Ross-Stallings 2007) or is considered to be a kind of torture or violence, even though nearly all accounts describe the practice as applying only to enemies who were already dead. For example, one researcher asserted that "human body mutilations such as these *must* be regarded as violent acts designed to disable the body and soul of the victim" (Mensforth 2007:223, emphasis added).[2] This distinction is revealing. Certainly, the modern practices of embalming and autopsy would count as torture were they performed on live people. Equating the modification of a corpse with torture or violence only muddies the interpretation of trophy taking.

This is not to deny that scalps were sometimes taken from live people, which is well documented in the ethnohistoric and archaeological literature (Jacobi 2007; Mensforth 2007; Oneroad and Skinner 2003:95; Wallis 1947:105; Weltfish 1965:294; Willey 1990). In such cases, the practice would certainly have been torture, although the motive behind it—acquiring the scalp—was primarily a religious obligation, as will be seen (e.g., Dorsey 1904b:

166). Many people who suffered live scalping survived the experience; some died soon after from infection; and some lived on only to be slain and scalped again later. In some groups, surviving a scalping meant social isolation (Weltfish 1965:294), but in others it was not particularly limiting (Oneroad and Skinner 2003:95; Wallis 1947:105). In any case, knowingly scalping a live person is different from scalping a corpse. One is torture, the other is not. Scalping the dead was the expected and usual procedure in some cultures.

Similarly, "a pile of broken skulls and bones" on an Inuit battlefield or the scalps of enemies slain by Chilcotin warriors and left in streams, but not carried back to the Chilcotin settlement, might be better interpreted as trophy *leaving*, as opposed to trophy *taking* (Maschner and Reedy-Maschner 2007:37). This might seem a minor distinction, but it is emblematic of the lack of precise definitions employed when members of one culture undertake to discuss the "shocking" practices of another. Besides the question of *taking*—and, presumably, curating the body part(s)—one must ask what constitutes a trophy, and, indeed, whether this concept exists outside European-based cultures. If a war chief uses a bag of bones as a pillow (Lovisek 2007:52), is that a trophy? It would seem more congruent with the definition of a charm or fetish than a trophy, more akin to a Catholic saint's relic than to putting an enemy's head on a post at the town gates.

Historical documents record two instances of scalping done purely to acquire battle trophies. These scalp takers acquired and publicly displayed scalps simply to gain attention, to appear heroic to their compatriots, and to warn potential enemies. Neither of these instances of scalp taking were informed by the scalp takers' religious beliefs or their mourning for slain loved ones. The first incident was the killing and scalping of Cheyenne men, women, and children at Sand Creek, Colorado, and the display of their scalps at saloons and a theater in Denver by a local militia under the command of John Chivington in 1864 (United States Congress 1865). The second was the scalping of Dead Arm, a nephew of the Lakota Ghost Dance leader Kicking Bear, by white cowboys near Pine Ridge, South Dakota, in 1890 (Rapid City Journal 1890). The newspaper reported that a city founder and power broker, Tom Sweeney, acquired the scalp, presumably for display alongside other "curios" in his large store in Rapid City. The lack of public outcry suggests that these were not isolated events, but these should suffice as examples of European-derived attitudes toward the bodies of enemies. The eagerness of anthropologists and museum curators to acquire Indian skulls in the nineteenth and early twentieth centuries is a broader example of the European-based treatment of the bodies of vanquished enemies, although in this case, the bodies included those of noncombatants and those taken from graves (Lovisek 2007:59).

What constitutes a "trophy"? It is not helpful to define any human body part as a trophy without regard to the context in which it was acquired, curated, used, and eventually discarded. Under some definitions, a child's baby tooth, the skull of a venerated ancestor kept in a shrine, and the head of an executed criminal placed on a pike on London Bridge would all count as trophies. A more exact definition is any "memorial of a victory or conquest." In this sense, the scalps displayed at Denver and Rapid City qualify as trophies and had no other clear function. This definition also includes enemy scalps taken by American Indians, but it does not preclude that those scalps served other functions in indigenous societies. As will be seen, the assertion that scalps were merely or primarily trophies is contradicted by a large body of ethnographic literature.

Lest this chapter be viewed as "denialist" (Demarest 2007:394), please note that I do not dispute that scalping was part of many Native American cultures both before and after European contact. The existence of precontact scalping is well established by studies of bone pathologies (Andrushko et al. 2005; Axtell and Sturtevant 1980; Chacon and Dye 2007a:6; Howard and Janetski 1992; Owsley and Jantz 1994; Willey 1990; Willey and Bass 1978). Further, that the practice was widespread and similar throughout much of North America argues for a long history. At the same time, archaeologists are not immune to finding what they expect to find in their data. As Mark Seeman (2007:173) noted, "it is difficult to conclusively recognize the results of [precontact] trophy taking . . . and it is easy to confuse them with other practices." To avoid misunderstandings about the meaning of scalping, the practice is considered here within a larger system of beliefs.

Patterns of Scalping

Although scalps might be taken opportunistically, deliberate scalp raids are well documented in the ethnohistoric literature. The parent of a slain warrior might approach a dead son's companions to elicit a vow from them to take an enemy scalp for the benefit of the deceased loved one, who at that time would be "traveling the spirit road"—that is, whose spirit was on a journey of four days, months, or years, along a road represented by the Milky Way (Bek 1938:354; Hall 1997; Kidd 1986:72; Skinner 1926:202; Smith 1937). Generally, the young men of the group were called together and offered a pipe. If they accepted it and smoked, they were obligated to remain in a state of mourning for their dead companion until they were able to take a scalp for him, generally during the following spring or summer. The deceased's family remained in mourning as well. Usually this vow was made in honor of a warrior killed in combat; however, such avowed scalp raids were also sometimes undertaken in honor of an individual who had died of illness or accident. This widespread practice is the origin of the belief that scalping was done for retribution or revenge. Certainly, such motives played into the custom, but the rationale is more complicated than simple vengeance. For example, in most Native American cultures, any enemy scalp would suffice; it need not be from the same group that caused the death of the beloved warrior. The scalp of a woman or child would do, and no shame was attached to killing them, since it was considered to be the larger society's obligation to protect its vulnerable members.

In many areas of North America, warriors—and sometimes noncombatants as well—removed the scalp of an enemy corpse. The scalp was later stretched on a hoop, scraped clean of loose flesh, and painted (in red, in red and black halves, or in red with a black X dividing the design into four parts) (Blair 1911:I:158; Grinnell 1910; Howard 1977:104, 180; Lowie 1935:218; Skinner 1926:204; Wallis 1947:18–21). The hair was combed and decorated with feathers or other items. The scalp was affixed to the end of a slender staff and carried into the camp upon the return of the war party (Blair 1911:I:158; Eastman 1995:1050 [1849]; Grinnell 1910; Howard 1977:104, 180; Mishkin 1940:29; Walker 1980:272). As the war party approached its home camp, the warriors painted their faces black as a sign that they were setting aside mourning (Grinnell 1910; Mishkin 1940:29; Wallis 1947:21, 31). If any of the war party had been killed, the surviving warriors did not paint their faces but entered camp in a subdued manner to show they continued in mourning.

After the war party's formal entry into the home camp, they presented the scalp (or, more rarely, the entire head) to the female mourners of the slain person in whose honor the war party had been raised (Blair 1911:II:158; Clark 1885:326; Curtis 1909:36; Driver 1969:299, 320; Eastman 1995:1050 [1849]; Grinnell 1910; Howard 1977:180; Lambert 2007:72; Smith 1937; Wallis 1947:21). The women danced the scalps around a center pole—forked near the top and preferably of cottonwood. This ceremony was frequently referred to as a Scalp Dance or Victory Dance; however, its main significance lay in ending the family's or warrior society's period of mourning. In the Great Plains, acquisition of the scalp facilitated a safe passage of the deceased loved one's soul to the afterlife. This is the real meaning of the Victory or Scalp Dance. The women who performed this ceremony might affix scalps and other enemy body parts to the central pole, or they might carry them on the sticks prepared earlier by the returning war party. The dancers might also don their deceased loved one's war bonnet or other accoutrements. The Victory or Scalp

Dance was, in fact, an enactment of the travels of the loved one's soul along the spirit road, accompanied by the soul represented by the scalp. The scalp was carried aloft or fastened to the forked central pole by those closest to the deceased, usually his mother, sister, or wife (Walker 1980:272; Wallis 1947: 21). Forked poles and forked staffs are a recurrent theme in this ceremony and in the related Spirit Release ceremony (Dorsey 1889:146; Fletcher 1884:298, 303, 304; Hassrick 1964:302) and probably represent the spirit road, as does the Sun Dance pole in Lakota tradition (Buechel and Manhart 1998:232–233; Catches and Catches 1997:116–117).

This ceremony—marking the acquisition of the scalp—might be repeated until the season changed, but its final performance marked the end of mourning (Curtis 1909:36, 1911:83; DeMallie 1984:370; Dorsey 1902, 1904a:15–16; Dorsey 1885; Eastman 1995:1050 [1849]; Grinnell 1910; Hall 1997; Hassrick 1964:89; Mathews 1961:764; Smith 1937). After the ceremony, the scalp might be retained by the mourning family for a short time or it might be burned or buried (Eastman 1995:1050 [1849]; Howard 1977:104; Kidd 1986:167; Wallis 1947:21). Sometimes, it would be saved until it could be deposited inside enemy territory, where it was believed to cause death and disease (Dorsey 1894:484). At times, scalps were suspended from poles around the village, but rarely were they afforded long-term care or curation (Kidd 1986:167; Lambert 2007:83; Wallis 1947:21).

The Significance of Hair

In many Native American cultures, hair or the crown of the head is believed to be a repository of an individual's soul, essence, or one of several souls (Carrasco 1990:69; Codere 1950:107; Cybulski 1978:28–31; Dorsey 1894: 484; Engelbrecht 2003:43; Hassrick 1964:90; Lovisek 2007:53–55).[3] Certainly, the argument that scalps were preferred "trophies" because they are portable and easy to prepare for permanent display (Mensforth 2007:225) lacks credence: any piece of skin, fingers, toes, and so on would be equally portable and easier to detach. The ethnohistoric literature consistently noted that scalps were typically discarded (buried or burned) once the Victory Dance ceremony was over; thus, permanent display was not a consideration.

Two portions of the scalp are afforded special importance: the area above the forehead at the location of an infant's anterior fontanel and the hair whorl at the upper back of the head (Dorsey 1889:143–145; Fletcher 1884:297; Fletcher and La Flesche 1911:124). The fontanel is often viewed as a portal through which the soul enters and leaves the body at birth and at death.

Babies were not scalped because their unfused skull bones implied that the soul had not yet permanently fixed itself in the individual. The shape of the fontanel—a square with rays extending from each corner—is replicated on the earth altars used in various Lakota ceremonies (e.g., Fletcher 1884:284; Hall 1997:100). The area of the scalp including the whorl was referred to as the scalp lock. Special attention was given to the scalp locks of boys and men; from an early age the scalp lock was carefully combed, roached, braided, and/or decorated (Clark 1885:328; Fletcher and La Flesche 1911:122, 128). Sometimes the ornaments attached to a scalp lock symbolized the man's accomplishments in war and in horse raiding. A warrior might take either the entire scalp or just the scalp lock (Wallis 1947:21).

As noted, the ethnohistoric literature clearly indicated that Native Americans viewed hair as the seat of one of the souls (Dorsey 1889:143, 1893:298, 1894:484; Fletcher and La Flesche 1911:124; Hassrick 1964:302; Lovisek 2007:53–55; Lynd 1864:155). A person in mourning often cut off his or her hair and deposited it with the body or at the grave site (Bek 1938:354; Blair 1911:I:70; Clark 1885:91; Fletcher and La Flesche 1911:124; Hassrick 1964:334; Hilger 1952:43, 162, 1970; Lowie 1935:68; Mallery 1893:519; Oneroad and Skinner 2003:93, 100; Standing Bear 1933:211; Trenholm 1970:63; Wallis 1947:32–34). In the Lakota and Dakota spirit-keeping ceremony, it was most often a lock of the deceased loved one's hair that formed the nucleus of the spirit bundle (Curtis 1908:20; Dorsey 1889:143, 1893:298, 1894:484; Fletcher 1884:297; Hassrick 1964:302; Howard 1966:16, 1977:102; Oneroad and Skinner 2003:98, 101). This ceremony obligated the family to a long period (usually more than a year) of ritualized mourning, which allowed them to keep the deceased's spirit with them for a longer time. At the end of the mourning period, the family sponsored a ceremony to release the soul. The Kansa and Cree peoples likewise kept a lock of hair from a dead loved one in order to keep his or her soul near (Dorsey 1894:421; Kidd 1986:64). In many Native American societies, children's hair was never cut since this might lead to disruption of the developing soul—in other words, it might shorten the child's life (Dusenberry 1962:87; Hilger 1952:43; Wallis 1947:27). It was the cutting off of the children's hair that, as much as anything, dismayed the parents and children forced into the residential school system (Standing Bear 1933:189; Utley 1963:37; Wallis 1947:25–27).

The scalp appears in religious contexts because the hair it retained was viewed as representing or embodying the soul. In the Lakota Sun Dance, the small branches at the top of the center pole were left untrimmed because they were thought to be like the hair or scalp of the tree and thus the seat of its soul or spirit (Walker 1980:183). The Omahas' Sacred Pole was provided with a human scalp (Fletcher and La Flesche 1911:218–219). The Arikaras had a formal name-taking ceremony during which the scalp of an enemy woman was used as an offering (Dorsey 1904b:166). The Pawnees also made offerings of scalps (Dorsey 1905:498). The use of scalps as religious offerings is also reported for southeastern North America and Mesoamerica (Carrasco 1990:69; Driver 1969:324). During the Blackfoot Sun Dance, a participant might offer a severed finger joint or, "still dearer," a lock of hair (Kidd 1986:180). Finally, scalps (and skulls) are included in sacred bundles in some Plains Indian societies (Bowers 1965:342, 345, 432; Thomas 1941), and a few scalps were among the hundreds of offerings left at a sacred cave in the northern Great Plains (Over 1946).

The Scalp as a Psychopomp

The belief that the dead travel to the afterworld along the path seen in the sky as the Milky Way is widespread in North America. Many groups believed that they could help their deceased loved ones along this path by providing a psychopomp—a guide or servant to accompany the soul along its way. Like the belief in the Milky Way as the spirit road to the afterworld, the concept of the psychopomp has parallels in Eurasia. Odin/Woden, Hermes, and St. Michael take this role in some European traditions. In the Americas, the guide is either a dog or one of the two or four souls of a deceased person—generally, that soul embodied by the hair (Blair 1911:I:293; DeMallie 1984: 227–230; Oneroad and Skinner 2003:98; Taylor 1994:154). As noted, mourners donated their own cut hair to the deceased person, sometimes along with that of his or her horse, but the ideal psychopomp was the soul represented by an enemy scalp.

In Lakota tradition, it was considered best if another person's *nagi* (ghost or soul) accompanied that of a deceased loved one on its journey to the spirit world (Walker 1980:71). This ghost could be that of someone who died at the same time or that of a slain enemy. The former would be a traveling companion, the latter a servant (Walker 1917:86; 1980:123). As the Lakota religious specialists explained to James Walker (1917:86), if a deceased person killed and scalped an enemy "he has thereby gained control of the spirit of the enemy whose spirit cannot enter on the spirit trail until the one who controls it does so, and even then it must serve the controlling spirit to the end of the trail." Those honored in the *hunka* (adoption) ceremony were instructed that if a fellow *hunka* were killed in war, the initiate was not to rest until he had "provided a companion for his spirit" (Walker 1980:237). The Blackfoot had a similar tradition of providing a spirit servant for a deceased loved one, especially a warrior (Henry and Thompson 1897:332–333; Kidd 1986:162). Among the Osages, surviving warriors vowed to take a scalp for each dead comrade so that they "would be recognized" in the spirit world (Mathews 1961:462). When such raids were outlawed in historic times, the mourners substituted either hair cut from a Pawnee who agreed to let the warriors track him and cut a lock of his hair; a strand of long hair purchased from a white woman with long, blonde tresses (Mathews 1961:739); or their own cut hair accompanied by the head of a deer (Dorsey 1902:411). These were deposited on the grave of the dead warrior(s), much as mourners placed their own hair with the body. Among the Fox and Sauk peoples, warriors "gave away" the spirits of the enemies they had killed in war in order to serve their deceased comrade in the afterlife (Nicholas Perrot, cited in Blair 1911:I:206). An Omaha man in mourning might lay his deceased child's moccasins beside the body of an enemy he had killed "in the belief that the dead man would recognize and befriend the child as it slowly made its way toward its relatives in the other world" (Fletcher and La Flesche 1911:594).

Conclusions

Were scalps trophies of war? That depends on the definitions of "trophy" and "war." Concerning the latter, scalps were sometimes taken in large-scale aggressive warfare, such as occurred at Crow Creek (Willey 1990). In most cases, however, scalps were obtained through small raids or skirmishes involving between 4 and perhaps 50 warriors (Mishkin 1940; Smith 1937). These were one-time expeditions that ceased fighting and returned home as soon as the participants killed and scalped an enemy. Without minimizing the violence of such actions, they can hardly be considered war in the sense of sustained, bureaucratized, high-casualty conflicts.

As to the question of trophies, scalps seem not to have served that role, at least not primarily. Scalps were generally presented to a grieving family, used in ceremonies for a few days or weeks, and then buried or burned. Some were attached to a horse's bridle to show that it had run down an enemy; however, that would make it a trophy only for the horse. Scalps were carried in triumph into the village, but this was more a signal that the expedition had been successful than a personal acclamation. It is significant that the entire war party painted their faces black and rode into the village together, carrying the scalp(s) on a long pole: the expedition was considered a team effort. If any special acclaim or blame was accrued, that lay with the leader, not the warrior(s) taking a scalp. Significantly, no formal Victory Dance was held when a war party returned with horses but not scalps (Mishkin 1940:31).

The foremost function of scalps, then, appears to have been to symbolize the soul of the slain enemy that would accompany a deceased loved one to the afterlife. Scalp raids were organized at the request of the mourning family and were conducted to accomplish the task of obtaining a psychopomp for their dead son, father, or husband. While a warrior would be honored for carrying out this obligation, he had many other ways of gaining prestige: counting coup, serving as a scout or war party leader, and capturing horses or eagles. In general, taking a scalp carried less prestige than counting first coup (Grinnell 1910). In the Kiowa system of ranking warriors' deeds, taking a scalp was not even considered (Mishkin 1940:39).

Secondary functions also reflected beliefs about the soul and the afterlife. Some scalps were kept in sacred bundles and some were used as religious offerings, neither of which seems consistent with an interpretation of scalps as trophies of war. It appears that all scalps received special, ritualized treatment: careful removal of any adhering flesh and its ceremonial deposition, stretching the skin onto a hoop to dry, and painting it in colors and patterns that represented blood and/or the universe. While some groups did view scalped enemies as in some way disabled in the afterlife, this belief appears to have been restricted in its distribution, with more groups either not mentioning such a result or asserting that a scalped person fared as well as or better than an unscalped person in the journey to the afterlife.

Was scalping a byproduct of an unending cycle of revenge feuds (Welch and Stekler 1994:140–141)? At first glance, it might seem so. The death of a warrior necessitated the death of another to get the first one across to the afterlife, and so on. But the cycle could be broken in two ways: first, the family did not have to request that a scalp be presented to them, and second, any scalp would do. It need not be from the same person, family, clan, or nation as the person who had killed the beloved warrior (Mishkin 1940:28–31). The war party simply endeavored to take a scalp from whichever enemy the warriors first encountered in or near their own camp. In a true cycle of vengeance, one specific group trades deaths with another. Furthermore, as Axtell and Sturtevant (1980:470) pointed out, Europeans adopted and promoted the practice of scalping in the Americas through a system of offering bounties for enemy scalps even though Christianity prohibited it (see also Driver 1969: 520; Mooney 1910). Like so much else in European-based cultures, scalps became commodities, something to be exchanged for money or goods. By contrast, Native Americans continued an apparently ancient practice of scalping because their religion demanded it. Scalps provided necessary companions for deceased family members or comrades. Taking a scalp was necessary not for revenge per se but to end the period of mourning and allow a return to normal life (Beier 1998).

At this point, it is fair to ask, does researchers' misapprehension of scalping matter? Is there a problem with referring to the practice of scalping as the "taking and displaying of human body parts as trophies" (Chacon and Dye, ed. 2007)? I would argue that in the interests of a less-biased anthropology and history, the answer is yes. Native Americans have rightly questioned why archaeologists choose to look at only certain aspects of ancient cultures, and why some archaeology seems to reduce human beings to little more than food-getting, material-culture-producing, warring creatures. Recognizing that scalp taking met multiple cultural or personal imperatives is a step toward appreciating the complexity of individual people and of cultures. Referring to a vast array of disparate mortuary practices, including scalping, as "trophy taking" would seem to preclude any motivation not related to personal or group aggrandizement or to terrorism directed toward the group's enemies (Chacon and Dye 2007b:618–625).

Marshall Beier (1998) noted that white America tends to view the Native Americans of the past as lacking social control and living a Hobbesian existence of perpetual warfare. This bias may lead researchers to interpret observed behaviors in ways that reinforce the stereotypes and that justify conquest and colonization. As he noted, "an important part of any colonial project is the remaking of the colonized to suit the colonizer's preferred—and often requisite—image of them" (Beier 1998:37).

In recent years, archaeologists have become increasingly adept at bringing a more emic perspective to studies of ancient cultures. Through the careful use of ethnohistorical and historical records (i.e., taking the time to separate Native American accounts from the nonnative interpretations of them), the close examination of iconography, considering artifacts and features in their broader context, and simply recognizing the centrality of religion to the lifeways of Native American nations, Americanist archaeology has begun to fill in the gaps and set the record straight.

Notes

1. George Bird Grinnell (1910) stated that scalps were merely trophies and of no great importance; however, he then described elaborate religious practices surrounding them.

2. This belief seems largely to have been limited to the Iroquois. One clue that some other groups believed being scalped prevented proper passage into the spirit

world is the Pawnee fear of the ghosts of scalped people who, along with those who survived scalping, were believed to lurk around and cause mischief (Weltfish 1965: 294). However, other groups asserted that a scalped warrior proceeded directly to the afterlife (Clark 1885:71).

3. Karl Schlesier (1987:19, 28–29) noted that northern Siberians also believed in four souls, one residing in the head or hair; these groups also practiced scalping and believed that scalping an enemy would prevent his or her rebirth, and they also practiced "soul keeping" by retaining a lock of a dead loved one's hair.

16

Contextualizing the Precolumbian Postmortem "Life" of Modified Human Remains

Maria Ostendorf Smith

In precolumbian North America, human skeletal elements that are interpreted as objects of material culture are not uncommon, but they are infrequent. That is, they are typically individual cases in a single archaeological context. Documentation is often minimal, descriptive, and usually confined to site reports. As Johnston's (this volume) overview notes, modified human bones are often peremptorily labeled "trophy" items (i.e., demonstrations of raiding success or personal prowess in combat) (see Sundstrom, this volume) or as evidence of ancestor veneration. However, the chapters in this volume provide much-needed broader cosmological and sociocultural interpretations of these objects and underscore that the kinds and frequency of human bone artifacts vary temporally and regionally in the Midwest. Ascertaining cultural meanings in evidently diverse sociopolitical and economic contexts requires comprehensive deductive analysis that marshals mortuary patterning, nonutilitarian artifact identification and analysis, and ethnohistorical documentation of nuanced intercultural differences in mortuary ritual and the emic concepts of life, death, soul(s), rebirth, and more. Unfortunately, some of these basic data are irretrievable. Nevertheless, much can be gleaned from the contributions in this volume that can serve as a point of departure for the continuing assessment of the complex cultural context of modified human remains.

The results of my research in a geographic area that borders the Midwest (i.e., the Tennessee River valley) have revealed relevant observations that help to decouple warfare from the a priori interpretation that modified human remains are "trophies": (1) precolumbian intergroup violence is not synonymous with the retrieval of human body element (e.g., scalps, forearms, hands, heads) or human bone modification (Smith 1992, 1993a, 1993b, 1995, 1997, 2002, 2003); and (2) there are temporal and regional differences in postmortem body processing regarding dismemberment, the maintenance of body integrity, and the time between death and permanent interment, which are independent of the mortuary presence of modified human remains (Smith 1997). Therefore, cosmological and sociopolitical variables must also be considered when interpreting the postmortem social use and ultimate fate (i.e., interment or disposal) of the deceased. The temporal and geographic distribution of objects described in this volume (e.g., modified mandibles and maxillae, rondelles, drilled teeth [Blue; Cobb; Johnston; Lillie and Schermer; Nawrocki and Emanovsky; Schermer and Lillie], incised bone [Hedman; Lillie and Schermer], skull masks or rattles [Cook and Munson], drilled phalanges [Schermer and Lillie], long bone phalli [Lee and Johnston], and human bone tools [Cook and Munson; Hargrave and Cook; Hedman; Munson et al.; Zejdlik]) may offer key clues to determining some of these variables. The mortuary context is equally important (e.g., body staging [Carr and Novotny], as grave inclusions, or disposal in refuse pits).

My goal here is to marshal the information generated by the volume authors and to generate a broader interpretive framework. To accomplish this, I critically assess archaeological perspectives (processualist, postprocessualist); examine the ethnographic record of the cultural uses of human bone objects; construct an outline of Native American cosmology as it relates to the postmortem life (soul) of bone objects; and then thread all this information together in a temporal framework. The information generated in this volume will undoubtedly contribute to generating plausible cultural or cosmological explanations for the postmortem life of modified human remains.

The Shifting Etic Theoretical View

Much of the mortuary interpretation after circa 1970 was based on the presumptions that mortuary complexity mirrors social complexity and that funeral rituals reflect the social role of the deceased (Binford 1971; Brown 1971; Peebles and Kus 1977; Saxe 1970). This framework, referred to as the Saxe-Binford model, presumed a linear evolution to a hierarchical social organization that included ascribed elites (e.g., chief, paramount chief) with interment location and the number and kinds of grave accompaniments as the sociopolitical horizon marker. It would theoretically follow that the primary interpretation of extraneous—particularly, processed or objectified—human bone in graves was either as some sort of ritual affirmation of legitimacy or as a status (e.g., ancestor veneration) marker or sign of achievement or prowess (e.g., "trophy" items). In the twenty-first century, theoretical shifts (i.e., post-processualism, agency theory) and new research initiatives have challenged the explanatory power of the Saxe-Binford perspective (see McGuire 1988, 1992; and Sullivan and Mainfort 2010 for a review) with interpretive frameworks primarily developed as a counterpoint to the New Archaeology of the 1970s and 1980s (Dobres and Robb 2000). However, postprocessualism and agency theory are often frustratingly rife with cross-disciplinary (and often obscure) jargon, including adverbs rarely seen outside of an unabridged dictionary. Their application to archaeological problem solving is often questionable, since the theories seem to be less interpretively useful than intent on applying labels for (arguably, etic) conceptualizations. However, to their credit, these theories have enabled the mining of a broader interpretive database and the theoretical inclusion of the agent (the individual human) as a cultural catalyst (see Fowler 2004; Hamilakis et al. 2002; Joyce 2005).

The broader interpretive database in post–Saxe-Binford mortuary analysis now often includes ethnohistoric information (e.g., Brown 2003, 2007; Byers 2009) to illuminate horizontal roles and relationships (heterarchy) and cosmological (metaphysical) considerations. In this light, the modification of human remains into meaningful artifacts (as vital actors or inert props) by indigenous peoples represents one aspect of a complex interplay between the physical and metaphysical realms (Brown 2010; Pauketat 2010). Cosmological interpretations have benefited from recent strides in interpreting precolumbian iconography (Brown 2007; Galloway 1989; Hall 1989; King 2007; Knight 2006; Knight et al. 2001; Reilly and Garber 2007; Townsend and Sharp 2004) particularly since Cahokia has been argued as the apparent source of what is referred to as the Southeastern Ceremonial Complex (SECC) (Brown and Kelly 2000). Significantly for the discussion here, a cosmological connection has also been suggested between the SECC and the earlier Hopewell phenomenon (Brown 2007).

The Chronically Missing Emic View

Shamanism, the spirit world, mortuary rituals, ceremonies of renewal, and, of course, warfare are some of the factors that explain postmortem use of human remains. Most of these factors are aspects of cosmology and religion, according to ethnohistorical records. Many ethnohistories, particularly nineteenth-century attempts, lack the detail to answer questions regarding the postmortem social and ritual use of the dead. However, much ethnographic information has yet to be distilled, and some accounts may yet provide the needed information to explain the various forms of postmortem bone modification and their mortuary and nonmortuary recovery contexts. The more recent primary ethnographic sources commonly mined for cosmological, ritual, or practical meaning are studies of the presumptive cultural descendants of the prehistoric peoples in question. This, however, is a geographically wide and culturally heterogeneous ethnographic net. These sources geographically and inferentially include various and long-distinct Algonquian, Iroquoian, and (Dhegiha and Chiwere) Siouan speakers (Bushnell 1920, 1927; Curtin 1922; Dorsey 1906; Dorsey and Kroeber 1903; Fletcher and La Flesche 1911; Halbert 1900; Hewitt 1903; La Flesche 1921; Leland 1884; Mooney 1900; Radin 1948, 1949; Swanton 1929) whose histories were irretrievably affected by European contact.

The Euro-American cultural-historical interaction with Native Americans was agonistic, which resulted in disproportionately more etic Eurocentric information about dismemberment and warfare-related body-part retrieval (see Chacon and Dye, ed. 2007; Sundstrom, this volume) than about the varied mortuary customs of socially marginalized Native American cultures. The retrieval of war-related "trophies," which range from scalps to disarticulated appendages, was widely practiced among the indigenous peoples of the Midwest, the Southeast, and the Plains, and this routinely included public display as part of post-raiding ceremonies (e.g., Chacon and Dye 2007a; Grinnell 1910; May 2004; Sagard-Théodat 1939). It is unclear how long body parts were displayed. Some researchers observed that they were discarded (Evers 1997). Seventeenth-century eyewitness accounts of captives' treatment by the Iroquois described the discarding of killed captives (e.g., they were thrown into a river) or their consumption by the captors (Williamson 2007). However, various Plains Indian groups hung scalps with scaffold burials or sewed scalp strands onto items of clothing (e.g., leggings, "war shirt"). Unfortunately, it is unclear how the physical disposal of the remains of war captives or war-retrieved osseous body parts translates into a presence in archaeological contexts as midden debris or as grave inclusions (if ever) (Jamieson 1983; Williamson 2007).

Although prowess in warfare is a pervasive benchmark for manhood and social advancement, apparently the primary motive for raiding among the Native American peoples of the Eastern Woodlands was avenging group members' deaths (Bailey and Young 2001; Williamson 2007; Young and Hoffman 2001). Indeed, Iroquois warfare was codified as "mourning wars." The protracted torture to the point of death of certain war captives functioned to facilitate the celestial journeys of the souls of community members who had died violently (Jamieson 1983; Trigger 1969). This torture was cosmologically necessary since those who died violently were apparently excluded from the Feast of the Dead mortuary rituals (Jamieson 1983; Richter 1992; Williamson 2007). These post-raiding mourning war activities included the social complexities of scalp adoption (scalp = life essence) and the captive's adoption and "rebirth" into the village community before his tortured death.

How pervasive this was is unknown, but it was also true of the Quapaw culture of the Mississippi valley (Young and Hoffman 2001). Clearly, neither the body element nor the victim were dehumanized or objectified, which adds metaphysical complexity to their characterization as simply a war trophy (see Sundstrom, this volume). The ethnographic record reinforces this in instances where tattooing or special adornments (feathers, paint) are the pervasive tangible markers of prowess in war (e.g., Brown and Irwin 2001; M. Wedel 2001).

Underscoring the interpretive complexity, Owsley and colleagues (2007) observed that little ethnographic information has been recorded concerning the retention or modification (e.g., incising, engraving) of the bony body parts except for the occasional mention of necklaces made from human phalanges. It has been argued that these were not necessarily warfare retrievals, since many Plains Indian groups practiced self-inflicted finger joint amputation as part of a vision quest (and acquisition of metaphysical power) or as part of the mourning process (e.g., Bushnell 1920, 1927; Parks 2001; Stewart 2001; Wood and Irwin 2001). Indeed, Starr (1891) referred to these necklaces as "mourning attire."

Ancestor veneration has long been a viable processualist (Saxe-Binford) interpretation for the archaeological occurrences of eccentric unmodified or modified human body parts in graves. However, the actual ethnographic evidence for such mortuary inclusions is missing. Certainly this omission was not caused by a lack of postmortem opportunities to acquire bone elements, since burning, defleshing, and interim taphonomic contexts (e.g., scaffolding, charnel houses, temporary burials) are common (Barrett and Skinner 1932; Bushnell 1920, 1927; Dorsey 1906; Dorsey and Kroeber 1903; Halbert 1900; Hudson 1976; Lorenz 2000; Williamson 2007). Ethnographic studies of Siouan-, Iroquoian-, and Algonquian-speaking peoples have described a widespread postmortem (but pre–final interment) social role for human (but not inanimate) remains (i.e., "soul bundles" or "death bundles") that apparently functioned as a kind of leveling mechanism (Hall 1997; Palmer 2008). For example, a practice referred to as "retaining the ghost" was employed among cultures (e.g., Santee/Mdewakanton, Sesseton/Sisseton, Wahpeton, Brulé) that dispossessed the deceased's family of all material belongings associated with the deceased (Bushnell 1927). Strands of hair ("the ghost") cut off from the dead loved one were wrapped to become part of a bundle to which, over the course of time, gifts were anonymously added by community members. The material wealth redistribution function is evident because, at some future time, the goods in the ghost gift bundle were given to the deceased's family. According to the synthesis by Hall (1997), the final interment (soul release) may have been the occasion for such redistribution.

There are other postmortem roles for human body elements that can be marshaled to explain precolumbian midden or grave retrieval (Crawford and Kelley 2005). Although the source of the cremains is unclear, the ashes of the dead were used as part of the fire rekindling at the New Fire/Green Corn ceremony of the Choctaw people (Halbert 1900). Among the Mandan and Assiniboine people, a place of solace, for communing with the dead and vision questing, was created in an open space by arranging buffalo skulls and human skulls of the community's dead in a circle facing a central medicine pole (Bushnell 1927; Lowie 1910). Anonymous human bones have been included in tribal medicine bundles, such as the "waterbuster bundle" of the Hidatsa people and the "skull bundle" of the Mandan people. The origin of the bones is obscure but they functioned at least as mnemonic devices tied to the mythic origins of the bundles (e.g., Bowers 1965; Dorsey 1904c; Wood and Irwin 2001). Although contact with the spirit of the deceased (placative, supplicative, nurturing, vision quest) is apparent, the behaviors have not been recorded as venerative or related to lineage validation.

In addition to a limited ethnographic record, any socioreligious or cosmological interpretations of precolumbian human bone objects are additionally hamstrung by disjunctions and cultural transitions between the ethnographic present and the archaeological past (Echo-Hawk 2000; Mason 2000). The primary disjunction is European contact, but there is certainly evidence of precolumbian cultural discontinuities caused by diasporas and territorial abandonment (e.g., see Cobb and Butler 2002 for a discussion of Stephen Williams's (1990) A.D. 1450–1550 vacant quarter hypothesis). Such discontinuities resulted in a loss of community or ethnic affiliation that was central to mortuary ritual and the meaning of objects and behaviors. Interpretation is also confounded by the fusion of different belief systems (syncretism) (e.g., Bowers 1965; Stewart 2001) and the cultural drift of ritual, symbol, and cosmology over the centuries, which may have been abrupt and personality (agent) driven (e.g., revitalization movements led by the Seneca prophet Handsome Lake; the Shawnee prophet Tenskwatawa; the Paiute Jack Wilson a.k.a. Wovoka of the Ghost Dance movement; and the Kickapoo prophet Kenekuk) (Callender et al. 1978; Edmunds 1985; Kehoe 2006; Parker 1912), stress driven (e.g., famine, flood, epidemic, tornado), or phenomenon driven (e.g., the supernova of A.D. 1054) (Pauketat 2009).

Transitions and/or disjunctions are clearly evident in the fact that, until this volume, the ethnographic record of the contiguous United States apparently has not recorded the use of carved or incised human bones. Adding to the interpretive complexity, the iconography of supernatural beings (thunderer, birdman, sun/star) incised in precolumbian human bones (Lillie and Schermer, this volume) and the shell and ceramic objects painted or incised with disembodied heads, skulls, and limb elements have little or no ethnographic context. Although an ethnographically derived meta-analysis provides a basic mythological and ritual framework, the cosmological meaning of this precolumbian body part imagery is still actively debated by archaeologists (Brown 1997, 2007; Hall 1989, 2000; Hudson 1976; King 2007; Knight 2006; Knight et al. 2001; Reilly and Garber 2007; Townsend and Sharp 2004). The missing emic information also includes the purpose of these manufactured objects, whether the items functioned as esoteric power objects or channels of power, and how and when this power may be lost (if midden discard is any indication). Despite the lack of ethnographic context for the use of modified human bones, a fundamental observation can be made: human bone objects are not divorced from larger cosmological or social functions.

The Visible and the Invisible Native American Physical World

According to Lankford (2007b:8), "the basic beliefs of an ancient North American international religion are already known, at least in the forms in which they yet survive." Although there is much cultural heterogeneity in Native American religions, four concepts can be distilled to frame the postmortem role of human remains in the prehistoric Midwest: (1) the Native American physical world did not segregate the natural from the supernatural; (2) the organization of the universe and continued human existence comprised a dual, opposition-balanced whole maintained by cosmologically defined human behavior; (3) esoteric power had to be acquired and revitalized to create balance and to affect the outcome of conditions or events; and (4) death was not a terminus.

Axiomatically, the Native American cosmos was composed of the physical world and a complex spirit world of heroes, monsters, and other beings as well as the soul(s) of humans and animals (Carr and Novotny, this volume; Hall 1997; Hudson 1976; Lankford 1987, 2007b, 2008; Swanton 1929). These had to be managed, bargained with, placated, or petitioned by individuals, medicine societies, and shamans in order to obtain esoteric power that would affect outcomes (e.g., illness, warfare) and preserve the status quo (e.g., human and agricultural fecundity). Power could also be derived from, among other things, vision quests, fasting, and pain or sacrifice (including deprivation and self-mutilation) (Crawford and Kelley 2005). The Native American cosmos was divisible into three realms of several layers each: the celestial above, a realm below of water and the subterranean, and the floating (on water) earth disk in between (Hudson 1976; Lankford 2007b). Celestial bodies were routinely identified as power-laden sentient beings (e.g., the planet Venus = Morning Star = Red Horn [Menominee] = Birdman [SECC]; the constellation Scorpio = Great Serpent) or physical objects (e.g., Orion = hand = portal; Milky Way = path of souls) whose cycles and configurations were explained by a wide range of narratives (Brown 2007; Hall 1989; Lankford 2007b). The worlds were connected by a cosmic tree (axis mundi). Certain humans (e.g., shamans) and animals could travel between the realms along the axis, ostensibly to bring back power for human use. Human survival and continuity needed powers from both worlds. The axis mundi made tangible was apparently the ubiquitous village dance pole, a sacred object in the center of the also sacred dance circle where public rituals were performed (Lankford 2007b).

The celestial realm included the path of souls (the Milky Way), the westward trail taken by the spirits of the dead toward their final destination south to the land lorded over by the Great Serpent (the constellation Scorpio), who was also the principal power of the below realm (Lankford 2008). The path was accessed via a celestial portal of specific stars (the constellation Orion) that were visualized as a hand (Lankford 2007b). The journey was difficult and, for various reasons, not always successfully completed.

The cosmos was envisioned as a persistent dual opposition between the spirit forces of the above and below realms with the earth disk and humanity in the middle. All was well when the realms were in balance, and this balance was maintained by human behavior. That is, the fortunes and misfortunes of humans in the prehistoric Native American natural world were not achievement driven, capricious, or random circumstances but consequences of both the careful observance of ritual and the use of esoteric power or transgressions that upset the power balance. The performance of sacred ceremonies had to be accurate for success and survival. Understandably, ceremonies relating to human physical perpetuity (fecundity, renewal, adoption) and postmortem continuity (journey on the path of souls) were of particular importance. In this cosmology, the shaman, by definition an intermediary between the earth realm and the spirit world, played important and multiple roles, such as resource person (keeper of cosmological knowledge), healer, purveyor of hunting magic, ritual leader, and spirit guide (psychopomp). Communities may have had one or several purview-specific shamans or semi-lay specialists as well as medicine societies (Crawford and Kelley 2005; Hall 1997).

In-depth studies of precolumbian iconography, the growing interest in archaeoastronomy (Brown and Dye 2007; Brown and Kelly 2000; Galloway 1989; King 2007; Knight et al. 2001; Lankford 1987, 2008; Reilly and Garber 2007; Townsend and Sharp 2004), careful reanalyses of Cahokian and Hopewellian mortuary patterns (Carr and Case 2005; Case and Carr 2008; Pauketat 2009), and ethnography-based cosmology have offered credible explanations of several iconographic images of Woodland and Mississippian period mortuary practices of the Midwest and the Southeast (Brown 2007). In particular, the presence of the cosmologically complex celestial hero Morning Star/Birdman/Red Horn has been equated with continuity, the regeneration of human life, and warfare (as the first warrior) (Brown 2007; Radin 1948). Seen at Cahokia's Mound 72 and other contexts (e.g., Cahokia Submound 51, Halliday, East St. Louis), this ceremonial behavior included pageantry, cosmological reenactments, human sacrifice, and the use of the postmortem human body as a ritual tool (Brown 2010; Pauketat 2009). Based on the contributions in this volume (Carr and Novotny) and elsewhere (Carr and Case 2005), this ritual use of mortal remains dates to at least the Middle Woodland period (ca. 100 B.C.–ca. A.D. 500) and very likely earlier (Lockhart et al. 2009; Schmidt et al. 2010).

The Disembodied and Embodied Postmortem Soul(s)

What sociopolitical or cosmological role(s) human mortal remains may have played was arguably anchored in Native American self-perceptions, much of which we can certainly intellectually recognize. Humans do not possess the physical strength, keen eyes, claws, or canines of other animals. Humans require extracorporeal support to survive: clothing, shelter, tools, and weapons. Human survival also is not without effort or failure. Unlike the Aristotelian and Judeo-Christian anthropocentric and hierarchical *scala naturae*, or ladder of life, humans' preeminence on the landscape in the minds of Native American peoples is of questionable merit and only possible because of the benevolence of animals (both predators and prey), human trickery or mischief (e.g., twins narratives), the benevolence of celestial beings (e.g., shell and copper are gifts of the Great Serpent), or the murder or sacrifice of spiritual beings (e.g., Selu, the mother of corn) (Hudson 1976; Lankford 2007b, 2008; Pauketat 2009). Also, unlike the ladder of life, humans and animals share a lateral kinship, which includes attributing to animals and inanimate objects some human conditions, such as sentience and postmortem souls (spirits, ghosts).

This extension of soul and sentience predictably impacted the domestic use of animal parts and how they were discarded (Lankford 2007b, 2008).

This certainly could apply to the postmortem use of human parts and how they were discarded (i.e., in midden/refuse areas). Therefore, understanding the Native American concept of the soul is an important interpretive tool. The seminal study of this topic was undertaken by Åke Hultkrantz (1953, 1979). He determined that although as many as four human souls were recognized, most indigenous peoples recognized at least two: a free or mind soul and the mortal life force of a body soul. Other human souls were described as hovering entities, which could be merely vexing, dangerous, or sources of esoteric power. There were certainly some practical uses for a multiple soul cosmology. For example, the body soul of an individual who died by deliberate violence could harass his or her slayer(s). Emotional and social voids could be filled by soul adoption (absorption of the free soul into a living recipient).

The Mind Soul

This was the sentient self and was often described as residing in the head (and its proxy, the scalp). This was the self that left the body in dreams and at mortal death traveled across the path of souls to the realm of the dead. The path journey was extremely difficult, could result in failure, and could not be successfully navigated alone. According to T. S. Smith (1995:58), in most Native American cultures, the sentient soul was accompanied by a spirit guide (psychopomp). Between death and the completion of the journey along the path of souls, this soul (with proper powers) could return to the body or be reborn into a new body (e.g., soul adoption) (Hall 1997; Lankford 2007b). This applied laterally to animals as well. For example, before tracking, a Cherokee or a Menominee hunter would recite a specific chant or enter into a reciprocal bargain that could return the game animal to life (Dieterle 2005; Speck et al. 1993).

From albeit limited ethnographic narratives of the Southeast, Midwest, Northeast, and eastern Plains, the only human body part that was, reflected, or could become a sentient power being was the human head, the arguable seat of the mind soul. Other human body parts (e.g., the femur) could become power objects, but apparently it was the human head that could act as an independent sentient entity. It appeared in Iroquois narratives as an independent troublesome monster of unknown origin (Coppée 1900; Johnson 1881). In the Midwest (Menominee) the disembodied head occurred in metaphorical narratives relating to Morning Star or Evening Star (Radin 1948), and in certain Plains groups (Pawnee, Arapaho) it was an aspect of astronomical allegories relating to the Pleiades star cluster (Dieterle 2005; Dorsey 1906; Dorsey and Kroeber 1903; Welsch 1981). The celestial being Red Horn (as either

Morning Star or Evening Star) or Birdman of the Southeastern Ceremonial Complex was often depicted with reactive (i.e., winking, blinking, outsticking tongue) human heads as ear ornaments or gorgets. In both Menominee and Pawnee narratives, the head (or skull) had independent powers (it spit fire or spit objects of value) and would aggressively pursue humans. In some of the narratives, the disembodied head/skull was the ghost or soul of a deceased individual (Dieterle 2005; Radin 1948). The soul (i.e., the disembodied head) of a beheaded enemy could become the slave of the killer (Chacon and Dye 2007a). This concept of "soul capture" apparently had a broad cultural distribution (as likely did a soul capture avoidance or soul capture retrieval ceremony). The captured soul was apparently also a source of power. In one narrative, the slayer of the brother of Red Horn was made immortal by the possession of the disembodied head (Brown and Dye 2007).

In the disembodied head narratives of the Menominee and Pawnee tribes, the head could also be "killed" with death-dealing objects (arrow, bow, celt) (Dieterle 2005; Dorsey 1906; Dorsey and Kroeber 1903; Radin 1948). It is unclear whether this narrative was intended to suggest that destroying a skull in the material world killed the mind soul or if a realm-wandering casualty of the path of souls could ultimately be killed. Sacred objects (e.g., medicine bundles) in ethnographic accounts could certainly be killed, for example, by contact with a menstruating woman or simply contact with the ground (Bellin 2007). In the American Southeast, Midwest, and Southwest, objects (like the arguable stepped-fret skull rattle described by Cook and Munson, this volume) and vessels could be "killed" by deliberately breaking them (Brody et al. 1983; Prentice 1986; Walthall 1990).

The ethnographic information suggests that modified head/face elements (as part or all of the mind soul) could have been power objects, which may (in the time between death and final interment) or may not (after final interment) have a soul. The head/face objects from mortuary contexts may have been power objects of captured souls (cosmologically more than a war trophy, or cosmologically a group member [i.e., adopted by the captors]) or of select group members who (at physical death, young or old) accrued esoteric powers and functioned as psychopomps on the difficult journey along the path of souls. Modified head/face objects recovered from midden/refuse contexts may also have been power objects, which were either "killed" or their power purposefully and totally spent and rendered useless.

The Body Soul

The mortal or bodily life force, often characterized as actively or potentially malevolent, was often described as residing in the marrow cavity (Hall 1997;

Hultkrantz 1953; Lankford 2007b). It is clear from ethnography that there was considerable intercultural variability concerning the postmortem potency or immortality of the mortal soul as it related to natural decay, postmortem body processing, and accidental or deliberate mutilation.

Powdered or cremated remains factored into rituals of rebirth in the Midwest (Winnebago/Ho Chunk) and the Southeast (Choctaw) (Halbert 1900; Radin 1948). In the Pawnee culture, the consumption of the unrecoverable war dead by carrion eaters was a mark of honor (Dieterle 2005). In the traditional Cherokee culture, an incomplete body could not traverse the path of souls (Mooney 1900), whereas the long bones and cranium were all that was retrieved for final interment after Plains Indian scaffold burials (Dorsey and Kroeber 1903; Lowie 1910; Parks 2001). Indeed, in the Choctaw tribe, soft tissue was discarded or burned in the postmortem defleshing by the "bone pickers" (Halbert 1900). Perhaps cosmologically facilitating a permanent exit, in the Menominee culture it was believed that broken bones denied the free soul a return to its mortal self (Dieterle 2005). This may have been the reason for the placement of burned animal bone elements where the radius and ulna should have been in a Late Archaic burial from the Robinson site of west-central Tennessee (Smith 1993a). As noted above, the ritual consumption of victims was observed among the Iroquois and suspected for other groups (Jamieson 1983). Given the great ethnographic diversity of attitudes toward the body soul, and absent the material culture correlates of particular attitudes toward body integrity, it is difficult to be confident of the interpretation of modified long bones in archaeological contexts.

In most Euro-American cultures, birth is traditionally seen as the beginning of mortal life and death as the end. In most Native American cosmologies, death was universally a release of a sentient soul but it was clearly not considered to be a complete or permanent corporeal exit. More important, the process of death, birth, and rebirth in the form of soul adoption and reincarnation intertwined.

An epiphany for me was Williamson's (2007) explanation of the cosmological significance of the deliberately painful and mutilating violent death of Iroquoian war captives, including the concept of pain itself. Not only did the physical pain provide power to facilitate the journey of the community's violently killed pilgrims along the path of souls, but it was transformative (a rebirth) for the soon-to-be-killed war captive. This complex intertwining may explain the complexity of Red Horn/Birdman of the SECC, the deity associated with rebirth and war. This may also explain the frequent depiction of Birdman with a disembodied head (e.g., the Braden gorget) (Brown and Dye 2007). Death, rebirth, and religion have been intimate partners for millennia, and ritualized and actualized sacrifices are demonstrable in virtually every culture. This complexity also puts the infamous 1725 funeral of Tattooed Serpent, a Natchez Great Sun (Hudson 1976; Lorenz 2000; White et al. 1971), into cosmological perspective. The eighteenth-century Natchez Indians of Mississippi were arguably the last Mississippian culture in the United States (Hudson 1976; Lorenz 2000; White et al. 1971). The elaborate funeral rite of Tattooed Serpent included a mass suicide of retainers and family members. This gesture was horrifying to European onlookers. Although it was certainly sociopolitically magnanimous of the volunteers, it could be argued that it was not without personal gain for the sacrificed. With the Great Sun as psychopomp, the successful completion of the journey along the path of souls was assured. Another self-serving factor for the self-sacrificing was the capability of the sentient soul to reincarnate either by the efforts of grieving family members or by personally harnessing the power of the Great Sun. In other words, sacrifice of the mortal self may have been seen as a pragmatic cosmological choice, and it may have been particularly important with the advent of European contact. The stress of culture change and the introduction of new diseases may have been perceived as gross imbalances between the sky and the below world realms. The funeral of the Great Sun may therefore have been culturally atypical but predictable if esoteric power was perceived to be insufficient to return balance but enough for the mind souls that piggybacked on Tattooed Serpent in order to successfully navigate the path of souls.

Precolumbian mortuary practices in the Midwest and elsewhere are highly variable across space and time. They may consist of single-decedent primary, secondary, or cremation interments. They may be protracted multiple-stage processes with a single public interment ritual. They may or may not be intertwined with ceremonies of renewal that may or may not include pageantry, reenactments, and human sacrifice (Carr and Novotny, this volume). According to this soul cosmology, delay between the time of death and final interment means the decedent still possesses (at least) two souls. This undoubtedly impacts the spiritual status of places of temporary interment and may also impact the spiritual status of places of body processing, such as fire pits (for cremation) and midden areas, where the dead are dismembered. With incomplete ethnographic data, the archaeological mortuary contexts of these human bone objects are critical to, if not providing an explanation, certainly framing one. However, it is clear that there was an overarching cosmology with a smorgasbord of appropriate ritual options, some portion of which was utilized by different cultures across time and space.

Recovery Contexts: Clues and Ambiguities of the Postmortem Life of Skeletal Objects

The archaeological context of modified human remains, as many authors in this volume know, is often frustratingly incomplete and indeterminate. This contextual difficulty seems to fall into three main categories: lack of temporal control, lost provenience, and an ambiguous mortuary pattern that includes midden/refuse disposal.

A reality of archaeological recovery is that human remains often cannot be assigned to particular cultural horizons, particularly if there are no grave accompaniments. Even then, single cultural horizons may encompass several centuries of inevitable social change. Multicomponent sites, such as Aztalan (Wisconsin), are particularly complex since the successions of site occupants churn the middens of their predecessors (Zejdlik, this volume). Socio-religious meanings, traditions, and values may, as the Cahokia phenomenon illustrates (Pauketat 2009), change across a few generations (e.g., Chapman 2005; O'Shea 1984). Unless it is archaeologically detectable, mortuary change may mask as internal mortuary complexity.

The second category—lost cultural context—is pervasive in many of the chapters in this volume. This may include plow zone recovery, poor within-site preservation, incompletely reported cultural context, and, all too often, nonarchaeological aspects, such as looting and/or private collections. The most infamous of the looted sites is the Slack Farm site (Munson et al., this volume). The Quandahl rockshelter in Iowa, which yielded the single suspendible mandible described by Schermer and Lillie (this volume), was also extensively looted. The cache of hemimandibles from the heavily looted Hopewell Mount Vernon (General Electric) site also has no context beyond its general association with the mound (Nawrocki and Emanovsky, this volume). The lack of precision in the field notes challenges the veracity of the cache of nested mandibles from the Red Wing area (Blue, this volume). Poor preservation forestalls an accurate assessment of the modified human teeth from the Red Wing locality (Blue, this volume). Lee and Johnston (this volume) report that only one of eight stone or bone phalli from the prehistoric Midwest and interior Southeast (Kentucky, Tennessee) was recovered in situ. This phallus (Hopewell Mound group, Shetrone's Mound 17) was, not surprisingly, recovered with objects and materials interpreted to be of cosmological significance (e.g., copper, silver, and meteoric iron). More tantalizing is the co-associated cache of celts described by Greber and Ruhl (1989) as phallic in appearance. Precolumbian phallic "charm stone" (plummet?) necklaces have been recovered from California, New York, and Florida mortuary contexts (Reiger 1999). The recovery in the late 1990s of hematite phallic pendants at the Martz rockshelter in Pennsylvania adds an important in situ example (Means 1999). There is a possibility that both the phalli and phallic celts and the presumptive plummets are power objects and are associated with renewal and rebirth ceremonies. For example, Brown and Dye (2007) argued that the hair lock of the birdman image is a phallic symbol. Given a Victorian legacy in Euro-American culture, anything overtly sexual would have been omitted in the early ethnographies, and the symbolic sexual imagery of postcontact Native American peoples would have been suppressed by the overarching Euro-Christian behavioral norms. The recent recognition of vulvar imagery in rock art from southwestern Illinois and southeastern Missouri (Diaz-Granados and Duncan 2004; Duncan and Diaz-Granados 2004) certainly suggests that representations of male and female sexual parts had a culturally endorsed symbolic meaning. Whether and how the meaning of either male or female representational imagery is tied to ceremonies of renewal is unclear. There are undoubtedly more cases and contexts of modified human bones that have not been reported, preventing the emergence of the full contextual picture.

The third interpretive issue is the in situ contexts of the modified remains. Based on the contributions to this volume, they occur in two contexts: formal mortuary (mound, bounded cemetery, circumresidential) and informal village middens (bone scatter, refuse pit). Some of the modified bones display the wear and tear of long-term use. Many have drill holes that suggest suspension. Many of the modified bones may have been acquired soon after death since they display the multiple cut marks associated with defleshing. Certainly many are deliberately engraved or incised with symbols and images (Lillie and Schermer, this volume) similar to those seen in SECC iconography.

The Middle Woodland Period: Four Interpretations

The Hopewell tradition (broadly dated 200 B.C.–A.D. 500) in Illinois, eastern Iowa, Indiana, and Ohio is archaeologically well known for a complex and rich material culture. There are four current interpretations of the meaning of Hopewell modified human remains: trophy taking, ancestor veneration, memento mori, and ritual objects (Cobb, this volume; Johnston, this volume; Konigsberg and Frankenberg 1993). Based on the chapters in this volume, several facts emerge that are relevant to framing the use of modified human remains. First, Hopewell had an exceptionally symbol-rich, complex mortuary pattern. Second, Hopewell exhibited the most extensive use of modified human remains in eastern North American prehistory. Third, the osteological signatures of intergroup violence (e.g., embedded projectiles and perimortem cranial trauma) are not typically found in Hopewell mortuary contexts (Johnston, this volume; Seeman 2007). Fourth, Hopewell iconography appears to be dominated by themes pertaining to shamanism, renewal (celestial themes), and animal spirits (Brown 1997, 2007; Brown and Dye 2007; Byers 2004; Carr and Novotny, this volume; Seeman 2004, 2007).

In the ethnographic literature, warfare is undoubtedly the primary source of retrieved body parts, and these do provide tangible proof of prowess (trophy taking), but there is an apparently consistent pattern of great cosmological value(s) for the dismembered elements (e.g., appeasement of the dead, power object in mortuary ritual) (Sundstrom, this volume). Evidence that could potentially be marshaled to support the principal function of Hopewell modified body elements as war trophies include direct evidence of intergroup violence (e.g., embedded projectile points), ethnographic evidence of warfare-related body part retrieval, evidence of public display (e.g., drilled holes for suspension, arm or wrist bands made of jaws interred with some deceased), the mortuary association of aggressive power elements of carnivores (e.g., teeth, jaws, claws), or, given an absence of direct evidence of violence, the possibility that any victims of violent death may have been ineligible for community interment (e.g., Williamson 2007).

While there are contextual aspects of these modified Hopewell remains that suggest a war trophy, there are other aspects that are inconsistent with such a primary function. Specifically, in addition to the absence of embedded projectile points, there is a dearth of war paraphernalia as grave accompaniments; there are modified body elements included with female burials or from females; and there are inclusions of nonhuman (presumptively) ritual objects. Additionally, the imagery on carved or incised pipes noted by Seeman (2007) to suggest warfare (i.e., a dog consuming a human head on the "Great Pipe," Seip Mound, Ohio; a raven consuming a human head on the "Hungry Pipe," Gibson Mound, Illinois; a raptor pecking at a human hand on a Mound City, Ohio, pipe) or on effigy boatstones (i.e., a falcon with a human head on top of a raptor's head from the Hopewell Mound group) can be alternatively interpreted as metaphors (mind = head) or as narratives about soul flight and impediments along the treacherous and casualty-ridden path of souls. For example, the hand is the portal to the path of souls (the constellation Orion) that must be passed through, and a dog and a raptor are two of several dangerous, soul-defeating obstacles en route (Brown 1997; Carr and Novotny, this volume; Lankford 2007b).

The contexts might also suggest "revered ancestors" (Webb and Snow

1945; Willoughby and Hooton 1922), but this interpretation is not strongly supported by the data marshaled in this volume (Johnston; Nawrocki and Emanovsky) nor by the ethnographic overview provided earlier. However, a kin-related explanation with merit suggested by several authors relates to the frequent accompaniment of the modified jaws with animal "power" parts: they may have had totemic or eponymic meaning (Case and Carr 2008; Johnston 2002). The interpretation of memento mori is not supported in the contexts of modified human element recovery in middens or with caches of objects, but drilled phalanges (Baby 1961; Schermer and Lillie, this volume), as mentioned earlier, may have functioned as memento "mourning attire."

The strongest case that can be made is for the ritual use(s) of the modified human remains. These uses were arguably varied and, based on Native American cosmology, there is good reason to presume that these were (temporarily or permanently) objects of power. The most frequently selected skeletal element for modification is the skull. The most frequently observed elements are ground maxillae and mandibles. These have a specific distribution across Illinois, Indiana, Ohio, and possibly Iowa and overlap the use of similarly modified animal jaws (Cobb, this volume; Johnston, this volume, Nawrocki and Emanovsky, this volume; Seeman 2007). Also based on Native American cosmology, which argues synonymy between humans and animals, the emphasis on the mouth area may reflect voice or song, exit portals of the soul, portals of consumption or disgorgement (e.g., purgative purification rituals such as "black drink"), or aggression (biting, tooth baring) and warfare. What is quite striking is the lack of co-association of modified mandibles and maxillae with grave inclusions of domestic use (e.g., awls, fleshers, scrapers). Instead, mandibles and maxillae are accompanied by items such as flakes of copper (copper = gift of the Great Serpent) (see Lankford 2007b), bear teeth, mica, quartz, pearls (a power metaphor for stars?) (see Carr and Novotny, this volume), effigy objects, and pipes (Cobb, this volume), which strengthens the interpretation that the modified remains are ritual and power objects.

Other modified crania and cranial elements are differentially represented geographically. There were five perforated (possibly for suspension) crania at Tremper Mound in Ohio, but none in Illinois, Iowa, or the Mount Vernon site in southern Indiana (Cobb, this volume; Nawrocki and Emanovsky, this volume; Schermer and Lillie, this volume). Human calotte vessels (bowls) reported for the Middle Woodland are apparently extremely rare; there is a "killed" skull bowl from the Middle Woodland Hopewell Mound group (Seeman 1988, 2007). Calotte vessels have been recovered in Late Archaic contexts in the riverine Southeast (Jacobi 2007; Smith 1997). In post-Hopewell contexts, a child's cranium from a Fort Ancient (A.D. 1000–1650) context in Indiana (Munson et al., this volume) and the calotte fragments from the Oneota (ca. A.D. 1300–1700) Utz site (central Missouri) (Lillie and Schermer, this volume) may have been vessels. Cranial elements that have been found with greater frequency are excised round frontal or parietal squamae (rondelles, disks, gorgets), such as those described by Schermer and Lillie (this volume) in Iowa contexts. These have also been found in the Ohio Hopewell site of Turner. Other Middle Woodland contexts include a single unprovenienced rondelle from eastern Tennessee (Williams 1975), and in western Tennessee, Pinson Mounds (the largest Middle Woodland habitation in the Southeast) yielded two incised rondelles that evidently were worn at the knee as rattles (Mainfort 1986). There is a patchy post-Hopewell distribution. One rondelle with a central perforation was recovered from the Stirling phase (A.D. 1100–1200) St. Thomas site near Cahokia (Krutchen and Vanderford 2005). From the central Ohio River valley, Munson and Cook (this volume) report that there is one rondelle with an engraved image of a raptor that was interred with an infant from an Adena culture (1000–200 B.C.) context (Florence Mound, Ohio) and another from the Angel site (A.D. 1050–1400). Two rondelles and two disembodied crania were recovered from a burned house feature in a Red Wing (A.D. 1050–1300), Minnesota, context (Blue, this volume). Contextually pertinent, human bone rondelles used as rattles have been identified in historic and protohistoric Iroquoian contexts (Williamson 2007).

Presumably metaphorically interrelated are the rondelle-sized perforations in crania from Ohio Hopewell contexts. Perforated crania and perforated long bone metaphyses are found in the Great Lakes area of Minnesota and Michigan in the Middle Woodland (Laurel, 200 B.C.–A.D. 900) and later horizons (Black Duck, A.D. 800–1400) (Greenman 1967; Helms 2008; Hinsdale and Greenman 1936; Torbenson et al. 1992). The holes in the bones from the Upper Midwest have been independently interpreted as evidence of soul release (Helms 2008; Torbenson et al. 1992). However, not every bone displays soul portals and the infrequency of rondelles suggests more as yet undetected or indiscernible cosmological complexity. Rondelles may have been the precursors to the shell gorgets of later prehistory. If so, there may have been some synonymy of function and meaning that was time transcendent.

Although the manufacturing focus in the Middle Woodland appears to be mandibles and maxillae, other less frequently modified body elements include long bone flutes (radius), blowing tubes, and the aforementioned drilled phalanges (e.g., Baby 1961; Schermer and Lillie, this volume). Because of the rarity of modified human postcranial elements, these are also likely ritual or sacred objects.

The human sources of the raw material may have been war captives, community members, or both. Whoever they were, they were of enough social significance to merit time-consuming postmortem processing and subsequent retention for some community or personal benefit. The complex material remains associated with the Hopewell mortuary behavior has suggested that the interment events had multiple functions (Carr and Novotny, this volume). This behavior does indeed look like it cemented what were arguably mutually beneficial heterarchical social relationships, served as a stage for rituals of fertility and renewal (Carr and Novotny, this volume), and facilitated the journey of the mind souls of the deceased along the difficult path of souls. For example, mind souls from (adopted) war captives, from deceased and/or sacrificed young men and women, or from empowered individuals (shamans) could serve as the necessary psychopomp for the path of souls. The retention, use, and decommissioning of an object may also relate to the occasional crisis renewal or rebalance rituals that required more power to counter episodic survival-threatening events (e.g., tornado, flood, famine, epidemic) caused by ritual transgressions.

The archaeological inability to distinguish a trophy from an honored decedent is perhaps in itself meaningful. With respect to Hopewell imagery that exhibits what has been interpreted as both war-like and renewal-like messages (Brown 1997, 2007; Lankford 2007b), Seeman suggested that "ambiguities and overlaps in these themes very well may have been intentional" (2007:181). Indeed, I am struck by Williamson's (2007) observation that in the Iroquoian language, a single term (*aireskoi*) was used to refer to a spiritual force that equated war and fertility. If Red Horn (Birdman) does indeed have Hopewell roots, then the conflation of war (or mortal death) and rebirth has a deep time line.

The Early to Middle Mississippian Period: What Is the Meaning of Midden Disposal?

Compared to the Middle Woodland, the modified human remains from the Midwest after A.D. 1000 are less common and contextually more complex. As mentioned, rondelles and calotte bowls infrequently still occur. The socioreligious and iconographic impact of the Cahokia phenomenon is still being unraveled (Pauketat 2009). Like Hopewell, it includes reenactment tableaus. It, too, leaves us with a conflated imagery of renewal and, if not warfare, certainly mortal death (Galloway 1989; King 2007; Reilly and Garber 2007; Townsend and Sharp 2004). Like the Woodland phenomenon, we have pieces of the cultural whole, but there are more pieces (e.g., warfare, midden/refuse disposal). There is also apparently greater regional and intraregional sociocultural heterogeneity (e.g., Mississippian, Oneota, Fort Ancient, Caddo). The examples included in this volume illustrate this quite effectively.

There are at least four factors that are relevant to framing the interpretation of late prehistoric modified human remains. First, there is ample direct evidence (embedded projectile points, massacre episodes) of intergroup violence. Second, there is irrefutable evidence of widespread perimortem scalping and evidence that the victims have not been excluded from standard mortuary treatment. Third, because of hypothesized endemic violence, the common interpretation of (at least) the nonmodified human body element grave inclusions is that they represent prowess-verifying trophy items. Fourth, there is a referential (but arguably not the only) cosmological framework (e.g., SECC) to marshal (King 2007; Pauketat 2009).

A regional overview of the data provides the foundation. The Angel site, Indiana (A.D. 1050–1400); Red Wing, Minnesota (A.D. 1050–1300); much of the Aztalan site, Wisconsin (A.D. 1000–1200); and Cahokia (A.D. 1050–1400) temporally overlap and share many recovery contexts and the kinds of modified objects retrieved. One of these common denominators is the presence of human remains in midden contexts. At the Angel site, a political and religious center, the midden yielded a stepped-fret human skull mask or rattle that appears to have been ritually killed, and additional cranial fragments that may also have been a killed rattle (Cook and Munson, this volume). The linkage by Cook and Munson of the stepped-fret mask or rattle to Mississippian severed head iconography (e.g., Rogan plates, Etowah) suggests a connection to Red Horn/Birdman renewal rituals. Two other human bone objects from this site were also found in midden contexts. Cook and Munson argue that they may have been deliberately, perhaps ritually, used for hide processing (a flensing tool or a beamer). The midden-recovered tibia from the Aztalan site is interpreted by Zejdlik (this volume) as some form of hide-processing tool. In this context, however, Zejdlik suggests an opportunistic use of a chance recovery. At Aztalan, in addition to primary burials, bundle burials, and charnel house cremations, there are scattered human remains, some with cut marks, in refuse pits, in fire pits, and across the occupation area. The mortuary pattern in the Red Wing area of Minnesota appears to be mound (primary or secondary interment) or a midden bone scatter. The bones in the scatter also display cut marks, and some clearly have been burned. It is in the midden context that most of the modified human teeth were recovered as well as at least one mandible perforated for suspension (Blue, this volume). These sites temporally overlap Cahokia, which is the apparent source of the iconography (e.g., birdman) that defines the Mississippian period (Lankford 2007b). The mortuary practices at Cahokia are elaborate and include primary inhumation, sacrifice, and cremation. As Hargrave and Cook report in this volume, there is also modified human bone (ulna awl, femur dibble) and deliberate long bone breakage from refuse contexts. Pauketat et al. (2002) identified the material from the Submound 51 feature as representing feasting debris and the deconstruction and burning of one or more temple/charnel houses.

Additional information derives from the Oneota culture, which pre- and postdates the aforementioned sites and is the Mississippian cultural equivalent in Wisconsin, Iowa, and northern Illinois. Intergroup violence and scalp taking have been identified in Oneota sites in Illinois (Milner et al. 1991). Human bone modification occurs sporadically in Oneota contexts in Illinois, Indiana, Wisconsin, and Missouri and, not surprisingly, is primarily cranial (Hedman, this volume). Iowa Oneota mortuary treatment consists of primary and secondary burials in four contexts: discrete cemeteries away from villages, intrusions into Woodland mounds, in villages as midden, or as storage pit debris. In the sites described by Lillie and Schermer (this volume), there are cut marks indicative of mortuary processing and evidence of burning; however, all of the deliberately modified remains are from nonmortuary contexts. In western Iowa, a cranial fragment with incised images of a forked eye, a sun/star, and an anthropomorphic figure was recovered from an eroding bank at a habitation site, either from village midden or refuse deposits.

What then are the possible meanings of isolated human bones in midden or refuse debris? They could be charnel house debris that included killed ritual objects. The osseous material may initially have been disposed of at the village margins and, over time and because of village growth, it became incorporated into the living space. But if warfare is indeed endemic in later prehistory, captives may certainly have been a source for at least some human bone midden debris and may have played varied cosmological roles (including psychopomp). The dance circle with its dance pole (the axis mundi) is sacred space and a fixture in the center of aggregate Native American communities. Ritual ceremonies are performed there. Therefore the images on, for example, the Braden B shell cup (Phillips and Brown 1978:Plate 57) have meaning vis-à-vis dismemberment mortuary treatment. In this image the axis mundi (as a striped dance pole) is flanked by a motif identified as a sky symbol (the celestial realm); on the opposite side is the Great Serpent (the below world realm) (Reilly and Garber 2007). In between is a tangle of disembodied heads, skulls, a hand, broken long bones, and mace heads associated with Birdman. Tongue-like protrusions extend from the mouths of the heads and at breaks in the bones, which Lankford (2007b) interpreted as soul release. The hand could be the sky portal to the path of souls. The beaded forelocks of the heads suggest they are males (Brown 2007; Lankford 2007b). The skull (perhaps meaning a heretofore retained object) has incised markings that could indicate scalping (suggesting a warfare origin). Is this a depiction of the ritualized dispatching of a war captive (as a soul capture or adopted soul) or a psychopomp to the path of souls (Brown 2007)? It could certainly suggest a one-way trip if bone breakages (releasing the malevolent body soul) reflect a cosmological "kill" that prevents reincarnation.

Complex mortuary rituals and SECC iconography (as a proxy for ritual and perhaps as a cosmological point of departure for non-Mississippian cultures) may co-vary with midden bone scatter. Since the heyday of SECC iconography was circa A.D. 1240–1350, there may be unexplored temporal patterns that require more publications of modified human bones and their recovery contexts. This volume is a move in that direction. Continued research may link imagery with mortuary patterns.

Late Prehistoric Contexts: Some Common Threads

The Caborn-Welborn phase (A.D. 1400–1700), the Huber phase of the Upper Mississippian (A.D. 1400–1700) (represented by the Hoxie Farm and Anker sites, Illinois), and the Classic phase of the Oneota (A.D. 1350–1650) (represented by the McKinney site, Iowa) temporally overlap. As Munson and colleagues (this volume) report, the Caborn-Welborn phase of the lower Ohio River valley succeeds the Mississippian period Angel culture.

Caborn-Welborn burials are most often primary interments found in rowed cemeteries, house floors, and village middens. There is evidence of status-based differential interment and intergroup violence (a case of scalping) (Munson et al., this volume). Modified human bone is found in three contexts: an unprovenienced cemetery (two mandibles, possible grave inclusion), the midden of a house basin (a clavicle and a cranial fragment from a possible disturbed house floor mortuary context), and the midden at the village margin (a clavicle and an ulna, discarded?). Although the meaning is obscured owing to the unfortunate recovery contexts (looting, construction projects), the unusual suite of modified bones poses new questions concerning meaning and use. The protohistoric Oneota Anker site brings together elements seen in the Hopewell period: multiple animal jaws and modified human bones. Hedman (this volume) argues that the context is consistent with ritual medicine (power) bundles similar to those of the Algonquian/Siouan Grand Medicine Society (Midewiwin), which had both male and female members. More archaeological information needs to be gathered from this time period since it is recent enough for the ethnographic record to be relevant.

Several overarching facts do emerge. Birth (rebirth, soul adoption) and death (mortality, body soul) have complex meanings in the precontact Native American cosmology. It is also clear from ethnography that the postmortem body is not inert (body soul) and has a culturally variable definition of its integrity (e.g., dismemberment for interment vs. dismemberment as ineligible for interment). The word "trophy" needs definition or qualifiers, since it is too broadly defined and inadequate to reflect the real indigenous world of animate objects and nonhuman beings (see Sundstrom, this volume). Perhaps some thought should be given to agency theory in order to coin a meaningful alternative. At least two objective patterns emerge about the modification and use of human body parts: differential use and differential value.

Differential Use: Human Bone Is Not Raw Material for Secular Use

Human skeletal remains, like other animal bones, are potentially retrievable sources of raw material for the construction of utilitarian tools, such as axe and adze handles, fish hooks, and hoes. Given that many of the peoples in the Midwest engaged in mortuary behavior that would make those usable elements available (e.g., defleshing and cremation), it can be concluded that human bones are not routinely harvested as raw material. Therefore, when human bones are retrieved that do appear to have been used as utilitarian implements, the explanation could be an inadvertent or ritual use.

Sometimes the ritual significance is deducible given the survival needs of food producers (Byers 2004; Carr and Case 2005; Case and Carr 2008). Some may be objects of power for specific uses and mirror the backbone of Native American cosmology: the quest for cosmic balance. For example, human bone fleshers or beamers may be a cosmic balance-maintaining reciprocal bargain for the use of animal pelts with ritual importance (e.g., bear skin). This cosmological balance may (etically) explain the human bone inclusions in the primary headless adult male burial from the Bluff Creek site, northern Alabama (Jacobi 2007; Ross-Stallings 2007), often referred to as the "bone picker" or the "dentist." He was interred with 131 human teeth and 5 human bone (fibulae, radius) awls located linearly on the right side of his body. With a trophy-taking perspective of human bone retrieval and usage, Jacobi interpreted the scenario as a punitive decapitation and stabbing (with the awls). In light of the chapters in this volume, an alternative interpretation could be the retrieval of the head of a powerful shaman (a likely successful traveler on the path of souls) for community use (as a psychopomp, among other things). The awls, given their linear arrangement on the body, may have been fasteners for a fur cloak in which the individual was interred. The awls, in other words, could have functioned as pins. If cosmic balance is the spiritual goal of indigenous peoples, then the reciprocal bargain may have mandated the use of human bone in a functional capacity in exchange for the privilege of using the skin. This interpretation of the "bone picker" may be fanciful and entirely speculative, but it serves to illustrate the need for more careful descriptive and contextual mortuary and ethnographic data.

Differential Value: Not All Body Elements Are Eligible for Postmortem Use

If being human were the criteria for postmortem use, all human bones would be eligible as secular mementos or power objects. The human bones routinely occurring as cultural objects are those that are quintessentially human and taphonomically easily retrievable: the cranium, face, teeth, and hands. It cannot be argued that trunk elements are inaccessible since the deliberate dismemberment processing of humans would be no more difficult than dismembering a large-bodied game animal. Indeed, in the Plains, bison and elk ribs have been used as rasps, knife handles, and fish hooks (Brooks 2004:341; W. Wedel 2001). Given that only a little modification would enable the stringing of, say, cervical vertebrae, these elements are evidently not wanted.

The nonhuman bone elements used in Hopewell mortuary contexts have been argued to be "power parts," that is, the jaws, claws, and teeth (Seeman 2007). They are also the signature parts that distinguish animals from each other. The human cranium and limb elements may also underscore human uniqueness and have great metaphorical significance.

The fact that these modified human bone elements are apparently rare suggests that there are specific circumstances when their fashioning, use, and disposal are merited. These may be stress-related circumstances that do not have archaeological signatures. The elements may also reflect a continuity of ritual and meaning with simply a change in the metaphor (e.g., rondelles fashioned of shell [gorgets] instead of a human calotte) that we do not perceive. Finally, recognizing the fact that the Native American sense of self with respect to the natural world is not the *scala naturae* of the Euro-American, human bone objects may have been perceived as inherently less power-laden than those of, for example, the bear or the eagle. In other words, the human centric etic view may have elevated the importance of human bone objects and their puzzled-over midden/refuse disposal.

Several avenues of research have opened with the presentations and discussions of modified human bone in this volume. First, more of these modified human bones need to be reported for the purpose of establishing a timeline, which would reveal regional patterns and identify cultural continuities.

Many human bone artifacts may have been dismissed as trophy items and not considered as a vital part of the nonutilitarian material culture. Indeed, undisturbed primary or secondary interments missing head or limb elements should be reassessed with respect to mortuary ritual. Some attention should be paid to the nature and content of nonutilitarian objects where there has never been evidence of modified human bone use. This includes a careful assessment of animal bone use. Modified human bones should be included in future assessments of iconography—not just in the assessment of imagery but also in analyses of objects such as effigies and the enigmatic head pots of northeastern Arkansas (Cherry 2009). There may be numerous undetected human bone objects misidentified as animal in many collections because of their midden or refuse area recovery.

When there is a more comprehensive temporal and regional framework, a follow-up volume would be useful. I have certainly been inspired to take a second look at the "head burials" of the Hamilton mortuary complex of eastern Tennessee and at the apparent absence of modified human bones in the southern Appalachian heartland of SECC shell gorget use.

Acknowledgments

I would like to thank the editors of this volume for asking me to participate as discussant in the 2008 MAC symposium entitled *Human Bone as Cultural Object: A Midwestern Perspective* and for inviting me to contribute to this volume.

References

Agogino, George A., and Eugene Galloway
1963 Osteology of the Four Bear Burials. *Plains Anthropologist* 8:57–60.

Ahler, Steven R., and Peter J. DePuydt
1987 *A Report on the 1931 Powell Mound Excavations, Madison County, Illinois*. Reports of Investigation No. 43. Illinois State Museum, Springfield.

Alex, Lynn M.
2000 *Iowa's Archaeological Past*. University of Iowa Press, Iowa City.

Alex, Robert
1974 University of Wisconsin–Milwaukee 1974 Summer Field School. *Newsletter of the Wisconsin Anthropological Society* 3(1):4–5.

Alt, Susan M.
2006 Cultural Pluralism and Complexity: Analyzing a Cahokian Ritual Outpost. Unpublished Ph.D. dissertation, Department of Anthropology, University of Illinois, Urbana.

Anderson, Duane C.
1971 Human Skeletal Remains in the Sanford Museum Collection. *Northwest Chapter of the Iowa Archeological Society Newsletter* 19(1):6–16.

Anderson, Kristen L.
1994 The Aztalan Site: A Human Skeletal Inventory and Excavation. Unpublished Master's thesis, Department of Anthropology, University of Chicago, Chicago.

Andrushko, Valerie A., Kate A. S. Latham, Diane L. Grady, Allen G. Pastron, and Phillip L. Walker
2005 Bioarchaeological Evidence for Trophy-Taking in Prehistoric Central California. *American Journal of Physical Anthropology* 127:375–384.

Ansell Research
2001 The Penis Size Survey. Electronic document, http://www.free-condom-stuff.com/education/research.html, accessed March 15, 2009.

Arnold, Bettina, and Nancy L. Wicker (editors)
2001 *Gender and the Archaeology of Death*. AltaMira, Walnut Creek, California.

Asch, David L.
1976 *The Middle Woodland Population in the Lower Illinois Valley: A Study in Paleo-*

demographic Methods. Archaeological Program Scientific Papers No. 1. Northwestern University, Evanston, Illinois.

Axtell, James, and William C. Sturtevant
1980 The Unkindest Cut; or, Who Invented Scalping. *William and Mary Quarterly*, 3rd ser. 37:451–472.

Baadsgaard, Aubrey, Alexis T. Boutin, and Jane E. Buikstra (editors)
2012 *Breathing New Life into the Evidence of Death: Contemporary Approaches to Bioarchaeology*. School for Advanced Research Press, Santa Fe, New Mexico.

Baby, Raymond S.
1954 Hopewell Cremation Practices. *Ohio Historical Society Papers in Archaeology* 1:1–7.
1956 A Unique Hopewellian Mask Headdress. *American Antiquity* 21:303–305.
1961 A Hopewell Human Bone Whistle. *American Antiquity* 27:108–110.

Bailey, Garrick A. (editor)
1995 *The Osage and the Invisible World from the Works of Francis La Flesche*. University of Oklahoma Press, Norman.

Bailey, Garrick A., and Gloria A. Young
2001 Kansa. In *Plains*, edited by Raymond J. DeMallie, pp. 462–475. Handbook of North American Indians, Vol. 13, William C. Sturtevant, general editor, Smithsonian Institution, Washington, D.C.

Baker, Frank C., James B. Griffin, Richard G. Morgan, Georg K. Neumann, and Jay L. B. Taylor
1941 Contributions to the Archaeology of the Illinois River Valley. *Transactions of the American Philosophical Society* 32(1). Philadelphia.

Balzer, Marjorie Madelstam
1996 Flights of the Sacred: Symbolism and Theory in Siberian Shamanism. *American Anthropologist* 98:305–318.

Barley, Nigel
1995 *Grave Matters: Encounters with Death around the World*. Waveland, Long Grove, Illinois.

Barnouw, Victor
1977 *Wisconsin Chippewa Myths and Tales and Their Relation to Chippewa Life*. University of Wisconsin Press, Madison.

Barrett, Samuel
1917 *Pomo Bear Doctors*. University of California Press, Berkeley.
1933 Ancient Aztalan. *Bulletin of the Public Museum of the City of Milwaukee* 13.
1952 Material Aspects of Pomo Material Culture. *Bulletin of the Public Museum of the City of Milwaukee* 20.

Barrett, Samuel A., and Alanson Skinner
1932 Certain Mounds and Village Sites of Shawano and Oconto Counties, Wisconsin. *Bulletin of the Public Museum of the City of Milwaukee* 10(5).

Basden, George Thomas
2009 *Among the Ibos of Nigeria*. Reprinted. Kessinger, Whitefish, Montana. Originally published 1921, Seeley, Service, London.

Beck, Lane A. (editor)

1995 *Regional Approaches to Mortuary Analysis.* Plenum, New York.

Beck, Stephen

2009 Maritime Mechanisms of Contact and Change: Archaeological Perspectives on the History and Conduct of the Queensland Labour Trade. Unpublished Ph.D. thesis, Department of Anthropology, Archaeology and Sociology, James Cook University, Townsville, Australia.

Beier, J. Marshall

1998 *Blackened Faces and Ticker-Tape Parades: Situating the Leviathan in Lakota and Euroamerican Conceptions of War.* Occasional Paper 54. Center for International and Security Studies, York University, York, Ontario, Canada.

Bek, William G. (translator)

1938 First Journey to North America in the Years 1822 to 1824 by Paul Wilhelm, Duke of Wuerttemberg. *South Dakota Historical Collections* 19:7–471.

Bellin, Joshua D.

2007 *Medicine Bundle: Indian Sacred Performance and American Literature, 1824–1932.* University of Pennsylvania Press, Philadelphia.

Benn, David W.

1989 Hawks, Serpents, and Bird-Men: Emergence of the Oneota Mode of Production. *Plains Anthropologist* 34(125):233–260.

Berres, Thomas E.

2001 *Power and Gender in Oneota Culture: A Study of a Late Prehistoric People.* Northern Illinois University Press, DeKalb.

Berres, Thomas E., David M. Stothers, and David Mather

2004 Bear Imagery and Ritual in Northeast North America: An Update and Assessment of A. Irving Hallowell's Work. *Midcontinental Journal of Archaeology* 29(1):5–42.

Berryman, Hugh E., Harry H. Mincer, and S. J. Moore

1991 Forensic Characteristics of Antemortem, Perimortem, and Postmortem Dental Fractures. American Academy of Forensic Sciences Program of the 43rd Annual Meeting. AAFS Publication 91-2. Fittje Brothers, Colorado Springs, Colorado.

Best, Elsdon

1934 *The Maori as He Was: A Brief Account of Maori Life as It Was in Pre-European Days.* Dominion Museum, Wellington, New Zealand.

Betancourt, Philip P.

1965 A Description of Certain Engraved Artifacts from the Utz Oneota Site. *Plains Anthropologist* 10(30):256–270.

Betts, Colin

2006 Pots and Pox: The Identification of Protohistoric Epidemics in the Upper Mississippi Valley. *American Antiquity* 71:233–260.

2007 Depopulation, Ethnohistory, and the Seventeenth Century Ioway(s). Paper presented at the Annual Midwest Archaeological Conference, South Bend, Indiana.

Binford, Louis

1971 Mortuary Practices: Their Study and Their Potential. In *Approaches to the Social Dimensions of Mortuary Practices*, edited by James A. Brown, pp. 6–29. Memoir 25. Society for American Anthropology, Salt Lake City, Utah.

Birch, Jennifer

2010 Coalescence and Conflict in Iroquoian Ontario. *Archaeological Review from Cambridge* 25:29–48.

Birmingham, Robert, and Leslie Eisenberg

2000 *Indian Mounds of Wisconsin*. University of Wisconsin Press, Madison.

Bishop Museum

2010 [1892] Preliminary Catalogue of the Bernice Pauahi Bishop Museum of Polynesian Ethnology and Natural History, Pt. III. Reprinted. Electronic document, http://hbs.bishopmuseum.org/pubs-online/pdf/sp1-3.pdf, accessed July 29, 2009.

Black, Glenn A.

1967 *Angel Site: An Archaeological, Historical and Ethnological Study*. 2 vols. Indiana Historical Society, Indianapolis.

Blackwell, Mark

2004 Extraneous Bodies: The Contagion of Live-Tooth Transplantation in Late-Eighteenth-Century England. *Eighteenth-Century Life* 28:21–68.

Blaine, Martha Royce

1995 *The Ioway Indians*. University of Oklahoma Press, Norman.

Blair, Emma Helen

1911 *The Indian Tribes of the Upper Mississippi Valley and Region of the Great Lakes*. 2 vols. Arthur H. Clark, Cleveland, Ohio.

Blom, Deborah E.

2005 Embodying Borders: Human Body Modification and Diversity in Tiwanaku Society. *Journal of Anthropological Archaeology* 24:1–24.

Blue, Kathleen T.

1997a 21GD4 Bryan Site, Drift Osteology Report, April 10, 1997. Manuscript on file, Hamline University Osteology Laboratory, St. Paul, Minnesota.

1997b SMM2416 21GD86 Ft. Sweney, Osteological Report. Manuscript on file, Hamline University Osteology Laboratory, St. Paul, Minnesota.

2006 Family or Foes? Intentional Modification of Skeletal Remains from the Red Wing Locality. Paper presented at the Midwest Archaeological Conference, Urbana, Illinois.

Bluhm, Elaine A., and Allen Liss

1961 *The Anker Site*. Bulletin 3:89–137. Illinois Archaeological Survey, Champaign.

Boddington, Andrew, Andrew N. Garland, and Robert C. Janaway

1987 *Death, Decay, and Reconstruction: Approaches to Archaeology and Forensic Science*. Manchester University, Manchester, United Kingdom.

Bonnemains, Jacqueline

1984 *Charles-Alexandre Lesueur en Amerique du Nord (1816–1837): Catalogue des*

Documents du Muséum d'Histoire Naturelle du Havre (2). Annales du Muséum du Havre No. 30. LeHavre, France.

Bonney, Heather, and Margaret Clegg

2011 Heads as Memorials and Status Symbols: The Collection and Use of Skulls in the Torres Strait Islands. In *The Bioarchaeology of the Human Head: Decapitation, Decoration, and Deformation*, edited by Michelle Bonogofsky, pp. 51–66. University Press of Florida, Gainesville.

Bonogofsky, Michelle

2011 Contextualizing the Human Head: An Introduction. In *The Bioarchaeology of the Human Head: Decapitation, Decoration, and Deformation*, edited by Michelle Bonogofsky, pp. 1–47. University Press of Florida, Gainesville.

Bonogofsky, Michelle (editor)

2006 *Skull Collection, Modification, and Decoration*. BAR International Series 1539. Archaeopress, Oxford, United Kingdom.

2011 *The Bioarchaeology of the Human Head: Decapitation, Decoration, and Deformation*. University Press of Florida, Gainesville.

Bonogofsky, Michelle, and Jeremy Graham

2011 Melanesian Modeled Skulls, Mortuary Ritual, and Dental X-Rays. In *The Bioarchaeology of the Human Head: Decapitation, Decoration, and Deformation*, edited by Michelle Bonogofsky, pp. 67–96. University Press of Florida, Gainesville.

Borden, Charles E. (editor)

1963 Current Research. *American Antiquity* 29:255–269.

Bowers, Alfred W.

1965 *Hidatsa Social and Ceremonial Organization*. Bureau of American Ethnology Bulletin 194. Smithsonian Institution, Washington, D.C.

Brain, Jeffrey P., and Philip Phillips

1996 *Shell Gorgets: Styles of the Late Prehistoric and Protohistoric Southeast*. Peabody Museum Press, Cambridge, Massachusetts.

Braun, David P.

1986 Midwestern Hopewellian Exchange and Supralocal Interaction. In *Peer Polity Interaction and Socio-political Change*, edited by Colin Renfrew and John F. Cherry, pp. 117–126. Cambridge University Press, Cambridge.

Braun, David P., James B. Griffin, and Paul F. Titterington

1982 *The Snyders Mounds and Five Other Mound Groups in Calhoun County, Illinois*. Technical Reports No. 13. Museum of Anthropology, University of Michigan, Ann Arbor.

Bray, Robert T.

1961 The Flynn Cemetery: An Orr Focus Oneota Burial Site in Allamakee County. *Journal of the Iowa Archeological Society* 10(4):15–25.

1963 Southern Cult Motifs from the Utz Oneota Site, Saline County, Missouri. *Missouri Archaeologist* 25:1–40.

1991 The Utz Site: An Oneota Village in Central Missouri. *Missouri Archaeologist* 52:1–146.

Brody, Jacob J., Catherine J. Scott, and Steven A. LeBlanc
1983 *Mimbres Pottery: Ancient Art of the American Southwest.* Hudson Hills Press, New York.

Brooks, Robert L.
2004 From Stone Slab Architecture to Abandonment. In *The Prehistory of Texas*, edited by Timothy Perttula, pp. 331–341. Anthropology Series No. 9. Texas A&M University, College Station.

Brose, David S., C. Wesley Cowan, and Robert C. Mainfort Jr. (editors)
2001 *Societies in Eclipse: Archaeology of the Eastern Woodlands Indiana* A.D. *1400–1700.* University of Alabama Press, Tuscaloosa.

Brose, David S., and N'omi Greber (editors)
1979 *Hopewell Archaeology: The Chillicothe Conference.* Kent State University Press, Kent, Ohio.

Brower, Jacob V., and William M. Sweney
1903 *Memoirs of Explorations in the Basin of the Mississippi*, Vol. 6. H. L. Collins, St. Paul, Minnesota.

Brown, Donald N., and Lee Irwin
2001 Ponca. In *Plains*, edited by Raymond J. DeMallie, pp. 416–431. Handbook of North American Indians, Vol. 13, William C. Sturtevant, general editor, Smithsonian Institution, Washington, D.C.

Brown, James A.
1971 The Dimensions of Status at Spiro. In *Approaches to the Social Dimensions of Mortuary Practices*, edited by James A. Brown, pp. 92–102. Memoir 25. Society for American Anthropology, Washington, D.C.

1975 Spiro Art and Its Mortuary Contexts. In *Death and the Afterlife in Pre-Columbian America*, edited by Elizabeth P. Benson, pp. 1–32. Dumbarton Oaks Research Library and Collections, Washington, D.C.

1979 Charnel Houses and Mortuary Crypts: Disposal of the Dead in the Middle Woodland Period. In *Hopewell Archaeology: The Chillicothe Conference*, edited by David S. Brose and N'omi Greber, pp. 211–219. Kent State University Press, Kent, Ohio.

1996 *The Spiro Ceremonial Center: The Archaeology of the Arkansas Valley Caddoan Culture in Eastern Oklahoma.* Memoir 29. Museum of Anthropology, University of Michigan, Ann Arbor.

1997 The Archaeology of Ancient Religion in the Eastern Woodlands. *Annual Reviews in Anthropology* 26:465–485.

2003 The Cahokia Mound 72-Sub1 Burials as Collective Representation. In *A Deep Time Perspective: Studies in Symbols, Meaning and the Archaeological Record: Papers in Honor of Robert L. Hall*, edited by John D. Richards and Melvin L. Fowler. Special issue, *Wisconsin Archeologist* 84:81–97.

2004 The Cahokian Expression: Creating Court and Cult. In *Hero, Hawk, and Open Hand: American Indian Art of the Ancient Midwest and South*, edited by Richard F. Townsend and Robert V. Sharp, pp. 104–123. Yale University Press, New Haven, Connecticut.

2006 Where's the Power in Mound Building? An Eastern Woodlands Perspective. In *Leadership and Polity in Mississippian Society*, edited by Brian M. Butler and Paul D. Welch, pp. 197–213. Occasional Paper 33. Center for Archaeological Investigations, Southern Illinois University, Carbondale.

2007 On the Identity of the Birdman within Mississippian Period Art and Iconography. In *Ancient Objects and Sacred Realms: Interpretations of Mississippian Iconography*, edited by F. Kent Reilly III and James F. Garber, pp. 56–106. University of Texas Press, Austin.

2010 Cosmological Layouts of Secondary Burials as Political Instruments. In *Mississippian Mortuary Practices: Beyond Hierarchy and the Representationist Perspective*, edited by Lynne P. Sullivan and Robert C. Mainfort Jr., pp. 30–53. University Press of Florida, Gainesville.

Brown, James A., and David H. Dye

2007 Severed Heads and Sacred Scalplocks: Mississippian Iconographic Trophies. In *The Taking and Displaying of Human Body Parts as Trophies by Amerindians*, edited by Richard J. Chacon and David H. Dye, pp. 278–298. Springer, New York.

Brown, James A., and John E. Kelly

2000 Cahokia and the Southeastern Ceremonial Complex. In *Mounds, Modoc, and Mesoamerica: Papers in Honor of Melvin L. Fowler*, edited by Steven R. Ahler, pp. 469–510. Scientific Papers Vol. 28. Illinois State Museum, Springfield.

Brown, James A., and Patricia J. O'Brien

1990 *At the Edge of Prehistory: Huber Phase Archaeology in the Chicago Area.* Illinois Department of Transportation, Center for American Archaeology, Kampsville, Illinois.

Bruhy, Patricia, and Lynne Goldstein

1981 Historic Indian Occupation. In *A Continuing Archaeological Survey of Portions of the Rick River Drainage in Jefferson County, Wisconsin*, edited by Lynne Goldstein, pp. 82–98. Report of Investigations No. 52. University of Wisconsin Archaeological Research Laboratory, Milwaukee.

Buechel, Eugene, and Paul I. Manhart

1998 *Lakota Tales and Texts in Translation.* Tipi Press, Chamberlain, South Dakota.

Buikstra, Jane E.

1976 *Hopewell in the Lower Illinois Valley: A Regional Approach to the Study of Human Biological Variability and Prehistoric Behavior.* Archaeological Program Scientific Papers No. 2. Northwestern University, Evanston, Illinois.

1981 Mortuary Practices, Palaeodemography and Palaeopathology: A Case Study from the Koster Site (Illinois). In *The Archaeology of Death*, edited by Robert Chapman, Ian Kinnes, and Klavs Randsborg, pp. 123–132. Cambridge University Press, Cambridge.

Buikstra, Jane E., and Douglas H. Ubelaker (editors)

1994 *Standards for Data Collection from Human Skeletal Remains.* Research Series No. 44. Arkansas Archaeological Survey, Fayetteville.

Burks, Jarrod

2009 The 1938 Excavations of the Florence Mound. *Pickaway Quarterly* 49(3): 6–11.

Bushnell, David I.

1920 *Native Cemeteries and Forms of Burial East of the Mississippi.* Bureau of American Ethnology Bulletin 71. Smithsonian Institution, Washington, D.C.

1927 *Burials of the Algonquian, Siouan and Caddoan Tribes West of the Mississippi.* Bureau of American Ethnology Bulletin 83. Smithsonian Institution, Washington, D.C.

Butt, Audrey

1967 To Dance among Bird-Women. In *Trances*, edited by Stewart Wavel, Audrey Butt, and Nina Epton, pp. 53–61. George Allen and Unwin, London.

Byers, A. Martin

2004 *The Ohio Hopewell Episode.* University of Akron Press, Akron, Ohio.

2005 The Mortuary "Laying-In" Crypts of the Hopewell Site: Beyond the Funerary Paradigm. In *Interacting with the Dead: Perspectives on Mortuary Archaeology for the New Millennium*, edited by Gordon F. M. Rakita, Jane E. Buikstra, Lane A. Beck, and Sloan R. Williams, pp. 124–141. University Press of Florida, Gainesville.

2009 *Cahokia: A World Renewal Cult Heterarchy.* University Press of Florida, Gainesville.

Callender, Charles, Richard K. Pope, and Susan M. Pope

1978 Kickapoo. In *Northeast*, edited by Bruce G. Trigger, pp. 656–667. Handbook of North American Indians, Vol. 15, William C. Sturtevant, general editor, Smithsonian Institution, Washington, D.C.

Carr, Christopher

2005 The Tripartite Ceremonial Alliance among Scioto Hopewellian Communities and the Question of Social Ranking. In *Gathering Hopewell: Society, Ritual, and Ritual Interaction*, edited by Christopher Carr and D. Troy Case, pp. 258–338. Kluwer Academic/Plenum, New York.

2008 Social and Ritual Organization. In *The Scioto Hopewell and Their Neighbors: Bioarchaeological Documentation and Cultural Understanding*, edited by D. Troy Case and Christopher Carr, pp. 151–288. Springer, New York.

Carr, Christopher, and D. Troy Case (editors)

2005 *Gathering Hopewell: Society, Ritual, and Ritual Interaction.* Kluwer Academic/Plenum, New York.

Carr, Christopher, Beau J. Goldstein, and Jaimin Weets

2005 Estimating the Sizes and Social Compositions of Mortuary-Related Gatherings at Scioto Hopewell Earthwork-Mound Sites. In *Gathering Hopewell: Society, Ritual, and Ritual Interaction*, edited by Christopher Carr and D. Troy Case, pp. 480–532. Kluwer Academic/Plenum, New York.

Carrasco, Davíd

1990 *Religions of Mesoamerica.* Harper and Row, San Francisco.

Case, D. Troy, and Christopher Carr (editors)
2008 *The Scioto Hopewell and Their Neighbors: Bioarchaeological Documentation and Cultural Understanding*. Springer, New York.

Catches, Pete, Sr., and Peter Catches
1997 *Oceti Wakan, Sacred Fireplace*. Oceti Wakan, Pine Ridge, South Dakota.

Cawley, Arthur C. (editor)
1993 *Everyman and Medieval Miracle Plays*. J. M. Dent, London.

Ceatus Media Group
2009 Your Dentistry Guide. Electronic document, http://www.yourdentistryguide.com, accessed July 28, 2009.

Chacon, Richard J., and David H. Dye
2007a Introduction to Human Trophy Taking: An Ancient and Widespread Practice. In *The Taking and Displaying of Human Body Parts as Trophies by Amerindians*, edited by Richard J. Chacon and David H. Dye, pp. 5–31. Springer, New York.
2007b Supplemental Data on Amerindian Trophy Taking. In *The Taking and Displaying of Human Body Parts as Trophies by Amerindians*, edited by Richard J. Chacon and David H. Dye, pp. 618–629. Springer, New York.

Chacon, Richard J., and David H. Dye (editors)
2007 *The Taking and Displaying of Human Body Parts as Trophies by Amerindians*. Springer, New York.

Chapman, John
2000 *Fragmentation in Archaeology: People, Places, and Broken Objects in the Prehistory of South-eastern Europe*. Routledge, London.

Chapman, Robert W.
2005 Mortuary Analysis: A Matter of Time? In *Interacting with the Dead: Perspectives on Mortuary Archaeology for the New Millennium*, edited by Gordon F. M. Rakita, Jane E. Buikstra, Lane A. Beck, and Sloan R. Williams, pp. 25–50. University Press of Florida, Gainesville.

Chapman, Robert, Ian Kinnes, and Klavs Randsborg (editors)
1981 *The Archaeology of Death*. Cambridge University Press, Cambridge.

Charles, Douglas K., and Jane E. Buikstra
2006 *Recreating Hopewell*. University Press of Florida, Gainesville.

Cherry, James F.
2009 *The Headpots of Northeast Arkansas and Southern Pemiscot County, Missouri*. University of Arkansas Press, Fayetteville.

Chesson, Meredith S. (editor)
2001 *Social Memory, Identity, and Death: Anthropological Perspectives on Mortuary Rituals*. Archaeological Papers of the American Anthropological Association No. 10. Arlington, Virginia.

Clark, William Philo
1885 *The Indian Sign Language*. Hammersly, Philadelphia.

Cobb, Charles R., and Brian M. Butler

2002 The Vacant Quarter Revisited: Late Mississippian Abandonment of the Lower Ohio Valley. *American Antiquity* 67:625–641.

Cobb, Charles R., and Eric Drake

2008 The Colour of Time: Head Pots and Temporal Convergences. *Cambridge Archaeological Journal* 18:85–93.

Cobb, Dawn E.

1999 Galt Site 11G161, Gallatin County, Illinois. Human Skeletal Remains Protection Act Investigations, Report No. 12. Submitted to the Illinois Historic Preservation Agency. Quaternary Studies Program Technical Report No. 99-0000-33. Illinois State Museum, Springfield.

Codere, Helen

1950 *Fighting with Property*. American Ethnological Society Monograph 18. Augustin, Locust Valley, New York.

Coggins, Clemency Chase, and Orrin C. Shane

1984 *Cenote of Sacrifice: Maya Treasures from the Sacred Well at Chichén Itzá*. University of Texas Press, Austin.

Cole, Fay-Cooper, and Thorne Deuel

1937 *Rediscovering Illinois: Archaeological Explorations in and around Fulton County*. University of Chicago Press, Chicago.

Collins, Newell E.

1943 Perforated Indian Skulls. *Wisconsin Archeologist* 24:49–53.

Conrad, Lawrence A.

1989 The Southeastern Ceremonial Complex on the Northern Middle Mississippian Frontier: Late Prehistoric Politico-Religious Systems in the Central Illinois River Valley. In *The Southeastern Ceremonial Complex: Artifacts and Analysis: The Cottonlandia Conference*, edited by Patricia Galloway, pp. 93–113. University of Nebraska Press, Lincoln.

1991 The Middle Mississippian Cultures of the Central Illinois River Valley. In *Cahokia and the Hinterlands: Middle Mississippian Cultures of the Midwest*, edited by Thomas E. Emerson and R. Barry Lewis, pp. 119–156. University of Illinois Press, Urbana.

Converse, Robert N.

1979 *The Glacial Kame Indians*. Archaeological Society of Ohio, Columbus.

Cook, Charles Weldon

1976 The Development of American Indian Ritual Drama as Evidenced in Hopi and Zuni Indians of the Southwestern United States. Unpublished Ph.D. dissertation, New York University, New York.

Coppée, Henry (editor)

1900 *The Classic and the Beautiful from the Literature of Three Thousand Years*. Carson and Simpson, Philadelphia.

Crawford, Suzanne J., and Dennis Francis Kelley (editors)

2005 *American Indian Religious Traditions: An Encyclopedia*. ABC-CLIO, Santa Barbara, California.

Curtin, Jeremiah
1922 *Seneca Indian Myths*. Dutton, New York.

Curtis, Edward S.
1908 *The North American Indian*, Vol. 3: *The Teton Sioux, the Yanktonai, the Assiniboin*. E. S. Curtis, Seattle.
1909 *The North American Indian*, Vol. 4: *The Apsaroke, or Crows, the Hidatsa*. E. S. Curtis, Seattle.
1911 *The North American Indian*, Vol. 6: *The Peigan, the Cheyenne, the Arapaho*. E. S. Curtis, Seattle.

Cybulski, Jerome S.
1978 Modified Human Bones and Skulls from Prince Rupert Harbour, British Columbia. *Canadian Journal of Archaeology* 2:15–32.

Dancey, William S., and Paul J. Pacheco (editors)
1997 *Ohio Hopewell Community Organization*. Kent State University Press, Kent, Ohio.

Daniélou, Alain
1995 *The Phallus: Scared Symbol of Male Creative Power*. Translated by Jon Graham. Inner Traditions, Rochester, Vermont.

DeMallie, Raymond J. (editor)
1984 *The Sixth Grandfather: Black Elk's Teachings Given to John G. Neihardt*. University of Nebraska Press, Lincoln.

Demarest, Arthur A.
2007 Ethics and Ethnocentricity in Interpretation and Critique: Challenges to the Anthropology of Corporeality and Death. In *The Taking and Displaying of Human Body Parts as Trophies by Amerindians*, edited by Richard J. Chacon and David H. Dye, pp. 591–617. Springer, New York.

Denig, Edwin Thompson
1930 *Indian Tribes of the Upper Missouri*. Edited by J. N. B. Hewitt. Bureau of American Ethnology Bulletin 46, pp. 375–628. Smithsonian Institution, Washington, D.C.

Denman, Leslie van Ness
1953 *Sha'A La K'o Mana, Hopi Shungopavi*. Grabhorn, San Francisco, California.

Deuel, Thorne
1952 Hopewellian Dress in Illinois. In *The Archaeology of Eastern United States*, edited by James B. Griffin, pp. 165–175. University of Chicago Press, Chicago.

Diamond, Beverly, M. Sam Cronk, and Franziska von Rosen
1994 *Visions of Sound: Musical Instruments of First Nations Communities in Northeastern America*. Wilfrid Laurier University Press, Waterloo, Canada.

Diaz-Granados, Carol, and James R. Duncan
2000 *The Petroglyphs and Pictographs of Missouri*. University of Alabama Press, Tuscaloosa.
2004 Reflections of Power, Wealth and Sex in Missouri Rock-Art Motifs. In *The Rock-Art of Eastern North America: Capturing Images and Insight*, edited

by Carol Diaz-Granados and James R. Duncan, pp. 14–158. University of Alabama Press, Tuscaloosa.

Dickson, Don F.

ca. 1945 Catalog of Relics in the Dickson Mounds Museum. Manuscript on file, Dickson Mounds Museum, Lewistown, Illinois.

Dictionary.com

2013 Dictionary.com Unabridged. Random House. Electronic document, http://dictionary.reference.com/browse/pearly white, accessed February 22, 2013.

Dieterle, Richard L.

2005 The Encyclopedia of Hočąk (Winnebago) Mythology. Electronic document, http://hotcakencyclopedia.com, accessed October 2010.

Dobbs, Clark A.

1993 *The Archaeology of 21GD158: A 13th Century Native American Village at the Red Wing Locality*. Reports of Investigations No. 250. Institute for Minnesota Archaeology, Minneapolis.

Dobres, Marcia-Anne, and John Robb (editors)

2000 *Agency in Archaeology*. Routledge, New York.

Dobyns, Henry F.

1992 Native American Trade Centers and Contagious Disease Foci. In *Disease and Demography in the Americas*, edited by John W. Verano and Douglas H. Ubelaker, pp. 215–222. Smithsonian Institution Press, Washington, D.C.

Dorsey, George A.

1902 The Osage Mourning-War Ceremony. *American Anthropologist*, n.s. 4:404–411.

1904a *Mythology of the Wichita*. Publication 21. Carnegie Institution of Washington, Washington, D.C.

1904b *Traditions of the Arikara*. Publication 14. Carnegie Institution of Washington, Washington, D.C.

1904c *Traditions of the Skidi Pawnee*. Houghton, Mifflin, London.

1905 A Pawnee Personal Medicine Shrine. *American Anthropologist*, n.s. 7:496–498.

1906 *The Pawnee Mythology*. Publication 59. Carnegie Institution of Washington, Washington, D.C.

Dorsey, George A., and Alfred L. Kroeber

1903 *Traditions of the Arapaho*. Anthropology Series 5, Publication 81. Field Columbian Museum, Chicago.

Dorsey, James Owen

1885 Mourning and War Customs of the Kansas. *American Naturalist* 19:670–680.

1889 Teton Folk-Lore. *American Anthropologist* 2:143–158.

1893 Indian Doctrine of Souls. *Journal of American Folk-Lore* 6:298.

1894 *A Study of Siouan Cults*. Bureau of American Ethnology Annual Report 11, pp. 351–544. Smithsonian Institution, Washington, D.C.

Dougherty, Sean P., and Cheryl Ann Munson

2001 Preliminary Analysis of Disturbed Human Remains Identified during the 2001 Surface Survey of the Murphy Site (12P01), Posey County, Indiana, Appendix III. In *Archaeological Survey, Test Excavation, and Public Education in*

Southwestern Indiana by Cheryl Ann Munson. Prepared for Indiana Department of Natural Resources, Division of Historic Preservation and Archaeology, and the National Park Service, U.S. Department of Interior. Department of Anthropology, Indiana University, Bloomington.

Driver, Harold E.

1969 *Indians of North America*. 2nd ed., rev. University of Chicago Press, Chicago.

Drooker, Penelope Ballard

1998 *The View from Madisonville: Protohistoric Western Fort Ancient Interaction Patterns*. Memoirs 31. Museum of Anthropology, University of Michigan, Ann Arbor.

Drooker, Penelope B., and George R. Hammell

2004 Susannah Swan's "Wampum Bag." In *Perishable Material Culture in the Northeast*, edited by Penelope B. Drooker, pp. 197–215. Bulletin 500. New York State Museum, Albany.

Duday, Henri

2006 l'Archaeothanatologie ou l'Archéologie de la Mort (Archaeothanatology or the Archaeology of Death). Translated by Christopher J. Knusel. In *Social Archaeology of Funerary Remains*, edited by Rebecca Gowland and Christopher J. Knusel, pp. 30–56. Oxbow, Oxford.

Duday, Henri, and Claude Masset

1987 *Anthropologie Physique et Archaeologie*. CNRS, Paris.

Duday, Henri, Patrice Courtaud, Eric Crubezy, Pascal Sellier, and Anne-Marie Tillier

1990 L'anthropologie "de Terrain": Reconnaissance et Interprétation des Gestes Funéraires. In *Anthropologie et Archéologie: Dialogue sur les Ensembles Funéraires*, edited by Eric Crubezy, Henry Duday, Pascal Sellier, and Anne-Marie Tillier. Special issue, Bulletin et Mémoires de la Société d'Anthropologie de Paris 2:29–50.

Duncan, James R., and Carol Diaz-Granados

2000 Of Masks and Myths. *Midcontinental Journal of Archaeology* 25:1–26.

2004 Empowering the SECC: The Old Woman and Oral Tradition. In *The Rock-Art of Eastern North America: Capturing Images and Insight*, edited by Carol Diaz-Granados and James R. Duncan, pp. 190–215. University of Alabama Press, Tuscaloosa.

Duncan, William N.

2005 Understanding Veneration and Violation in the Archaeological Record. In *Interacting with the Dead: Perspectives on Mortuary Archaeology for the New Millennium*, edited by Gordon F. M. Rakita, Jane E. Buikstra, Lane A. Beck, and Sloan R. Williams, pp. 207–227. University Press of Florida, Gainesville.

Durkheim, Emile

1965 *The Elementary Forms of Religious Life*. Reprinted. Free Press, New York. Originally published 1915, George Allen and Unwin, London.

Dusenberry, Verne

1962 *The Montana Cree: A Study in Religious Persistence*. University of Oklahoma Press, Norman.

Dye, David H.

2004 Art, Ritual, and Chiefly Warfare in the Mississippian World. In *Hero, Hawk, and Open Hand: American Indian Art of the Ancient Midwest and South*, edited by Richard F. Townsend and Robert V. Sharp, pp. 190–205. Yale University Press, New Haven, Connecticut.

2007 Ritual, Medicine, and the War Trophy Iconographic Theme in the Mississippian Southeast. In *Ancient Objects and Sacred Realms: Interpretations of Mississippian Iconography*, edited by F. Kent Reilly III and James F. Garber, pp. 152–173. University of Texas Press, Austin.

Dye, David H., and Camille Wharey

1989 Exhibition Catalog. In *The Southeastern Ceremonial Complex: Artifacts and Analysis: The Cottonlandia Conference*, edited by Patricia Galloway, pp. 319–378. University of Nebraska Press, Lincoln.

Eastman, Mary Henderson

1995 [1849] *Dahcotah; or, Life and Legends of the Sioux*. Wiley, New York. Reprinted. Afton Historical Society Press, Afton, Minnesota.

Echo-Hawk, Roger

2000 Ancient History in the New World: Integrating Oral Traditions and the Archaeological Record in Deep Time. *American Antiquity* 65:267–290.

Edgar, Blake

1999 The Symbol and the Spear. *California Wild* 52:3. California Academy of Sciences.

Edmunds, R. David

1985 *The Shawnee Prophet*. University of Nebraska Press, Lincoln.

Eggan, Fred

1930 Preliminary Report on Mound F11, Morton Group, Fulton County. Manuscript on file, Dickson Mounds Museum, Lewistown, Illinois.

Electronic Human Relations Area Files Collection of Ethnography (eHRAF)

1987 EP04 SAAMI File. Electronic document, http://www.hti.umich.edu/bin/ehraf/hraf-idx?type=toc&rgn=BOOK&byte=158302806, accessed December 8, 1999.

Eliade, Mircea

1972 *Shamanism: Archaic Techniques of Ecstasy*. Princeton University Press, Princeton, New Jersey.

Elliott, Josephine Mirabella, and Jane Thompson Johansen

1999 *Charles-Alexandre Lesueur: Premier Naturalist and Artist*. University of Southern Indiana Foundation, Endowment for New Harmony Studies, Evansville.

Emanovsky, Paul

2002 A Taphonomic Analysis of Ohio Hopewellian Modified Animal Jaws from Tremper Mound. Unpublished Master's thesis, Program in Human Biology, University of Indianapolis, Indianapolis, Indiana.

Emerson, Kjersti, and Kristin Hedman

2007 Upper Mississippian Mortuary Practices in Northern Illinois and the Upper Illinois River Valley. Paper presented at the Annual Midwest Archaeological Conference, Notre Dame, Indiana.

Emerson, Thomas E.

1982 *Mississippian Stone Images in Illinois.* Circular 6. Illinois Archaeological Survey, Urbana.

1997a *Cahokia and the Archaeology of Power.* University of Alabama Press, Tuscaloosa.

1997b Cahokia Elite Ideology and the Mississippian Cosmos. In *Cahokia: Ideology and Domination in the Mississippian World,* edited by Timothy Pauketat and Thomas E. Emerson, pp. 190–228. University of Nebraska Press, Lincoln.

2003 Crossing Boundaries between Worlds: Changing Beliefs and Mortuary Practices at Cahokia. *Wisconsin Archeologist* 84(1–2):73–80.

Emerson, Thomas E., Kenneth B. Farnsworth, Sarah U. Wisseman, and Randall E. Hughes

2013 The Allure of the Exotic: Reexamining the Use of Local and Distant Pipestone Quarries in Ohio Hopewell Pipe Caches. *American Antiquity* 78:48–67.

Emerson, Thomas E., and Eve Hargrave

2000 Strangers in Paradise? Recognizing Ethnic Mortuary Diversity on the Fringes of Cahokia. *Southeastern Archaeology* 19:1–23.

Emerson, Thomas E., Randall E. Hughes, Mary R. Hynes, and Sarah U. Wisseman

2003 The Sourcing and Interpretation of Cahokia-Style Figurines in the Trans-Mississippi South and Southeast. *American Antiquity* 68:287–313.

Emerson, Thomas E., and Douglas K. Jackson

1984 *The BBB Motor Site.* American Bottom Archaeology, FAI-270 Site Reports No. 6. University of Illinois Press, Urbana.

Emerson, Thomas E., Brad Koldehoff, and Timothy R. Pauketat

2000 Serpents, Female Deities, and Fertility Symbolism in the Early Cahokian Countryside. In *Mounds, Modoc, and Mesoamerica: Papers in Honor of Melvin L. Fowler,* edited by Steven R. Ahler, pp. 511–522. Scientific Papers Vol. 28. Illinois State Museum, Springfield.

Emerson, Thomas E., George R. Milner, and Douglas K. Jackson

1983 *The Florence Street Site (11-S-458).* American Bottom Archaeology, FAI-270 Site Reports No. 2. University of Illinois Press, Urbana.

Emerson, Thomas E., and Timothy R. Pauketat

2002 Embodying Power and Resistance at Prehistoric Cahokia. In *The Dynamics of Power,* edited by Maria O'Donovan, pp. 105–125. Occasional Paper No. 30. Center of Archaeological Investigations, Southern Illinois University, Carbondale.

Engelbrecht, William

2003 *Iroquoia: The Development of a Native World.* Syracuse University Press, Syracuse, New York.

Esarey, Duane

1986 Red Ochre Mound Building and Marion Phase Associations: A Fulton County, Illinois Perspective. In *Early Woodland Archeology,* edited by Kenneth B. Farnsworth and Thomas E. Emerson, pp. 231–243. Kampsville Seminars in Archeology 2. Center for American Archeology, Kampsville, Illinois.

Esarey, Duane, Michael D. Wiant, Dawn E. Harn, Terrance J. Martin, Marjorie B. Schroeder, and Robert E. Warren

1998 *The Liverpool Lake Site: A Late Woodland Village on the Chautauqua Unit of the Illinois River National Wildlife Refuges, Mason County, Illinois*. Quaternary Studies Program. Illinois State Museum, Springfield.

Evers, Edward

1880 *The Ancient Pottery of Southeastern Missouri.* Contributions to the Archaeology of Missouri, Archaeological Section of the St. Louis Academy of Science. Pt. 1, Pottery. George A. Bates, Naturalists' Bureau, Salem, Missouri.

Evers, John C.

1997 *Plains History and Culture: Essays on Continuity and Change.* University of Oklahoma Press, Norman.

Farnsworth, Kenneth B.

2004 *Early Hopewell Mound Explorations: The First Fifty Years in the Illinois River Valley.* Studies in Archaeology 3. Illinois Transportation Archaeological Research Program, University of Illinois, Urbana.

Farnsworth, Kenneth B., and Karen Atwell

2013 *Excavations at the Blue Island and Naples-Russell Mounds and Related Hopewellian Sites in the Lower Illinois Valley.* Studies in Archaeology. Illinois State Archaeological Survey, Champaign.

Farquharson, Robert. J.

1876 Recent Archaeological Discoveries at Davenport, Iowa, of Copper Axes, Cloth, etc. Supposed to Have Come Down to Us from a Pre-Historic People, Called the Mound-Builders. *Proceedings of the Davenport Academy of Natural Sciences* 1:117–143.

1880 Amulets and Post-Mortem Trepanation. *American Antiquarian* 3:330–331.

Field, Stephanie, Anne J. Goldberg, and Tina Lee

2005 Gender, Status, and Ethnicity in the Scioto, Miami, and Northeastern Ohio Hopewellian Regions, as Evidenced by Mortuary Practices. In *Gathering Hopewell: Society, Ritual, and Ritual Interaction*, edited by Christopher Carr and D. Troy Case, pp. 386–404. Kluwer Academic/Plenum, New York.

Finney, Fred A., and James B. Stoltman

1991 The Fred Edwards Site: A Case of Stirling Phase Culture Contact in Southwestern Wisconsin. In *New Perspectives on Cahokia: Views from the Periphery*, edited by James B. Stoltman, pp. 229–254. Prehistory Press, Madison, Wisconsin.

Fishel, Richard L.

1999 *Bison Hunters of the Western Prairies: Archaeological Investigations at the Dixon Site (13WD8), Woodbury County, Iowa.* Report 21. Office of the State Archaeologist, University of Iowa, Iowa City.

Fisher, Alton K.

1977a *Human Bones from Lane Farm Mound Group Site, 13AM104.* Research Papers 2(6):20–21. Office of the State Archaeologist, University of Iowa, Iowa City.

1977b *Additional Human Remains from the Lane Farm Mound Group, 13AM104.* Research Papers 2(13):10–16. Office of the State Archaeologist, University of Iowa, Iowa City.

Fitzsimmons, James L., and Izumi Shimada

2011 *Living with the Dead: Mortuary Ritual in Mesoamerica.* University of Arizona Press, Tucson.

Fletcher, Alice C.

1884 *The White Buffalo Ceremony of the Uncpapas; The Elk Mystery or Festival, Ogallala Sioux; The Religious Ceremony of the Four Winds or Quarters, as Observed by the Santee Sioux; The Shadow or Ghost Lodge: A Ceremony of the Ogallala Sioux.* Annual Reports 16 and 17. Peabody Museum of American Archaeology and Ethnology, Cambridge, Massachusetts.

1903 Pawnee Star Lore. *Journal of American Folklore* 16:10–15.

Fletcher, Alice C., and Francis La Flesche

1911 *The Omaha Tribe.* Bureau of American Ethnology Annual Report 27. Smithsonian Institution, Washington, D.C.

1992 *The Omaha Tribe,* Vol. II. Reprinted. University of Nebraska Press, Lincoln. Originally published 1911, 27th Annual Report of the Bureau of American Ethnology 1905–1906, Government Printing Office, Washington, D.C.

Fletcher, Robert

1882 *Prehistoric Trephining and Cranial Amulets.* U.S. Geographical and Geological Survey of the Rocky Mountain Region, Department of the Interior, Washington, D.C.

Fogelson, Raymond D., and Paul Kutsche

1961 Cherokee Economic Cooperatives: The Gadugi. In *Symposium on Cherokee and Iroquois Culture,* edited by William N. Fenton and John Gulick, pp. 87–123. Bureau of American Ethnology Bulletin 180. Smithsonian Institution, Washington, D.C.

Fokken, Michael

1979 Human Skeletal Material from the McKinney Site 13LA1. In *Reports on Human Remains and Burial Mound Investigations in Louisa and Clay Counties, Iowa.* Research Papers 4(5):1–3. Office of the State Archaeologist, University of Iowa, Iowa City.

Ford, James A.

1936 *Analysis of Indian Village Site Collections from Louisiana and Mississippi.* Anthropological Study 2. Louisiana Geological Survey, New Orleans.

Fortier, Andrew C. (editor)

2007 *The Archaeology of the East St. Louis Mounds Center,* Pt. II: *The Northside Excavations.* Illinois Transportation Archaeological Research Report No. 22. Illinois Transportation Archaeological Research Program, University of Illinois, Urbana.

Foster, Lance Michael

1994 *Sacred Bundles of the Ioway Indians.* Unpublished Master's thesis, Department of Anthropology, Iowa State University, Ames.

Fowler, Chris

2004 *The Archaeology of Personhood.* Routledge, London.

Fowler, Melvin L.

1997 *The Cahokia Atlas: A Historical Atlas of Cahokia Archaeology.* Studies in Archaeology No. 2. Illinois Transportation Archaeological Research Program, University of Illinois, Urbana.

Fowler, Melvin L., Jerome Rose, Barbara Vander Leest, and Steven R. Ahler

1999 *The Mound 72 Area: Dedicated and Sacred Space in Early Cahokia.* Reports of Investigations No. 54. Illinois State Museum, Springfield.

Frazer, James G.

1922 *The Golden Bough.* Macmillan, New York.

Freeman, Joan E.

1966 Price Site III, RI4: A Burial Ground in Richland County, Wisconsin. *Wisconsin Archeologist* 47:33–75.

Fricker, Ian, Eve A. Hargrave, and Kristin M. Hedman

2003 Late Prehistoric Mortuary Behavior at the Hoxie Farm Site. Paper presented at the Annual Midwest Archaeological Conference, Milwaukee, Wisconsin.

Frisbie, Charlotte Johnson

1980 *Southwestern Indian Ritual Drama.* University of New Mexico Press, Albuquerque.

Fugle, Eugene M.

1962 Mill Creek Culture and Technology. *Journal of the Iowa Archeological Society* 11(4):1–26.

Furst, Peter M.

1973–1974 The Roots and Continuities of Shamanism. *ArtsCanada* 30(184–187): 33–69.

Galloway, Patricia K. (editor)

1989 *The Southeastern Ceremonial Complex: Artifacts and Analysis: The Cottonlandia Conference.* University of Nebraska Press, Lincoln.

Gardner, Andrew

2004 Introduction: Social Agency, Power, and Being Human. In *Agency Uncovered: Archaeological Perspectives on Social Agency, Power, and Being Human*, edited by Andrew Gardner, pp. 1–15. UCL Press, London.

Garland, A. Neil, and Rob C. Janaway

1987 The Taphonomy of Inhumation Burials. In *Burial Archaeology: Current Research, Methods, and Developments*, edited by Charlotte A. Roberts, Frances Lee, and John Bintliff, pp. 14–38. British Archaeological Reports International Series 211. University of London, London.

Gass, Jacob

1877a A Connected Account of the Explorations of Mound No. 3, Cook's Farm Group. *Proceedings of the Davenport Academy of Natural Sciences* 2:92–98.

1877b Report of Exploration of Mound No. 10, Cook's Farm Group. *Proceedings of the Davenport Academy of Natural Sciences* 2:141–142.

Geary, Patrick J.

1990 *Furta Sacra: Thefts of Relics in the Central Middle Ages*. Princeton University Press, Princeton, New Jersey.

Geller, Pamela L.

2009 Identity and Difference: Complicating Gender in Archaeology. *Annual Review of Anthropology* 38:65–81.

2011 Getting a Head Start in Life: Pre-Columbian Maya Cranial Modification from Infancy to Ancestorhood. In *The Bioarchaeology of the Human Head: Decapitation, Decoration, and Deformation*, edited by Michelle Bonogofsky, pp. 241–261. University Press of Florida, Gainesville.

Gibbon, Guy

1979 *Mississippian Occupation of Red Wing Area*. Minnesota Prehistoric Archaeology Series No. 13. Minnesota Historical Society, St. Paul.

Gifford, Diane P.

1981 Taphonomy and Paleoecology: A Critical Review of Archaeology's Sister Disciplines. *Advances in Archaeological Method and Theory* 4:365–438.

Giles, Bretton T.

2013 A Contextual and Iconographic Reassessment of the Headdress on Burial 11 from Hopewell Mound 25. *American Antiquity* 78:502–519.

Gillespie, Susan D.

2001 Personhood, Agency, and Mortuary Ritual: A Case Study from the Ancient Maya. *Journal of Anthropological Archaeology* 20:73–112.

Gilliland, Marion S.

1975 *The Material Culture of Key Marco, Florida*. University Press of Florida, Gainesville.

Goldstein, Lynne G.

1980 *Mississippian Mortuary Practices*. Scientific Papers No 4. Northwestern University Archeological Program, Evanston, Illinois.

1987 *The Southeastern Wisconsin Archaeology Project 1986–87 and Project Summary*. Report of Investigations No. 8. University of Wisconsin–Milwaukee Archaeological Research Laboratory, Milwaukee.

1995 Landscapes and Mortuary Practices: A Case for Regional Perspectives. In *Regional Approaches to Mortuary Analysis*, edited by Lane A. Beck, pp. 101–121. Plenum, New York.

2000 Mississippian Ritual as Viewed through the Practice of Secondary Disposal of the Dead. In *Mounds, Modoc, and Mesoamerica: Papers in Honor of Melvin L. Fowler*, edited by Steven R. Ahler, pp. 193–206. Scientific Papers Vol. 28. Illinois State Museum, Springfield.

2010 Aztalan Mortuary Practices Revisited. In *Mississippian Mortuary Practices: Beyond Hierarchy and the Representationist Perspective*, edited by Lynne P. Sullivan and Robert C. Mainfort Jr., pp. 90–112. University Press of Florida, Gainsville.

Goldstein, Lynne, and Donald H. Gaff

2002 Recasting the Past: Examining Assumptions about Aztalan. *Wisconsin Archeologist* 83:98–110.

Gonzalez-Whippler, Migene

1991 *The Complete Book of Amulets and Talismans*. Llewellyn, Woodbury, Minnesota.

Goodall, Jane

1986 *The Chimpanzees of Gombe: Patterns of Behavior*. Belknap, Cambridge.

Goodrich, Thomas

1997 *Scalp Dance: Indian Warfare on the High Plains, 1865–1879*. Stackpole, Mechanicsburg, Pennsylvania.

Goose, Denys H.

1963 Tooth Mutilation in West Africans. *Man* 63:91–93.

Gosden, Chris, and Yvonne Marshall

1999 The Cultural Biography of Objects. *World Archaeology* 31:169–178.

Gowland, Rebecca, and Christopher Knusel

2006 *Social Archaeology of Funerary Remains*. Oxbow, Oxford.

Gradwohl, David M.

1973 Final Report on Investigation of Archaeological Sites in Red Rock Reservoir, Iowa, as Covered in Contracts 14-10-0232–820 and 14-10-0232-1164 between the National Park Service and Iowa State University. Iowa State University Archaeological Laboratory. Copies on file, Iowa State University Archaeological Laboratory, Ames.

Greber, N'omi B.

1991 A Study of Continuity and Contrast between Central Scioto Adena and Hopewell Sites. *West Virginia Archeologist* 43(1–2):1–26.

Greber, N'omi B., and Katharine C. Ruhl

1989 *The Hopewell Site: A Contemporary Analysis Based on the Work of Charles C. Willoughby*. Westview, Boulder, Colorado.

2000 *The Hopewell Site: A Contemporary Analysis Based on the Work of Charles C. Willoughby*. Rev. ed. Eastern National, Ft. Washington, Pennsylvania.

Green, Thomas J., and Cheryl Ann Munson

1978 Mississippian Settlement Pattern in Southwestern Indiana. In *Mississippian Settlement Patterns*, edited by Bruce D. Smith, pp. 293–330. Academic, New York.

Green, William

1993 Examining Protohistoric Depopulation in the Upper Midwest. *Wisconsin Archeologist* 74:290–323.

1996 Enclosure, Renewal, and the Vision of the Thunderer: A Structural and Symbolic Perspective on Ancient Monuments at the Mouth of the Turkey River, Northeastern Iowa. Paper presented at the 54th Annual Plains Anthropological Conference, Iowa City. Copy on file, Office of the State Archaeologist, University of Iowa, Iowa City.

Green, William (editor)

1995 *Oneota Archaeology: Past, Present, and Future*. Report 20. Office of the State Archaeologist, University of Iowa, Iowa City.

Green, William, and Roland L. Rodell

1994 The Mississippian Presence and Cahokian Interaction at Trempeleau, Wisconsin. *American Antiquity* 59:334–359.

Greenman, Emerson F.

1967 *The Younge Site: An Archaeological Record from Michigan*. Reprinted. Occasional Contributions No. 6. Museum of Anthropology, University of Michigan, Ann Arbor. Originally published 1937, Museum of Anthropology, University of Michigan.

Griffin, James B.

1946 Culture Change and Continuity in Eastern United States Archaeology. In *Man in Northeastern North America*, edited by Frederick S. Johnson, pp. 37–95. Papers of the Robert S. Peabody Foundation for Archaeology No. 3. Phillips Academy, Andover, Massachusetts.

1960 A Hypothesis for the Prehistory of the Winnebago. In *Culture in History*, edited by Stanley Diamond, pp. 809–865. Columbia University Press, New York.

Griffin, James B., and Dan F. Morse

1961 The Short-Nosed God from the Emmons Site, Illinois. *American Antiquity* 26:560–563.

Grinnell, George Bird

1910 Coup and Scalp among the Plains Indians. *American Anthropologist*, n.s. 12: 296–310.

1923 *The Cheyenne Indians*, Vol. 1. Yale University Press, New Haven, Connecticut.

1972 *Blackfoot Lodge Tales: The Story of a Prairie People*. Corner House, Williamstown, Massachusetts.

Guerini, Vincenzo

1909 *A History of Dentistry: From the Most Ancient Times until the End of the Eighteenth Century*. Lea and Febiger, Philadelphia.

Hackenschmidt, Sebastian

2005 A Material Matter: Marcel Broodthaers' Use of Bones as a Surrealist Intervention against the Political Cult of the Dead. *Image and Narrative* 13. Electronic document, http://www.imageandnarrative.be/inarchive/surrealism/hackenschmidt.htm, accessed April 24, 2012.

Hagar, Stansbury

1906 Cherokee Star-Lore. In *Boas Anniversary Volume: Anthropological Papers Written in Honor of Franz Boas*, edited by Berthold Laufer, pp. 345–366. G. E. Stechert, New York.

Haglund, William D., and Marcella H. Sorg (editors)

1997 *Forensic Taphonomy: The Postmortem Fate of Human Remains*. CRC Press, Boca Raton, Florida.

2002 *Advances in Forensic Taphonomy: Method, Theory, and Archaeological Perspectives.* CRC Press, Boca Raton, Florida.

Halbert, Henry S.

1900 Funeral Customs of the Mississippi Choctaws. *Mississippi Historical Society Publications* 3:353–366.

Halifax, Joan

1979 *Shamanic Voices: A Survey of Visionary Narratives.* Dutton, New York.

Hall, K. R. L.

1963 Some Problems in the Analysis and Comparison of Monkey and Ape Behavior. In *Classification and Human Evolution*, edited by Sherwood Washburn, pp. 273–300. Aldine, Chicago.

Hall, Robert L.

1976 Ghosts, Water Barriers, Corn, and Sacred Enclosures in the Eastern Woodlands. *American Antiquity* 41:360–364.

1989 The Cultural Background of Mississippian Symbolism. In *The Southeastern Ceremonial Complex: Artifacts and Analysis: The Cottonlandia Conference*, edited by Patricia K. Galloway, pp. 239–278. University of Nebraska Press, Lincoln.

1991 Cahokia Identity and Interaction Models of Cahokia Mississippian. In *Cahokia and the Hinterlands: Middle Mississippian Cultures of the Midwest*, edited by Thomas E. Emerson and R. Barry Lewis, pp. 3–34. University of Illinois Press, Urbana.

1997 *An Archaeology of the Soul: North American Indian Belief and Ritual.* University of Illinois Press, Urbana.

2000 Sacrificed Foursomes and Green Corn Ceremonialism. In *Mounds, Modoc, and Mesoamerica: Papers in Honor of Melvin L. Fowler*, edited by Steven R. Ahler, pp. 245–253. Scientific Papers Vol. 28. Illinois State Museum, Springfield.

Hallowell, A. Irving

1926 Bear Ceremonialism in the Northern Hemisphere. *American Anthropologist*, n.s. 28:1–175.

1940 The Spirits of the Dead in Saulteaux Life and Thought. *Journal of the Royal Anthropological Institute* 70:29–51.

1960 Ojibwa Ontology, Behavior, and World View. In *Culture in History: Essays in Honor of Paul Radin*, edited by Stanley Diamond, pp. 19–52. Columbia University Press, New York.

Hamilakis, Yannis, Mark Pluciennik, and Sarah Tarlow (editors)

2002 *Thinking through the Body: Archaeologies of Corporeality.* Kluwer Academic/Plenum, New York.

Hamperl, H., and W. S. Laughlin

1959 Osteological Consequences of Scalping. *Human Biology* 31:800–889.

Hargrave, Eve

2005 Human Remains. In *The St. Thomas Site (11MS54), Madison County, Illinois,* edited by Jeffrey Krutchen. Research Reports No. 99. Illinois Transportation Archaeological Research Program, University of Illinois, Urbana.

Hargrave, Eve, and Kristin Hedman

2002 *The Halliday Site (11S27): Recent Investigations into Late Prehistoric Mortuary Behavior.* ITARP Research Reports No. 50. Illinois Transportation Archaeological Research Program, University of Illinois, Urbana.

Harn, Dawn E.

1998 Human Remains. In *The Liverpool Lake Site: A Late Woodland Village on the Chautauqua Unit of the Illinois River National Wildlife Refuges, Mason County, Illinois*, edited by Duane Esarey, Michael D. Wiant, Dawn E. Harn, Terrance J. Martin, Marjorie B. Schroeder, and Robert E. Warren, pp. 122–135. Quaternary Studies Program. Illinois State Museum, Springfield.

Harrington, Mark R.

1914 *Sacred Bundles of the Sac and Fox Indians.* Museum Anthropological Publications Vol. 9, No. 2. University Museum, University of Pennsylvania, Philadelphia.

Harrison, Charles E.

1878 Exploration of Mound No. 11, Cook's Farm Group, and Discovery of an Inscribed Tablet of Limestone. *Proceedings of the Davenport Academy of Natural Sciences* 2:221–224.

Harrison, Julia D.

1987 *The Spirit Sings: Artistic Traditions of Canada's First Peoples.* McClelland and Stewart, Toronto.

Harrison, Simon

2006 Skull Trophies of the Pacific War: Transgressive Objects of Remembrance. *Journal of the Royal Anthropological Institute* 12:817–836.

Harrod, Howard L.

2000 *The Animals Came Dancing: Native American Sacred Ecology and Animal Kinship.* University of Arizona Press, Tucson.

Hassrick, Royal B.

1964 *The Sioux.* University of Oklahoma Press, Norman.

Hathcock, Roy

1983 *The Quapaw and Their Pottery.* Hurley, Camden, Arkansas.

1988 *Ancient Indian Pottery of the Mississippi Valley.* 2nd ed. Hurley, Camden Arkansas.

Havill, Lorena M., and Cheryl Ann Munson

1998a Summary of Skeletal Inventory and Preliminary Analysis of Human Remains from the Surface of the Murphy Site (12Po1), Posey County, Indiana, Appendix III. In *Archaeological Investigations at Caborn-Welborn Phase Sites, 1997–1998, Posey County, Indiana*, edited by Cheryl Ann Munson. Prepared for Indiana Department of Natural Resources, Division of Historic Preservation and Archaeology and the National Park Service, U.S. Department of Interior. Department of Anthropology, Indiana University, Bloomington.

1998b Description of Disturbed Burials from the Murphy Site (12Po1), 1997–1998 Test Excavations, Posey County, Indiana, Appendix II. In *Archaeological Investigations at Caborn-Welborn Phase Sites, 1997–1998, Posey County, Indiana*, edited by Cheryl Ann Munson. Prepared for Indiana Department of Natural Resources, Division of Historic Preservation and Archaeology and the National Park Service, U.S. Department of Interior. Department of Anthropology, Indiana University, Bloomington.

Hedman, Kristin M.

2003 Incised Bone from the Hoxie Farm Site, Cook County, Illinois. Paper presented at the Annual Midwest Archaeological Conference, Milwaukee, Wisconsin.

2008 Human Bone as Ritual Object: Modified Human Bone from the Anker Site, Cook County, Illinois. Paper presented at the Annual Midwest Archaeological Conference, Milwaukee Wisconsin.

Hedman, Kristin M., and Douglas K. Jackson

2009 Mortuary Practices and Human Remains. In *Main Occupation Area Upper Mississippian Components at the Hoxie Farm Site, Cook County, Illinois*. Manuscript on file, Illinois Transportation Archaeological Research Program, University of Illinois, Urbana.

Hedman, Kristin M., and James LeFagre

2002 Incised Human Bone from the Hoxie Farm Site, Cook County, Illinois. Poster presented at the Annual Meeting of the Bioarchaeology and Forensic Anthropology Association, Indianapolis, Indiana.

Hegmon, Michelle

1992 Archaeological Research on Style. *Annual Review of Anthropology* 21:517–536.

Helms, Lindsey J.

2008 Perforation of Human Remains: Temporal, Regional, and Cultural Comparison of Mortuary Tapping in Minnesota. Unpublished undergraduate thesis, Hamline University, St. Paul, Minnesota.

Hendrie, Colin A., and Gayle Brewer

2012 Evidence to Suggest That Teeth Act as Human Ornament Displays Signaling Mate Quality. *PLOS ONE* 7(7). Electronic document, e42178.doi: 10.1371/journal.pone.0042178, accessed June 1, 2014.

Henn, Robert

1971 A Preliminary Report on the Leonard Site. *Proceedings of the Indiana Academy of Science* 80:67–73.

Henning, Dale R.

1970 Development and Interrelationships of Oneota Culture in the Lower Missouri River Valley. *Missouri Archaeologist* 32:1–180.

1982 Subsurface Testing Program: Proposed Perry Creek Dam and Reservoir Areas, Plymouth County, Iowa. Technical Report No. 82–05. Department of Anthropology, Division of Archeological Research, University of Nebraska, Lincoln.

1996 The Archeology of Two Great Oasis Sites in the Perry Creek Valley, Northwest Iowa. *Journal of the Iowa Archeological Society* 43:7–118.

Henry, Alexander, and David Thompson

1897 *New Light on the Early History of the Greater Northwest: The Manuscript Journals of Alexander Henry and David Thompson, 1799–1814*. 3 vols. Edited by Elliott Coues. F. P. Harper, New York.

Henschen, Folke

1966 *The Human Skull: A Cultural History*. Praeger, New York.

Herold, Elaine Bluhm, Patricia J. O'Brien, and David J. Wenner Jr.

1990 Part I: Hoxie Farm and Huber: Two Upper Mississippian Archaeological Sites in Cook County, Illinois. In *At the Edge of Prehistory: Huber Phase Archaeology in the Chicago Area*, edited by James A. Brown and Patricia J. O'Brien, pp. 1–119. Illinois Department of Transportation, Center for American Archaeology, Kampsville, Illinois.

Hester, Thomas R.

1969a Human Bone Artifacts from Southern Texas. *American Antiquity* 34:326–328.

1969b Archeological Investigations in Kleberg and Kenedy Counties, Texas, in August, 1967. State Building Commission Archeological Program Report 15. Austin. Electronic document, http://pdf885.xqhbooks.com/archeological-archaeological-investigations-in-kleberg-and-kenedy-counti_fsqu1.pdf, accessed July 27, 2014.

Hewitt, John N. B.

1895 The Iroquois Concept of the Soul. *Journal of American Folklore* 7:107–116.

1903 *Iroquoian Cosmology*. Bureau of American Ethnology Bulletin 21. Smithsonian Institution, Washington, D.C.

Hickerson, Daniel A.

1997 Historical Processes, Epidemic Disease, and the Formation of the Hasinai Confederacy. *Ethnohistory* 44:31–52.

Hilgeman, Sherri L.

2000 *Pottery and Chronology of the Angel Site, a Middle Mississippian Center in the Lower Ohio Valley*. University of Alabama Press, Tuscaloosa.

Hilger, M. Inez

1952 *Arapaho Child Life and Its Cultural Background*. Bureau of American Ethnology Bulletin 148. Smithsonian Institution, Washington, D.C.

1970 Notes on Crow Culture. *Baessler-Archiv*, n.s. 18:253–294.

Hill, Tom, and Richard W. Hill Sr.

1994 *Creation's Journey: Native American Identity and Belief*. National Museum of the American Indian, Smithsonian Institution, Washington, D.C.

Hillson, Simon

1996 *Dental Anthropology*. Cambridge University Press, New York.

Hinsdale, Wilbert B., and Emerson F. Greenman

1936 *Perforated Indian Crania in Michigan*. Occasional Contributions No. 5. Museum of Anthropology, University of Michigan, Ann Arbor.

Hochrein, Michael

2002 An Autopsy of the Grave: Recognizing, Collecting, and Preserving Forensic Geotaphonomic Evidence. In *Advances in Forensic Taphonomy*, edited by William D. Haglund and Marcella H. Sorg, pp. 45–70. CRC Press, Boca Raton, Florida.

Hodges, Denise C.

1989 Cranial Fragment from the Lowry Farm Site, 13MC4. In *Miscellaneous Reports on Iowa Archaeology*, edited by Mary C. Allen, pp. 58–59. Research Papers 14(3). Office of the State Archaeologist, University of Iowa, Iowa City.

1994 A Human Mandible from 13WD6, the Correctionville Site, Woodbury County, Iowa. In *Reports on Iowa Burial Projects: Osteology and Archaeology*, edited by Shirley J. Schermer and Robin M. Lillie, pp. 159–164. Research Papers 19(1). Office of the State Archaeologist, University of Iowa, Iowa City.

Holcomb, George R.

1952 An Analysis of Human Remains from Aztalan. Unpublished Master's thesis, Department of Anthropology, University of Wisconsin, Madison.

Holley, George R.

1989 *The Archaeology of the Cahokia Mounds ICT-II: Ceramics*. Illinois Cultural Resources Study 1. Illinois Historic Preservation Agency, Springfield.

Holley, George R., Kathryn E. Parker, Mikels Skele, Julie N. Harper, and Donald L. Booth

2001 The Knoebel Community Core (S-71, S-816). In *The Knoebel Locality, Scott Joint-Use Archaeological Project*, edited by George R. Holley, Kathryn E. Parker, Harold W. Watters Jr., Julie N. Harper, Mikels Skele, Jennifer E. Ringberg, Alan J. Brown, and Donald L. Booth, pp. 115–218. Office of Contract Archaeology, Southern Illinois University, Edwardsville.

Holliman, R. B.

1970 Evidence of a Prehistoric Physician in Virginia. *Virginia Medical Monthly* 97(10):642–644.

Hollinger, R. Eric

2005 Conflict and Culture Change in the Late Prehistoric and Early Historic American Midcontinent. Unpublished Ph.D. dissertation, Department of Anthropology, University of Illinois, Urbana-Champaign.

Hollinger, R. Eric, Carl R. Falk, Darcy Morey, and Holmes A. Semken Jr.

1999 *Report on the McKinney Oneota Village (13LA1) Subsistence Study*. University of Illinois, Urbana-Champaign. Submitted to State Historical Society of Iowa: Resource Enhancement and Protection Program/Historic Resources Development Program. Copy on file, Office of the State Archaeologist, University of Iowa, Iowa City.

Hollinger, R. Eric, and Joseph A. Vradenburg

1994 Report on Human Skeletal Remains from the Wever Site (13LE110). Draft

copy on file in Burial Project File No. 645. Office of the State Archaeologist, University of Iowa, Iowa City.
2004 Human Skeletal Remains. In *Oneota Occupations on the Wever Terrace: Archaeological Data Recovery for the U.S. 61 Wever Bypass, Lee County, Iowa DE-61-1(24)-2A-56*, Vol. III, pp. 409–438. Louis Berger Group, Marion, Iowa.

Holme, Bryan
1987 *Medieval Pageant*. Thames and Hudson, London.

Holmes, William H.
1883 *Art in Shell of the Ancient Americans*. Bureau of American Ethnology Annual Report 2, pp. 185–305. Smithsonian Institution, Washington, D.C.
1886 *Ancient Pottery of the Mississippi Valley*. Bureau of American Ethnology Annual Report 4, pp. 1–201. Smithsonian Institution, Washington, D.C.
1903 *Aboriginal Pottery of the Eastern United States*. Bureau of American Ethnology Annual Report 20. Smithsonian Institution, Washington, D.C.

Holtorf, Cornelius
2002 Notes on the Life History of a Pot Sherd. *Journal of Material Culture* 7:49–71.

Holtz-Leith, Wendy
2006 Archaeological Investigations at an Oneota Village in the Heart of La Crosse, Wisconsin: Data Recovery at the Seventh Street Interchange, USH 14/61, South Avenue, within the Sanford Archaeological District, La Crosse Wisconsin. WISDOT Project 1641-02–00/SHSW# 96-5002/Lc. Reports of Investigations No. 438. Mississippi Valley Archaeology Center, University of Wisconsin, La Crosse.

Horn, Andrew
1981 Ritual Drama and the Theatrical: The Case of Bori Spirit Mediumship. In *Drama and Theatre in Nigeria: A Critical Sourcebook*, edited by Yemi Ogunbiyi, pp. 181–202. Nigeria Magazine, Lagos.

Horse Capture, George P., and Emil Her Many Horses (editors)
2006 *A Song for the Horse Nation: Horses in Native American Cultures*. National Museum of the American Indian, Smithsonian Institution, Washington, D.C.

Hoskins, Janet
1998 *Biographical Objects: How Things Tell the Stories of People's Lives*. Routledge, New York.

Howard, James H.
1966 *The Dakota or Sioux Indians*. Anthropological Paper 2. University of South Dakota Museum, Vermillion, South Dakota.
1968 *The Southeastern Ceremonial Complex and Its Interpretation*. Memoir 6. Missouri Archaeological Society, Columbia.
1977 *The Plains-Ojibwa or Bungi*. Reprints in Anthropology, Vol. 7. J&L Reprints, Lincoln, Nebraska.
1981 *Shawnee! The Ceremonialism of a Native American Tribe and Its Cultural Background*. Ohio University Press, Athens.

Howard, Julie, and Joel C. Janetski
1992 Human Scalps from Eastern Utah. *Utah Archaeology* 5(1):125–132.
Howey, Meghan C. L., and John M. O'Shea
2006 Bear's Journey and the Study of Ritual in Archaeology. *American Antiquity* 71:261–282.
Howland, Henry R.
1877 Recent Archaeological Discoveries in the American Bottom. *Buffalo Society of Natural History Bulletin* 3(5):204–211.
Hoyme, Lucille E., and William E. Bass
1962 *Human Skeletal Remains from the Tollifero (Ha6) and Clarksville (Mc14) Sites, John H. Kerr Reservoir Basin, Virginia*. Bureau of American Ethnology Bulletin 182, pp. 329–400. Smithsonian Institution, Washington, D.C.
Hrdlička, Aleš
1941 Diseases of and Artifacts on Skulls and Bones from Kodiak Island. *Smithsonian Miscellaneous Collections* 101(4):1–14.
Hudson, Charles M.
1976 *The Southeastern Indians*. University of Tennessee Press, Knoxville.
Hudson, Jean
2004 A Sample of Animal Bone from Aztalan (47JE1), Wisconsin. *Wisconsin Archeologist* 85:50–59.
Hultkrantz, Åke
1953 *Conceptions of the Soul among North American Indians: A Study in Religious Ethnology*. Ethnographical Museum of Sweden, Stockholm.
1979 *The Religions of the American Indians*. University of California Press, Berkeley.
Hurley, William
1978 The Armstrong Site: A Silvernale Phase Oneota Village in Wisconsin. *Wisconsin Archeologist* 59(1):1–145.
Ifantidis, Fotis
2006 The Personal Ornaments from the Neolithic Settlement of Dispilio, Kastoria: Production and Function of an "Aesthetic Toolkit." Unpublished Master's thesis, Archaeology Department, Aristotle University of Thessaloniki, Greece.
Interesting Wisconsin Specimens
1956 *Wisconsin Archeologist* 37:24.
Issenman, Betty
1997 *Sinews of Survival: The Living Legacy of Inuit Clothing*. University of British Columbia Press, Vancouver.
Ives, John C.
1962 Mill Creek Pottery. *Journal of the Iowa Archeological Society* 11(3):1–59.
Jackson, Douglas K.
2010 The Anker Site Marine Shell Maskette and Mask Gorgets. *Illinois Archaeology* 22:359–378.

Jackson, Douglas K., and Thomas E. Emerson (editors)

2013 *The Hoxie Farm Site Fortified Village: Late Fisher Phase Occupation and Fortification in South Chicago.* Research Report No. 24. Illinois State Archaeological Survey, University of Illinois, Champaign.

Jackson, Douglas K., and Kristin M. Hedman

2009 Upper Mississippian Mortuary Practices at the Hoxie Farm Site, Cook County, Illinois. Paper presented at the Midwest Archaeological Conference, Iowa City, Iowa.

Jacobi, Keith P.

2003 The Malevolent "Un-Dead": Cross-Cultural Perspectives. In *Handbook of Death and Dying*, edited by Clifton D. Bryant, pp. 96–109. Sage, New York.

2007 Disabling the Dead: Human Trophy Taking in the Prehistoric Southeast. In *The Taking and Displaying of Human Body Parts as Trophies by Amerindians*, edited by Richard J. Chacon and David H. Dye, pp. 299–338. Springer, New York.

Jacobi, Keith P., and M. C. Hill

2000 Prehistoric Treatment of the Dead: Bone Handling in the Southeastern United States. Unpublished manuscript on file, Laboratory of Human Osteology, University of Alabama, Tuscaloosa.

Jamieson, James B.

1983 An Examination of Prisoner-Sacrifice and Cannibalism at the St. Lawrence Iroquoian Roebuck Site. *Canadian Journal of Archaeology* 7:159–175.

Jeffries, Richard W.

1976 *The Tunacunnhee Site: Evidence of Hopewell Interaction in Northwest Georgia.* Anthropological Papers No. 1. University of Georgia, Athens.

Jensen, Peter

1960 A Preliminary Report of the Excavation of Fort Sweney. Manuscript on file, State Historic Preservation Office, Minnesota Historical Society, St. Paul.

Johnsen, Teresa Marie

2003 Description and Analysis of Preserved Fabrics from the Northwest Mound at Aztalan: A Late Prehistoric Site in Southeastern Wisconsin. Unpublished Master's thesis, Department of Anthropology, University of Wisconsin, Milwaukee.

Johnson, Eileen

1989 Human Modified Bones from Early Southern Plains Sites. In *Bone Modification*, edited by Robson Bonnichsen and Marcella H. Sorg, pp. 431–471. Center for the Study of First Americans, Orono, Maine.

Johnson, Elias

1881 *Legends, Traditions and Laws, of the Iroquois, or Six Nations, and History of the Tuscarora Indians.* Union Printers and Publishers, Lockport, New York.

Johnston, Alexandra F., and Wim N. M. Hüsken (editors)

1997 *Civic Ritual and Drama.* Rodopi, Amsterdam.

Johnston, Cheryl

2002 Culturally Modified Human Remains from the Hopewell Mound Group. Unpublished Ph.D. dissertation, Department of Anthropology, Ohio State University, Columbus.

Johnston, Cheryl A., Stephen P. Nawrocki, Christopher C. Schmidt, and Matthew Williamson

1997 An Interregional Comparison of Culturally-Modified Hopewellian Human Remains. Paper presented at the 62nd Annual Meeting of the Society for American Archaeology, Nashville, Tennessee.

Joy, Jody

2009 Reinvigorating Object Biography: Reproducing the Drama of Object Lives. *World Archaeology* 41:540–556.

Joyce, Rosemary A.

2005 Archaeology of the Body. *Annual Review of Anthropology* 34:139–158.

Karsten, Rafael

1955 *The Religion of the Samek: Ancient Beliefs and Cults of the Scandinavian and Finnish Lapps*. Brill, Leiden.

Kehoe, Alice Beck

2005 Expedient Angled-Tang Endscrapers: Glimpsing Women's Work in the Archaeological Record. In *Gender and Hide Production*, edited by Lisa Frink and Kathryn Weedman, pp. 133–143. AltaMira, Walnut Creek, California.

2006 *The Ghost Dance: Ethnohistory and Revitalization*. 2nd ed. Waveland, New York.

Kellar, James H.

1967 Material Remains. In *Angel Site: An Archaeological, Historical, and Ethnographical Study*, by Glenn A. Black, pp. 431–489. Indiana Historical Society, Indianapolis.

Keller, Cynthia, and Christopher Carr

2005 Gender, Role, Prestige, and Ritual Interaction across the Ohio, Mann, and Havanna Hopewellian Regions, as Evidenced by Ceramic Figurines. In *Gathering Hopewell: Society, Ritual, and Ritual Interaction*, edited by Christopher Carr and D. Troy Case, pp. 428–460. Kluwer Academic/Plenum, New York.

Kelly, John E.

1997 Stirling Phase Socio-Political Activity at East St. Louis and Cahokia. In *Cahokia: Domination and Ideology in the Mississippian World*, edited by Timothy R. Pauketat and Thomas E. Emerson, pp. 141–166. University of Nebraska Press, Lincoln.

2000 The Grassy Lake Site: An Historical and Archaeological Overview. In *Mounds, Modoc, and Mesoamerica: Papers in Honor of Melvin L. Fowler*, edited by Steven R. Ahler, pp. 141–178. Scientific Papers Vol. 28. Illinois State Museum, Springfield.

Kidd, Kenneth E.

1986 *Blackfoot Ethnography*. Manuscript Series 8. Archaeological Survey of Alberta, Edmonton.

King, Adam

2004 Power and the Sacred: Mound C and the Etowah Chiefdom. In *Hero, Hawk, and Open Hand: American Indian Art of the Ancient Midwest and South*, edited by Richard F. Townsend and Robert V. Sharp, pp. 150–165. Yale University Press, New Haven, Connecticut.

King, Adam (editor)

2007 *Southeastern Ceremonial Complex: Chronology, Content, Context.* University of Alabama Press, Tuscaloosa.

Knight, Richard Payne

2006 [1865] A Discourse on the Worship of Priapus. In *Sexual Symbolism: A History of Phallic Worship* by Richard Payne Knight and Thomas Wright, pp. 1–122. Privately printed, London. 2006 facsimile ed. Dover, Mineola, New York.

Knight, Vernon J., Jr.

2006 Farewell to the Southeastern Ceremonial Complex. *Southeastern Archaeology* 25:1–5.

Knight, Vernon J., Jr., James A. Brown, and George E. Lankford

2001 On the Subject Matter of SECC Art. *Southeastern Archaeology* 20:129–153.

Knight, Vernon, Jr., and Vincas P. Steponaitis

2011 A Redefinition of the Hemphill Style in Mississippian Art. In *Visualizing the Sacred: Cosmic Visions, Regionalism, and the Art of the Mississippian World*, edited by George E. Lankford, F. Kent Reilly, and James F. Garber, pp. 210–239. University of Texas Press, Austin.

Knudson, Kelly J., Sloan R. Williams, Rebecca Osborn, Kathleen Forgey, and Patrick Ryan Williams

2009 The Geographic Origins of Nasca Trophy Heads Using Strontium, Oxygen, and Carbon Isotope Data. *Journal of Anthropological Archaeology* 28:244–257.

Koelikamp, Ted

1974 The Zorica Site. *Central States Archaeological Journal* 21:128–135.

Konigsberg, Lyle W., and Susan R. Frankenberg

1993 Missing Skulls and Missing Data in Ohio Hopewell. Paper presented at the 58th Annual Meeting of the Society for American Archaeology, St. Louis, Missouri.

Kopytoff, Igor

1986 The Cultural Biography of Things: Commoditization as Process. In *The Social Life of Things: Commodities in Cultural Perspective*, edited by Arjun Appadurai, pp. 64–91. Cambridge University Press, Cambridge.

Kraft, Herbert C.

1986 *The Lenape: Archaeology, History, and Ethnography.* New Jersey Historical Society, Newark.

Krutchen, Jeffrey D., and K. Shane Vanderford

2005 *The St. Thomas Site (11MS54), Madison County, Illinois.* Research Reports No. 99. Illinois Transportation Archaeological Research Program, University of Illinois, Urbana.

Lacer, Charles R.

1980 The Mann Site, Posey County, Indiana (12Po2). Unpublished manuscript on file, Department of Anthropology, Indiana University, Bloomington.

La Flesche, Francis

1921 *The Osage Tribe: Rite of the Chiefs, Sayings of the Ancient Men.* Bureau of American Ethnology Bulletin 36, pp. 35–604. Smithsonian Institution, Washington, D.C.

Lambert, Patricia

2007 Ethnographic and Linguistic Evidence for the Origins of Human Trophy Taking in California. In *The Taking and Displaying of Human Body Parts as Trophies by Amerindians*, edited by Richard J. Chacon and David H. Dye, pp. 65–89. Springer, New York.

Lankford, George E.

1987 *Native American Legends: Southeastern Legends: Tales from the Natchez, Caddo, Biloxi, Chickasaw, and Other Nations.* American Folklore Series. August House, Little Rock, Arkansas.

2004 World on a String: Some Cosmological Components of the Southeastern Ceremonial Complex. In *Hero, Hawk, and Open Hand: American Indian Art of the Ancient Midwest and South*, edited by Richard F. Townsend and Robert V. Sharp, pp. 206–217. Yale University Press, New Haven, Connecticut.

2007a *Reachable Stars: Patterns in the Ethnoastronomy of Eastern North America.* University of Alabama Press, Tuscaloosa.

2007b The "Path of Souls": Some Death Imagery in the Southeastern Ceremonial Complex. In *Ancient Objects and Sacred Realms: Interpretations of Mississippian Iconography*, edited by F. Kent Reilly III and James F. Garber, pp. 174–212. University of Texas Press, Austin.

2007c The Great Serpent in Eastern North America. In *Ancient Objects and Sacred Realms: Interpretations of Mississippian Iconograpy*, edited by F. Kent Reilly III and James F. Garber, pp. 107–135. University of Texas Press, Austin.

2008 *Looking for Lost Lore: Studies in Folklore, Ethnology, and Iconography.* University of Alabama Press, Tuscaloosa.

Lapham, Increase A.

2001 [1885] *The Antiquities of Wisconsin as Surveyed and Described.* Smithsonian Institution, Washington, D.C. 2001 facsimile ed. University of Wisconsin Press, Madison.

Larsen, Clark Spencer

2011 Foreword. In *The Bioarchaeology of the Human Head: Decapitation, Decoration, and Deformation*, edited by Michelle Bonogofsky, pp. xiii–xv. University Press of Florida, Gainesville.

Larsen, Lewis H., Jr.

1957 An Unusual Wooden Rattle from the Etowah Site. *Missouri Archaeologist* 19(4):6–11.

Lehmer, Donald J.

1954 *Archaeological Investigations in the Oahe Dam Area, South Dakota, 1950–51.* Bureau of American Ethnology Bulletin 158, River Basin Survey Papers 7. Smithsonian Institution, Washington, D.C.

Leland, Charles G.

1884 *The Algonquin Legends of New England: Myths and Folk Lore of the Micmac, Passamaquoddy, and Penobscot Tribes*. Riverside, Cambridge, Massachusetts.

LeMoine, Genevieve

1991 Use Wear Analysis of Bone Tools. *Archaeozoologia* 3:212–224.

1994 Use Wear on Bone and Antler Tools from the Mackenzie Delta, Northwest Territories. *American Antiquity* 59:316–334.

Lewis, Oscar

1942 *The Effects of White Contact on Blackfoot Culture, with Special Reference to the Role of the Fur Trade*. American Ethnological Society Monograph 6. Augustin, Locust Valley, New York.

Lillie, Robin M.

1990 Analysis of Human Skeletal Remains from 13DM3, Kingston Oneota Site, Des Moines County, Iowa. In *Reports on Iowa Burial Sites: Archaeology and Osteology*, edited by Mary C. Allen, pp. 84–85. Research Papers 15(5). Office of the State Archaeologist, University of Iowa, Iowa City.

1996a Human Skeletal Remains from the Howard Goodhue Site, 13PK1, Polk County, Iowa. In *Reports on Iowa Burial Projects: Osteology and Archaeology*, edited by Shirley J. Schermer and Robin M. Lillie, pp. 169–224. Research Papers 21(1). Office of the State Archaeologist, University of Iowa, Iowa City.

1996b Human Skeletal Remains from Northeast Iowa and the Henry P. Field Collections of Luther College. In *Reports on Iowa Burial Projects: Osteology and Archaeology*, edited by Shirley J. Schermer and Robin M. Lillie, pp. 9–32. Research Papers 21(1). Office of the State Archaeologist, University of Iowa, Iowa City, Iowa.

1996c Preliminary Report on Human Skeletal Fragments Recovered from the McKinney Site, 13LA1, Louisa County, Iowa. In *Reports on Iowa Burial Projects: Osteology and Archaeology*, edited by Shirley J. Schermer and Robin M. Lillie, pp.153–157. Research Papers 21(1). Office of the State Archaeologist, University of Iowa, Iowa City.

1998 Human Skeletal Remains from Deppe Mound Group, 13JK11, Jackson County, Iowa. Manuscript on file, Office of the State Archaeologist, University of Iowa, Iowa City.

1999 Human Remains. In *Bison Hunters of the Western Prairies: Archaeological Investigations at the Dixon Site (13WD8), Woodbury County, Iowa*, edited by Richard L. Fishel, pp. 109–116. Report 21. Office of the State Archaeologist, University of Iowa, Iowa City.

2002a A Culturally Modified Cranial Fragment from Lane Farm Mounds, 13AM104, Allamakee County, Iowa. In *Reports on Iowa Burial Projects: Osteology and Archaeology*, edited by Shirley J. Schermer and Robin M. Lillie, pp. 37–40. Research Papers 27(1). Office of the State Archaeologist, University of Iowa, Iowa City.

2002b A Mandibular Molar from Gillett Grove, 13CY2, Clay County, Iowa. In *Reports on Iowa Burial Projects: Osteology and Archaeology*, edited by Shirley J. Schermer and Robin M. Lillie, pp. 177–178. Research Papers 27(1). Office of the State Archaeologist, University of Iowa, Iowa City.

2002c Additional Human Skeletal Remains Recovered during 1970 and 1996 Excavations at the McKinney Site, 13LA1, Louisa County, Iowa. In *Reports on Iowa Burial Projects: Osteology and Archaeology*, edited by Shirley J. Schermer and Robin M. Lillie, pp. 55–66. Research Papers 27(1). Office of the State Archaeologist, University of Iowa, Iowa City.

Lillie, Robin M., and R. Eric Hollinger

2002 Two Human Parietal Fragments from the Schmeiser Site, 13DM101, Des Moines County, Iowa. In *Reports on Iowa Burial Projects: Osteology and Archaeology*, edited by Shirley J. Schermer and Robin M. Lillie, pp. 41–44. Research Papers 27(1). Office of the State Archaeologist, University of Iowa, Iowa City.

Lilly, Eli

1937 *Prehistoric Antiquities of Indiana*. Indiana Historical Society, Indianapolis.

Lithics Casting Lab

2012 Long-Nosed Copper God Mask, Calhoun County, Illinois. Electronic document, http://www.lithiccastinglab.com/gallery-pages/godmaskcopperlarge.htm, accessed February 10, 2012.

Lock, Margaret

1993 Cultivating the Body: Anthropology and Epistemologies of Bodily Practice and Knowledge. *Annual Review of Anthropology* 22:133–155.

Lockhart, Rachel. A., Christopher W. Schmidt, and Steven A. Symes

2009 Understanding Middle and Late Archaic Forelimb Removal: An Experimental Approach. Abstract. *American Journal of Physical Anthropology Supplement* 48:177.

Logan, Wilfred

1976 *Woodland Complexes in Northeastern Iowa*. Publications in Archeology 15. U.S. Department of the Interior, National Park Service, Washington, D.C.

Lorenz, Karl

2000 The Natchez of Southwest Mississippi. In *Indians of the Greater Southeast: Historical Archaeology and Ethnohistory*, edited by Bonnie G. McEwan, pp. 142–177. University Press of Florida, Gainesville.

Lovisek, Joan A.

2007 Human Trophy Taking on the Northwest Coast: An Ethnohistorical Perspective. In *The Taking and Displaying of Human Body Parts as Trophies by Amerindians*, edited by Richard J. Chacon and David H. Dye, pp. 45–64. Springer, New York.

Lowie, Robert H.

1910 *The Assiniboine*. Anthropological Papers Vol. 4, Pt. 1. American Museum of Natural History, New York.

1935 *The Crow Indians*. Farrar and Rinehart, New York.

Luby, Edward M., and Mark F. Gruber

1999 The Dead Must Be Fed: Symbolic Meanings of the Shellmounds of the San Francisco Bay Area. *Cambridge Archaeological Journal* 9:95–108.

Lurie, Nancy Oestreich

1989 Beaded Twined Bags of the Great Lakes Indians. In *Great Lakes Indian Art*, edited by David W. Penney, pp. 70–80. Detroit Institute of Arts. Wayne State University Press, Detroit, Michigan.

Lynd, James W.

1864 History of the Dakotas: James W. Lynd's Manuscripts. *Collections of the Minnesota Historical Society* 2(2):143–174.

MacAloon, John J.

1984 Olympic Games and the Theory of Spectacle in Modern Societies. In *Rite, Drama, Festival, Spectacle: Rehearsals toward a Theory of Cultural Performance*, edited by John J. MacAloon, pp. 241–280. Institute for the Study of Human Issues, Philadelphia.

MacCauley, Clay

1887 *The Seminole Indians of Florida*. Bureau of American Ethnology Annual Report 5, pp. 469–532. Smithsonian Institution, Washington, D.C.

Macdonald, William K.

1990 Investigating Style: An Exploratory Analysis of Some Plains Burials. In *Uses of Style in Archaeology*, edited by Margaret W. Conkey and Christine A. Hastorf, pp. 52–60. Cambridge University Press, Cambridge.

MacGregor, Gavin

1999 Making Sense of the Past in the Present: A Sensory Analysis of Carved Stone Balls. *World Archaeology* 31:194–213.

MacLean, J. Arthur

1931 Excavation of Albee Mound 1926–1927. *Indiana History Bulletin* 8(4):1–176.

MacNeish, Richard S.

1958 *An Introduction to the Archaeology of Southeast Manitoba*. Bulletin No. 157. National Museum of Canada, Department of Northern Affairs and National Resources, Ottawa.

Maher, Robert F.

1958 The Excavation and Reconstruction of the Southwest Pyramidal Mound at Aztalan. *Wisconsin Archeologist* 39:77–101.

Mainfort, Robert C., Jr.

1986 *Pinson Mounds, a Middle Woodland Ceremonial Center*. Research Series No. 7. Division of Archaeology, Tennessee Department of Conservation, Nashville.

Mainfort, Robert C., Jr., and Lynne P. Sullivan (editors)

1998 *Ancient Earthen Enclosures of the Eastern Woodlands*. University Press of Florida, Gainesville.

Malinowski, Bronislaw
1954 *Magic, Science, and Religion and Other Essays by Bronislaw Malinowski.* Doubleday Anchor, Garden City, New York.
Mallam, R. Clark
1978 The Quandahl Rockshelter Revisited. *South Dakota Archaeology* 2:5–17.
1979 A Cut and Perforated Human Mandible from the Quandahl Rockshelter, Winneshiek County, Iowa. *Journal of the Iowa Archeological Society* 26:30–36.
Mallery, Garrick
1893 *Picture-Writing of the American Indians.* Bureau of American Ethnology Annual Report 10. Smithsonian Institution, Washington, D.C.
Mann, Barbara A.
2003 *Native Americans, Archaeologists, and the Mounds.* Lang, New York.
Mann, Ceril B., Jr.
1983 Classification of Ceramics from the Lubbub Creek Archaeological Locality. In *Prehistoric Agricultural Communities in West Central Alabama,* Vol. II, edited by Christopher S. Peebles, pp. 2–121. University of Michigan, Ann Arbor.
Manseau, Peter
2009 *Rag and Bone: A Journey among the World's Holy Dead.* Holt, New York.
Mant, A. Keith
1987 Knowledge Acquired from Post-War Exhumations. In *Death, Decay, and Reconstruction: Approaches to Archaeology and Forensic Science,* edited by Andrew Boddington, Andrew N. Garland, and Robert C. Janaway, pp. 65–78. Manchester University Press, Manchester, United Kingdom.
Marcucci, Derrick J.
1997 *An Inventory and Assessment of Selected Prehistoric Mound Sites in Jackson County, Iowa.* Prepared for the Jackson County Historic Preservation Commission, HRDP Contract No. 96-103. Copy on file, Office of the State Archaeologist, University of Iowa, Iowa City.
Marshack, Alexander
1972 *The Roots of Civilization: The Cognitive Beginnings of Man's First Art, Symbol, and Notation.* McGraw-Hill, New York.
Martin, Debra L.
2000 Review of *Man Corn: Cannibalism and Violence in the Prehistoric American Southwest. American Antiquity* 65:199–201.
Martin, Debra L., Ryan P. Harrod, and Ventura R. Perez (editors)
2012 *The Bioarchaeology of Violence.* University Press of Florida, Gainesville.
Martin, Simon, and Nikolai Grube
2008 *Chronicle of the Maya Kings and Queens.* 2nd ed. Thames and Hudson, London.
Maschner, Herbert D. G., and Katherine L. Reedy-Maschner
2007 Heads, Women, and the Baubles of Prestige: Trophies of War in the Arctic and Subarctic. In *The Taking and Displaying of Human Body Parts as Trophies by Amerindians,* edited by Richard J. Chacon and David H. Dye, pp. 32–44. Springer, New York.

Masluk, Adrianna
1997 Analysis of Human Remains: Evidence for Prehistoric Competition in the Upper Mississippi Valley. Unpublished senior paper, Department of Anthropology, University of Wisconsin, La Crosse.

Mason, Ronald
2000 Archaeology and Native North American Oral Traditions. *American Antiquity* 65:239–266.

Mathews, John Joseph
1961 *The Osages: Children of the Middle Waters.* University of Oklahoma Press, Norman.

Matos Moctezuma, Eduardo
1988 *Obras Maestras del Templo Mayor.* Fomento Cultural Banamex, Banamex, Mexico.

Matternes, Hugh B.
2000 Social and Biological Structures in the Mound C Cemetery, Wickliffe Mound Group (15BA4). Unpublished Ph.D. dissertation, Department of Anthropology, University of Tennessee, Knoxville.

Matwychuck, Margo
1980 An Analysis of Northern Manitoba Cree and Ojibwa Bone Fleshers. *Manitoba Archaeological Quarterly* 4(3–4):2–66.

Mauss, Marcel
1938 Un Catégorie de l'Esprit Humain: La Notion de Personne, Celle de "Moi." *Journal of the Royal Anthropological Institute of Great Britain and Ireland* 68: 263–281.
1985 A Category of the Human Mind: The Notion of Person, the Notion of Self. Translated by W. D. Halls. Reprinted in *The Category of the Person: Anthropology, Philosophy, History*, edited by Michael Carrithers, Steven Collins, and Steven Lukes, pp. 1–25. Cambridge University Press, Cambridge. Originally published 1938.

Maxwell, Moreau S.
1950 Change in the Interpretation of Wisconsin's Prehistory. *Wisconsin Magazine of History* 33:427–443.

May, Stephanie A.
2004 Alabama and Koasati. In *Southeast*, edited by Raymond Fogelson, pp. 407–414. Handbook of North American Indians, Vol. 14, William C. Sturtevant, general editor, Smithsonian Institution, Washington, D.C.

Mazrim, Robert, and Duane Esarey
2007 Rethinking the Dawn of History: The Schedule, Signature, and Agency of European Goods in Protohistoric Illinois. *Midcontinental Journal of Archaeology* 32:145–200.

McElrath, Dale L., Joyce A. Williams, Thomas O. Maher, and Michael C. Meinkoth
1987 *Emergent Mississippian and Mississippian Communities at the Radic Site.* Ameri-

can Bottom Archaeology, FAI-270 Site Reports Vol. 17. University of Illinois Press, Urbana.

McGregor, John

1952 The Havana Site. In *Hopewellian Communities in Illinois*, edited by Thorne Deuel, pp. 43–91. Scientific Papers Vol. 5. Illinois State Museum, Springfield.

McGuire, Randall H.

1988 Dialogues with the Dead: Ideology and the Cemetery. In *The Recovery of Meaning in Historical Archaeology*, edited by Mark P. Leone and Parker B. Potter Jr., pp. 435–480. Smithsonian Institution Press, Washington, D.C.

1992 *Death, Society, and Ideology in a Hohokam Community*. Westview, Boulder, Colorado.

McKusick, Marshall

1964 *Men of Ancient Iowa: As Revealed by Archeological Discoveries*. Iowa State University Press, Ames.

1973 *The Grant Oneota Village*. Report No. 4. Office of the State Archaeologist, University of Iowa, Iowa City.

McNeill, Judith R.

2005 Putting the Dead to Work: An Examination of the Use of Human Bone in Prehistoric Guam. In *Interacting with the Dead: Perspectives on Mortuary Archaeology for the New Millennium*, edited by Gordon F. M. Rakita, Jane E. Buikstra, Lane A. Beck, and Sloan R. Williams, pp. 305–315. University Press of Florida, Gainesville.

Means, Bernard K.

1999 Monongahela Mortuary Practices in Somerset County, Pennsylvania: Observations and Implications. *Pennsylvania Archaeologist* 69(2):15–44.

Meinkoth, Michael C., Kristin Hedman, Mary Simon, Thomas Berres, and Douglas Brewer

1995 *The Sister Creeks Site Mounds: Middle Woodland Mortuary Practices in the Illinois River Valley*. Transportation Archaeological Research Reports No. 2. Illinois Transportation Archaeological Research Program, University of Illinois, Urbana.

Mensforth, Robert P.

2001 Warfare and Trophy Taking in the Archaic Period. In *Archaic Transitions in Ohio and Kentucky Prehistory*, edited by Olaf H. Prufer, Sara E. Pedde, and Richard S. Meindl, pp. 110–138. Kent State University Press, Kent, Ohio.

2007 Human Trophy Taking in Eastern North America during the Archaic Period: The Relationship to Warfare and Social Complexity. In *The Taking and Displaying of Human Body Parts as Trophies by Amerindians*, edited by Richard J. Chacon and David H. Dye, pp. 222–277. Springer, New York.

Meskell, Lynn

2005 Introduction: Object Orientations. In *Archaeologies of Materiality*, edited by Lynn Meskell, pp. 1–17. Blackwell, Malden, Massachusetts.

Metcalf, Peter, and Richard Huntington

1991 *Celebrations of Death.* Cambridge University Press, Cambridge.

Michelson, Truman

1930 *Contributions to Fox Ethnology,* Vol. II. Bureau of American Ethnology Bulletin 95. Smithsonian Institution, Washington, D.C.

Mills, William C.

1907 The Explorations of the Edwin Harness Mound. *Ohio Archaeological and Historical Quarterly* 16:112–193.

1909a Explorations of the Seip Mound. *Ohio Archaeological and Historical Quarterly* 18:269–321.

1909b *Exploration of the Seip Mound, Certain Mounds and Village Sites in Ohio,* Vol. 2, Pt. 1. F. J. Heer, Columbus, Ohio.

1916a Exploration of the Tremper Mound. *Ohio Archaeological and Historical Quarterly* 25:226–266.

1916b *Exploration of the Tremper Mound, Certain Mounds and Village Sites in Ohio,* Vol. 2, Pt. 3. F. J. Heer, Columbus, Ohio.

1917 Explorations of the Westenhaver Mound. *Ohio Archaeological and Historical Quarterly* 26:227–266.

Milner, George R.

1983 *The East St. Louis Stone Quarry Site Cemetery.* American Bottom Archaeology, FAI-270 Site Reports No. 1. University of Illinois Press, Urbana.

1984 Social and Temporal Implications of Variation among American Bottom Mississippian Cemeteries. *American Antiquity* 49:468–488.

1995 An Osteological Perspective on Prehistoric Warfare. In *Regional Approaches to Mortuary Analysis,* edited by Lane A. Beck, pp. 221–244. Plenum, New York.

1998 *The Cahokia Chiefdom: The Archaeology of a Mississippian Society.* Smithsonian Institution Press, Washington, D.C.

Milner, George R., Eve Anderson, and Virginia Smith

1991 Warfare in Late Prehistoric West-Central Illinois. *American Antiquity* 56: 581–603.

Milner, George R., Scott W. Hammerstedt, and Kirk D. French

2010 Chert Hoes as Digging Tools. *Antiquity* 84:103–113.

Milwaukee Public Museum

1921 Catalog Book No. 7. On file, Milwaukee Public Museum Anthropology Lab, Milwaukee, Wisconsin.

Miotshwa, Norma Princess Vumile

1988 A Study of Diverging and Converging Points between Ritual Drama and Contemporary Drama with Special Reference to Zulu Rituals. Unpublished Bachelor's thesis, University of Zululand, KwaDlangezwa, Zululand.

Mishkin, Bernard

1940 *Rank and Warfare among the Plains Indians.* Monograph 3. American Ethnological Society. Augustin, Locust Valley, New York

Moffat, Charles R., Brad Koldehoff, Kathryn E. Parker, Lucretia S. Kelly, Mary R. McCorvie, and Joseph Craig

1990 *Archaeological Data Recovery at Five Prehistoric Sites, Lake Red Rock, Iowa.* Report No. 133. American Resources Group, Carbondale, Illinois.

Mooney, James

1900 *Myths of the Cherokee.* Bureau of American Ethnology 1897–1898 Bulletin 19, Pt. 1. Smithsonian Institution, Washington, D.C.

1910 Scalping. In *Handbook of American Indians North of Mexico,* Vol. II, edited by Frederick Webb Hodge, pp. 482–483. Bureau of American Ethnology Bulletin 30. Smithsonian Institution, Washington, D.C.

Moore, Clarence B.

1905 Certain Aboriginal Remains of the Black Warrior River. *Journal of the Academy of Natural Sciences of Philadelphia* 13:123–244.

1907 Moundville Revisited. *Journal of the Academy of Natural Sciences of Philadelphia* 13:335–405.

1910 Antiquities of the St. Francis, White, and Black Rivers, Arkansas. *Journal of the Academy of Natural Sciences of Philadelphia* 14:292.

Moorehead, Warren K.

1891 Account of Explorations at Hopewell Group, Ohio for Department of Ethnology, W. C. E. Field notes on file. Field Museum of Natural History, Chicago.

1892 Unpublished, untitled document on file, Field Museum of Natural History, Chicago (file A17, folder 3).

1897 The Hopewell Group. *Antiquarian* 1:113–120, 153–158, 178–184, 208–214, 236–244, 254–264, 291–295, 312–316.

1906 Explorations at the Mouth of the Wabash. *Phillips Academy Bulletin* 3:62–86.

1922 *The Hopewell Mound Group of Ohio.* Anthropological Series Vol. 6, No. 5. Field Museum of Natural History, Chicago.

1968 *The Hopewell Mound Group of Ohio.* Reprinted. Kraus Reprint and Periodical Company, New York. Originally published 1922, Anthropological Series Vol. 6, No. 5, Field Museum of Natural History, Chicago.

Moorehead, Warren K., Jay L. B. Taylor, Morris M. Leighton, and Frank C. Baker

1928 *The Cahokia Mounds.* Bulletin Series Vol. 26, No. 4. University of Illinois, Urbana.

Morgan, Lewis H.

1901 *League of the Ho-De'-No-Sau-Nee or Iroquois,* Vol. I. Sage, New Haven, Connecticut.

Morrison, Kenneth

1984 The Sacred and the Profane: The Social Ideologies of Contact. In *The Embattled Northeast: The Elusive Ideal of Alliance in Abenaki-Euramerican Relations* by Kenneth Morrison, pp. 42–71. University of California Press, Berkeley.

2000 The Cosmos as Intersubjective: Native American Other-than-Human Persons. In *Indigenous Religions: A Companion,* edited by Graham Harvey, pp. 23–36. Cassell, London.

2002 *The Solidarity of Kin.* State University of New York Press, Albany.

Morse, Dan F.

1989 *Nodena: An Account of 90 Years of Archaeological Investigation in Southeast Mississippi County, Arkansas.* Research Series 30. Arkansas Archaeological Survey, Fayetteville.

Morse, Dan F., and Phyllis A. Morse

1965 The Hannah Site, Peoria County, Illinois. In *Middle Woodland Sites in Illinois.* Bulletin No. 5, pp. 129–146. Illinois Archaeological Survey, University of Illinois, Urbana.

Morse, Dan F., Phyllis A. Morse, and Merrill Emmons

1961 The Southern Cult: The Emmons Site, Fulton County, Illinois. *Central States Archaeological Journal* 8:124–140.

Moskowitz, Clara

2010 Stone Age Carving: Ancient Dildo? *Live Science.* Electronic document, http://www.livescience.com/9971-stone-age-carving-ancient-dildo.html, accessed July 22, 2010.

Munson, Cheryl Ann

1997 *Archaeological Survey and Testing of Mississippian Caborn-Welborn Phase Sites in Posey County, Indiana, 1996–1997: Investigations at the Hovey Lake and Murphy Sites and Environs.* Prepared for the National Park Service, U.S. Department of Interior, and the Indiana Department of Natural Resources, Division of Historic Preservation and Archaeology. Department of Anthropology, Indiana University, Bloomington.

1998 *Archaeological Investigations at Caborn-Welborn Phase Sites, 1997–1998, Posey County, Indiana.* Prepared for Indiana Department of Natural Resources, Division of Historic Preservation and Archaeology and the National Park Service, U.S. Department of Interior. Department of Anthropology, Indiana University, Bloomington.

2003 *Bone Bank: Archaeological Rescue Investigations at a Late Mississippian Site, Posey County, Indiana.* Prepared for Four Rivers Resource, Conservation, and Development Area, and Indiana Department of Natural Resources, Division of Historic Preservation and Archaeology. Department of Anthropology, Indiana University, Bloomington.

Munson, Cheryl Ann, and Della Collins Cook

2001 Residential Mortuary Practices and Skeletal Biology at the Mississippian Hovey Lake Site, Posey County, Indiana. *Midcontinental Journal of Archaeology* 26:1–52.

Munson, Cheryl Ann, Della C. Cook, and Terrance J. Martin

2001 Human Bone Modification from Three Caborn-Welborn Phase Sites. In *Indiana Academy of Sciences Program and Abstracts of the 117th Annual Meeting,* p. 17. Fort Wayne, Indiana.

Munson, Cheryl Ann, Sean P. Dougherty, and Lorena M. Havill

2001 Accidental Discovery and Data Recovery of Human Burials Impacted by Utility Line Trenches at the Murphy Site (12Po1), Posey County, Indiana,

Appendix IV. In *Archaeological Survey, Test Excavation, and Public Education in Southwestern Indiana* by Cheryl Ann Munson. Prepared for Indiana Department of Natural Resources, Division of Historic Preservation and Archaeology, and the National Park Service, U.S. Department of Interior. Department of Anthropology, Indiana University, Bloomington.

2002 Mitigative Investigations at the "Mouth of the Wabash" Murphy Site (12Po1), Posey County, Indiana. Paper presented at the 48th Annual Meeting of the Midwest Archaeological Conference, Columbus, Ohio.

Munson, Cheryl Ann, Marjorie M. Jones, and Bruce Eisterhold

1989 Surveying Mississippian Sites: 1987. Abstract in *Current Research in Indiana Archaeology and Prehistory: 1987 and 1988*, edited by Christopher S. Peebles, pp. 19–22. Research Reports 10. Glenn A. Black Laboratory of Archaeology, Indiana University, Bloomington.

Munson, Cheryl Ann, Marjorie Jones, and Robert Fry

1995 The GE Mound: An ARPA Case Study. *American Antiquity* 60:131–159.

Munson, Cheryl Ann, Marjorie M. Jones, Besse LaBudde, and Jocelyn C. Turner

2004 *Archaeology at the Hovey Lake Village Site*. 3rd ed. Historic Southern Indiana, University of Southern Indiana, Evansville.

Munson, Cheryl Ann, Marjorie Melvin Jones, and Bret J. Ruby

1989 The 1988 Archaeological Test Excavations at the Caborn Site, a Protohistoric Mississippian Village in Posey County, Indiana. Abstract in *Current Research in Indiana Archaeology and Prehistory: 1987 and 1988*, edited by Christopher S. Peebles, pp. 41–42. Research Reports 10. Glenn A. Black Laboratory of Archaeology, Indiana University, Bloomington.

Munson, Cheryl Ann, Dru E. McGill, Jocelyn C. Turner, Jonathan C. Criss, and Rexford C. Garniewicz

2008 Overview of Investigations at the Late Mississippian Hovey Lake Archaeological Site (12PO10), Posey County, Indiana. In *Abstracts of the Society for American Archaeology, 73rd Annual Meeting*, p. 401. Vancouver, Canada.

Munson, Cheryl Ann, Patrick J. Munson, Leslie L. Bush, and A. Gwynn Henderson

2004 Overview of the Bone Bank Archaeological Project, Posey County, Indiana: Rescue Investigations at a Late Mississippian Site. In *Abstracts of the 69th Annual Meeting of the Society for American Archaeology*, p. 244. Society for American Archaeology, Washington, D.C.

Munson, Cheryl Ann, and David Pollack

1998 Caborn-Welborn Phase. In *Archaeology of Prehistoric Native America: An Encyclopedia*, edited by Guy Gibbon, pp. 99–100. Garland, New York.

Munson, Cheryl Ann, David Pollack, and Mary Lucas Powell

1988 Slack Farm: Archaeology of a Looted Site. *Bulletin of the Society for American Archaeology* 6(6):1–2.

Munson, Cheryl Ann, and Susan Dale Spencer

2009 Analysis of the Late Mississippian Mann Cemetery, a Classic Caborn-Welborn Burial Ground. Paper presented at the 55th Annual Meeting of the Midwest Archaeological Conference, Iowa City, Iowa.

Munson, Cheryl Ann, and Thomas J. Green

1973 The Caborn-Welborn Complex of Southwestern Indiana. Paper presented at the 50th Annual Meeting of the Central States Anthropological Society, St. Louis, Missouri.

Nansel, Blane

1989 *Report on the 1989 Archaeological Field School and Teacher Workshop in Monona and Woodbury Counties, Iowa.* Research Reports Vol. 14, No. 2. Office of the State Archaeologist, University of Iowa, Iowa City.

National Museum of the American Indian

2012 Effigy Vessel from Bone Bank, Indiana. Electronic document, http://www.nmai.si.edu/searchcollections/item.aspx?irn=60672&catids=2&place=Bone%20Bank&src=1-3, accessed February 10, 2012.

Nawrocki, Stephen P.

1995 Taphonomic Processes in Historic Cemeteries. In *Bodies of Evidence: Reconstructing History through Skeletal Analysis*, edited by Anne Grauer, pp. 49–66. Wiley-Liss, New York.

1997 Analysis of the Human Remains. In *Hopewell in Mt. Vernon: A Study of the Mt. Vernon Site (12-Po-885)*, edited by General Electric, pp. 11–66. Distributed by Friends of APL, Mt. Vernon, Indiana.

2009 Forensic Taphonomy. In *Handbook of Forensic Anthropology and Archaeology*, edited by Soren Blau and Douglas Ubelaker, pp. 284–294. Left Coast Press, Walnut Creek, California.

Nawrocki, Stephen, John Pless, Dean Hawley, and Scott Wagner

1997 Fluvial Transport of Human Crania. In *Forensic Taphonomy*, edited by William Haglund and Marcella Sorg, pp. 529–552. CRC Press, Boca Raton, Florida.

Neitzel, Robert S.

1983 *The Grand Village of the Natchez Revisited: Excavations at the Fatherland Site, Adams County, Mississippi, 1972.* Archaeological Report No. 12. Mississippi Department of Archives and History, Jackson.

Nelson, Gretchen

1999 Osteological Analysis of the Adams Site (47Pi12), Pierce County, Wisconsin. Manuscript on file, Loucks and Associates, Maple Grove, Minnesota.

Nelson, Sarah M.

1993 Diversity of Upper Paleolithic "Venus" Figurines and Archeological Mythology. In *Gender in Cross-Cultural Perspective*, edited by Caroline B. Brettel and Carolyn F. Sargent, pp. 51–58. Prentice Hall, Englewood Cliffs, New Jersey.

Neumann, Georg K.

1950 Archeology and Race in the American Indian. Unpublished Ph.D. dissertation, Department of Anthropology, University of Chicago.

New York Times

1916 William Penn's Wampum Belts Recently Found Abroad. November 26. New York.

Nielsen, Inge
2002 *Cultic Theatres and Ritual Drama: A Study in Regional Development and Religious Interchange between East and West in Antiquity.* Aarhus University Press, Aarhus, Denmark.

Nilsson Stutz, Liv
2003 Embodied Rituals, Ritualized Bodies: Tracing Ritual Practices in Late Mesolithic Burials. *Acta Archaeologica Lundensia,* ser. 8:46.

Oakshott, Jane
2001 York Mystery Plays, 1998: The First Guild Production since 1559, Produced as Part of York Early Music Festival. Video recording. Films for the Humanities and Social Sciences, Princeton, New Jersey.

Obeyesekere, Gananath
1969 The Ritual Drama of the Sanni Demons: Collective Representations of Disease in Ceylon. *Comparative Studies in Society and History* 11:175–216.

O'Brien, Michael J.
1994 *Cat Monsters and Head Pots: The Archaeology of Missouri's Pemiscot Bayou.* University of Missouri Press, Columbia.

O'Brien, Michael J., and Gregory L. Fox
1994 Sorting Artifacts in Space and Time. In *Cat Monsters and Head Pots: The Archaeology of Missouri's Pemiscot Bayou* by Michael J. O'Brien, pp. 25–60. University of Missouri, Columbia.

O'Connell, Barbara
1995 Notes on SMM 2416 Ft. Sweney Modified Teeth. Unpublished data on file, Hamline University Osteology Laboratory, St. Paul, Minnesota.

O'Gorman, Jodie
1995 *The Tremaine Site Complex: Oneota Occupation in the La Crosse Locality, Wisconsin,* Vol. 3: *The Tremaine Site (47 Lc-95).* Archaeology Research Series, No. 3. Museum Archaeology Program, State Historical Society of Wisconsin, Madison.

Olsen, Sandra L., and Pat Shipman
1994 Cut Marks and Perimortem Treatment of Skeletal Remains on the Northern Plains. In *Skeletal Biology in the Great Plains: Migration, Warfare, Health, and Subsistence,* edited by Douglas W. Owsley and Richard L. Jantz, pp. 377–387. Smithsonian Institution Press, Washington, D.C.

Omojola, Alabode
2000–2001 From Ritual to Concert Opera: Style and Identity in Twentieth Century Yoruba Opera. *Bulletin of the International Committee on Urgent Anthropological and Ethnological Research* 41:121–136.

Oneroad, Amos E., and Alanson B. Skinner
2003 *Being Dakota: Tales and Traditions of the Sisseton and Wahpeton.* Edited by Laura L. Anderson. Minnesota Historical Society Press, St. Paul.

Orr, Ellison
1934 *Report of Reconnaissance Survey and Excavation of Indian Mound Groups and*

Cemeteries in Valley of Upper Iowa and Mississippi River under Project 1047 of the Iowa Planning Board, by Party under Dr. Charles R. Keyes, June 11 to Sept. 16, 1934. Orr Vol. 1, Effigy Mounds. Copy on file, Office of the State Archaeologist, University of Iowa, Iowa City.

1935 *Report of Surveys and Excavations of Mound Groups along the Mississippi River Bluffs and Terraces from McGregor to Clinton, Ia., under Project 1047 of the Iowa Planning Board, by Party under Dr. Charles R. Keyes, June 11 to Sept. 16, 1934.* Orr Vol. 3, Effigy Mounds. Copy on file, Office of the State Archaeologist, University of Iowa, Iowa City.

1937 *Survey and Excavation of Indian Mounds, Village Sites and Cemeteries in the Valleys of the Upper Iowa and Mississippi Rivers 1936.* Orr Vol. 5, Effigy Mounds. Copy on file, Office of the State Archaeologist, University of Iowa, Iowa City.

1942 *Sundry Archaeological Papers and Memoranda.* Orr Vol. 12, Effigy Mounds. Copy on file, Office of the State Archaeologist, University of Iowa, Iowa City.

Ortiz, Alfonso

1972 Ritual Drama and Pueblo World View. In *New Perspectives on the Pueblos*, edited by Alfonso Ortiz, pp. 135–161. University of New Mexico Press, Albuquerque.

O'Shea, John M.

1984 *Mortuary Variability: An Archaeological Investigation.* Academic, Orlando, Florida.

Ourada, Patricia K.

1990 *The Menominee.* Chelsea House, New York.

Over, William H.

1946 *The Indians Who Lived in Ludlow Cave.* Museum News 7(6). South Dakota State Museum, Vermillion.

Overholt, Thomas W., and J. Baird Callicott

1982 *Clothed-in-Fur and Other Tales: An Introduction to an Ojibwa World View.* University Press of America, Washington, D.C.

Owsley, Douglas W.

1994 Warfare in Coalescent Tradition Populations of the Northern Plains. In *Skeletal Biology in the Great Plains: Migration, Warfare, Health, and Subsistence*, edited by Douglas W. Owsley and Richard L. Jantz, pp. 333–343. Smithsonian Institution Press, Washington, D.C.

Owsley, Douglas W., Hugh E. Berryman, and William M. Bass

1977 Demographic and Osteological Evidence for Warfare at the Larson Site, South Dakota. *Plains Anthropologist Memoir* 13:119–131.

Owsley, Douglas W., Karin S. Bruwelheide, Laurie E. Burgess, and William T. Billeck

2007 Human Finger and Hand Bone Necklaces from the Plains and Great Basin. In *The Taking and Displaying of Human Body Parts as Trophies by Amerindians*, edited by Richard J. Chacon and David H. Dye, pp. 124–166. Springer, New York.

Owsley, Douglas W., and Richard L. Jantz (editors)

1994 *Skeletal Biology in the Great Plains: Migration, Warfare, Health, and Subsistence.* Smithsonian Institution Press, Washington, D.C.

Owsley, Douglas W., Robert W. Mann, and Timothy G. Baugh

1994 Culturally Modified Human Bones from the Edwards I Site. In *Skeletal Biology in the Great Plains: Migration, Warfare, Health, and Subsistence*, edited by Douglas W. Owsley and Richard L. Jantz, pp. 363–375. Smithsonian Institution Press, Washington, D.C.

Pacheco, Paul J. (editor)

1996 *A View from the Core: A Synthesis of Ohio Hopewell Archaeology.* Ohio Archaeological Council, Columbus.

Palmer, Jessica D.

2008 *The Dakota Peoples: A History of the Dakota, Lakota and Nakota through 1863.* McFarland, Jefferson, North Carolina.

Parker, Arthur Caswell

1912 *The Code of Handsome Lake, the Seneca Prophet.* Bulletin 163. New York State Museum, Albany.

Parker Pearson, Michael

1993 The Powerful Dead: Archaeological Relationships between the Living and the Dead. *Cambridge Archaeological Journal* 3:203–229.

1999 *The Archaeology of Death and Burial.* Texas A&M University Press, College Station.

Parker Pearson, Michael, and the Stonehenge Riverside Project

2012 *Stonehenge: Exploring the Greatest Stone Age Mystery.* Simon and Schuster, London.

Parks, Douglas R.

2001 Arikara. In *Plains*, edited by Raymond J. DeMallie, pp. 365–390. Handbook of American Indians, Vol. 13, William C. Sturtevant, general editor, Smithsonian Institution, Washington, D.C.

Parmalee, Paul W.

1959 Use of Mammalian Skulls and Mandibles by Prehistoric Indians of Illinois. *Transactions of the Illinois State Academy of Science* 52(3–4):85–95.

Pauketat, Timothy R.

1987 A Functional Consideration of a Mississippian Domestic Vessel Assemblage. *Southeastern Archaeology* 6:1–15.

1993 *Temples for the Cahokia Lords: Preston Holder's 1955–1956 Excavation of Kunnemann Mound.* Memoir 26. Museum of Anthropology, University of Michigan, Ann Arbor.

1998a Refiguring the Archaeology of Greater Cahokia. *Journal of Archaeological Research* 6:45–89.

1998b *The Archaeology of Downtown Cahokia: The Tract 15A and Dunham Tract Excavations.* Studies in Archaeology 1. Illinois Transportation Archaeological Research Program, University of Illinois, Urbana.

2003 Resettling Farmers and the Making of a Mississippian Polity. *American Antiquity* 68:39–66.

2009 *Cahokia: Ancient America's Great City on the Mississippi.* Viking, New York.

2010 The Missing Persons in Mississippian Mortuaries. In *Mississippian Mortuary Practices: Beyond Hierarchy and Representationist Perspective*, edited by Lynne P. Sullivan and Robert C. Mainfort Jr., pp. 14–29. University Press of Florida, Gainesville.

Pauketat, Timothy R. (editor)

2005 *The Archaeology of the East St. Louis Mound Center*, Pt. 1: *The Southside Excavations.* Transportation Archaeological Research Reports No. 21. Illinois Transportation Archaeological Research Program, University of Illinois, Urbana.

Pauketat, Timothy R., and Thomas E. Emerson

1991 The Ideology of Authority and the Power of the Pot. *American Anthropologist* 93:919–941.

Pauketat, Timothy R., and Thomas E. Emerson (editors)

1997 *Cahokia: Domination and Ideology in the Mississippian World.* University of Nebraska Press, Lincoln.

Pauketat, Timothy R., Lucretia S. Kelly, Gayle J. Fritz, Neal H. Lopinot, Scott Elias, and Eve Hargrave

2002 The Residues of Feasting and Public Ritual at Early Cahokia. *American Antiquity* 67:257–279.

Peacock, Thomas, and Marlene Wisuri

2002 *Ojibwe Waasa Inaabidaa: We Look in All Directions.* Afton Historical Society Press, Afton, Minnesota.

Pearce, J. E.

1938 Geographic Influence and Civilization with Special Reference to Indian Texas. *Texas Geographic Magazine* 2(1):1–13.

Peebles, Christopher S., and Susan M. Kus

1977 Some Archaeological Correlates of Ranked Societies. *American Antiquity* 42:421–448.

Peers, Laura, and Jennifer S. H. Brown

2000 "There Is No End to Relationship among the Indians": Ojibwa Families and Kinship in Historical Perspective. *History of the Family: An International Quarterly* 4:529–555.

Penney, David W.

1992 *Art of the American Indian Frontier: The Chandler-Pohrt Collection.* Detroit Institute of Arts. University of Washington Press, Seattle.

Pereira, Grégory

2005 The Utilization of Grooved Human Bones: A Reanalysis of Artificially Modified Human Bones Excavated by Carl Lumholtz at Zacapu, Michoacan, Mexico. *Latin American Antiquity* 16:293–312.

Perino, Gregory H.

1968 The Pete Klunk Mound Group, Calhoun County, Illinois: The Archaic and Hopewell Occupations. In *Hopewell and Woodland Site Archaeology in Illinois*, edited by James Brown, pp. 9–124. Bulletin No. 6. Illinois Archaeological Survey, University of Illinois, Urbana.

1971 *The Yokem Site, Pike County.* Bulletin No. 8, pp. 149–186. Illinois Archaeological Survey, Urbana.

Perkins, Raymond W.

1965 The Frederick Site. In *Middle Woodland Sites in Illinois*. Bulletin No. 5, pp. 68–95. Illinois Archaeological Survey, University of Illinois, Urbana.

Peterson, Les

1986 Brief Notes on Ft. Sweney, July 1986. Manuscript on file, Hamline University Osteology Laboratory, St. Paul, Minnesota.

Phillips, Philip

1970 *Archaeological Survey in the Lower Yazoo Basin, Mississippi, 1949–1955.* Papers of the Peabody Museum of American Archaeology and Ethnology Vol. 60. Harvard University, Cambridge, Massachusetts.

Phillips, Philip, and James A. Brown

1978 *Pre-Columbian Shell Engravings from the Craig Mound at Spiro, Oklahoma*, Pt. 1. Papers of the Peabody Museum Press, Cambridge, Massachusetts.

1980 *Pre-Columbian Shell Engravings from the Craig Mound at Spiro, Oklahoma*, Pt. 2. Papers of the Peabody Museum Press, Cambridge, Massachusetts.

Phillips, Ruth B.

1984 *Patterns of Power: The Jasper Grant Collection and Great Lakes Indian Art of the Early Nineteenth Century.* McMichael Collection, Kleinburg, Ontario.

1989 Dreams and Designs: Iconographic Problems in Great Lakes Twined Bags. In *Great Lakes Indian Art*, edited by David W. Penney, pp. 52–68. Detroit Institute of Arts. Wayne State University Press, Detroit, Michigan.

Phoenix Art Museum

2012 Sacred Word and Image: Symbols of Power—Sacred Spaces and Places. Special exhibit, January 4–March 25, Phoenix Art Museum, Phoenix, Arizona.

Pitt Rivers Museum

2009 Anthropology and World Archaeology, University of Oxford: Collections. Electronic document, http://www.prm.ox.ac.uk/collections.html, accessed March 3, 2009.

Pluckhahn, Thomas J.

2003 *Kolomoki: Settlement, Ceremony, and Status in the Deep South, A.D. 350 to 750.* University of Alabama Press, Tuscaloosa.

Pollack, David

2004 *Carbon-Welborn: Constructing a New Society after the Angel Chiefdom Collapse.* University of Alabama Press, Tuscaloosa.

Pollack, David, and Cheryl Ann Munson

1998 Caborn-Welborn Ceramics: Inter-Site Comparisons and Extra-Regional

Interaction. In *Current Archaeological Research in Kentucky*, Vol. 5, edited by Charles D. Hockensmith, Kenneth C. Carstens, Charles Stout, and Sara J. Rivers, pp. 163–202. Kentucky Heritage Council, Frankfort.

2003 The Angel to Caborn-Welborn Transition in Southwestern Indiana, Northwestern Kentucky, and Southeastern Illinois. In *Facing the Final Millennium: Studies in the Late Prehistory of Indiana, A.D. 700 to 1700*, edited by Brian G. Redmond and James R. Jones III, pp. 255–286. Department of Natural Resources, Division of Historic Preservation and Archaeology, Indianapolis.

Pollack, David, Cheryl Ann Munson, and A. Gwynn Henderson

1996 *Slack Farm and the Caborn-Welborn People*. Education Series 1. Kentucky Archaeological Survey, Lexington.

Porter, James W.

1974 Cahokia Archaeology as Viewed from the Mitchell Site: A Satellite Community at A.D. 1150–1200. Unpublished Ph.D. dissertation, Department of Anthropology, University of Wisconsin, Milwaukee.

Porubcan, Paula J.

2000 Human and Nonhuman Surplus Display at Mound 72, Cahokia. In *Mounds, Modoc, and Mesoamerica: Papers in Honor of Melvin L. Fowler*, edited by Steven R. Ahler, pp. 207–226. Scientific Papers Vol. 28. Illinois State Museum, Springfield.

Powell, Mary Lucas

1977 Prehistoric Ritual Skull Burials at the Crenshaw Site (3M16), Southwestern Arkansas. *Bulletin of the Texas Archeological Society* 48:111–118.

Pratt, William H.

1876 Report of Explorations of the Ancient Mounds at Toolesboro, Louisa County, Iowa. *Proceedings of the Davenport Academy of Natural Sciences* 1:106–111.

Prentice, Guy

1986 An Analysis of the Symbolism Expressed by the Birger Figurine. *American Antiquity* 51:239–266.

Quick, Edgar R.

1881 A Pre-Historic Cup Made from a Human Cranium. *Journal of the Cincinnati Society of Natural History* 3:296–297 and 4:257.

Quigley, Christine

2001 *Skulls and Skeletons: Human Bone Collections and Accumulations*. McFarland, Jefferson, North Carolina.

Radin, Paul

1945 *The Road of Life and Death: A Ritual Drama of the American Indians*. Pantheon, New York.

1948 *Winnebago Hero Cycles: A Study in Aboriginal Literature*. Publications in Anthropology and Linguistics Memoir 1. Indiana University, Bloomington.

1949 *The Culture of the Winnebago as Described by Themselves*. Waverly, Baltimore, Maryland.

1990 *The Winnebago Tribe*. Reprinted. University of Nebraska Press, Lincoln. Originally published 1923, Bureau of American Ethnology Annual Report 37, Smithsonian Institution, Washington, D.C.

Raemsch, Carol A.

1993 Mechanical Procedures Involved in Bone Dismemberment and Defleshing in Prehistoric Michigan. *Midcontinental Journal of Archaeology* 18:217–244.

Rafferty, Sean M.

2004 "They Pass Their Lives in Smoke, and at Death Fall into the Fire": Smoking Pipes and Mortuary Ritual during the Early Woodland Period. In *Smoking and Culture: The Archaeology of Tobacco Pipes in Eastern North America*, edited by Sean M. Rafferty and Rob Mann, pp. 1–41. University of Tennessee Press, Knoxville.

Rafferty, Sean, and Rob Mann (editors)

2004 *Smoking and Culture: The Archaeology of Tobacco Pipes in Eastern North America.* University of Tennessee Press, Knoxville.

Raglan, FitzRoy Richard Somerset

2003 *The Hero: A Study in Tradition, Myth, and Drama.* Reprinted. Courier Dover, New York. Originally published 1936, Methuen, London.

Rakita, Gordon F. M., Jane E. Buikstra, Lane A. Beck, and Sloan R. Williams (editors)

2005 *Interacting with the Dead: Perspectives on Mortuary Archaeology for the New Millennium.* University Press of Florida, Gainesville.

Ramenofsky, Ann F.

1987 *Vectors of Death.* University of New Mexico Press, Albuquerque.

Rapid City [South Dakota] *Journal*

1890 December 17 and 18.

Ravesloot, John C.

1988 Mortuary Practices and Social Differentiation at Casas Grandes, Chihuahua, Mexico. *Anthropological Papers of the University of Arizona* 49:1–113.

Redmond, Brian G.

1982 Drilled Skulls and Eyes of Clay: Late Woodland Burial Ceremonialism in the Western Lake Erie Basin. *Toledo Area Aboriginal Research Bulletin* 11:1–36.

Reiger, John F.

1999 Artistry, Status, and Power: How "Plummet" Pendants Probably Functioned in Pre-Columbian Florida—and Beyond. *Florida Anthropologist* 52:227–240.

Reilly, F. Kent, III

2004 People of the Earth, People of the Sky: Visualizing the Sacred in Native American Art of the Mississippian Period. In *Hero, Hawk, and Open Hand: American Indian Art of the Ancient Midwest and South*, edited by Richard F. Townsend and Robert V. Sharp, pp. 124–137. Yale University Press, New Haven, Connecticut.

2007 The Petaloid Motif: A Celestial Symbolic Locative in the Shell Art of Spiro. In *Ancient Objects and Sacred Realms: Interpretations of Mississippian Iconography*, edited by F. Kent Reilly III and James F. Garber, pp. 39–55. University of Texas Press, Austin.

Reilly, F. Kent, III, and James F. Garber (editors)
2007 *Ancient Objects and Sacred Realms: Interpretations of Mississippian Iconography.* University of Texas Press, Austin.

Ribick, Amy Kathleen
2004 Dickison Mounds 11-P477 and 11-478: A Reanalysis of Two Middle Woodland Burial Mounds from Illinois. Unpublished master's thesis, Department of Anthropology, Indiana University, Bloomington.

Richards, John D.
1992 Ceramics and Culture at Aztalan, a Late Prehistoric Village in Southeast Wisconsin. Unpublished Ph.D. dissertation, Department of Anthropology, University of Wisconsin, Milwaukee.
2007 Context and Process: Red Slipped Pottery in Cahokia's Northern Hinterlands. *Illinois Archaeology* 19:1–26.

Richards, John D., and Robert J. Jeske
2002 Location, Location, Location: The Temporal and Cultural Context of Late Prehistoric Settlement in Southeast Wisconsin. *Wisconsin Archeologist* 83: 32–54.

Richter, Daniel K.
1992 *The Ordeal of the Longhouse: The Peoples of the Iroquois League in the Era of European Colonization.* University of North Carolina Press, Chapel Hill.

Ritzenthaler, Robert
1958 Editor's Preface. *Wisconsin Archeologist* 39:1–2.

Ritzenthaler, Robert E., and George I. Quimby
1962 The Red Ochre Culture of the Upper Great Lakes and Adjacent Areas. *Fieldiana* 36(11):243–262.

Robbins, Louise M.
1974 Prehistoric People of the Mammoth Cave Area. In *Archeology of the Mammoth Cave Area*, edited by Patty Jo Watson, pp. 137–166. Studies in Archeology. Academic, New York.

Rodell, Roland L.
1991 The Diamond Bluff Site Complex and Cahokia Influence in the Red Wing Locality. In *New Perspectives on Cahokia: Views from the Periphery*, edited by James B. Stoltman, pp. 253–280. Prehistory Press, Madison, Wisconsin.

Rodrigues, Teresa
2005 Gender and Social Differentiation with the Turner Population, Ohio, as Evidenced by Activity-Induced Musculoskeletal Stress Markers. In *Gathering Hopewell: Society, Ritual, and Ritual Interaction*, edited by Christopher Carr and D. Troy Case, pp. 405–427. Kluwer Academic/Plenum, New York.

Rodriguez, William C., and William M. Bass
1985 Decomposition of Buried Bodies and Methods That May Aid in Their Location. *Journal of Forensic Sciences* 28:423–432.

Roksandic, Mirjana
2002 Position of Skeletal Remains as a Key to Understanding Mortuary Behavior.

In *Advances in Forensic Taphonomy: Method, Theory, and Archaeological Perspectives*, edited by William D. Haglund and Marcella H. Sorg, pp. 99–117. CRC Press, Boca Raton, Florida.

Ross-Stallings, Nancy A.

2007 Trophy Taking in the Central and Lower Mississippi Valley. In *The Taking and Displaying of Human Body Parts as Trophies by Amerindians*, edited by Richard J. Chacon and David H. Dye, pp. 339–370. Springer, New York.

Rowe, Chandler W.

1958 A Crematorium at Aztalan. *Wisconsin Archeologist* 39:101–110.

Rozik, Elik

2003 The Ritual Origin of Theatre: A Scientific Theory or Theatrical Ideology. *Journal of Religion and Theatre* 2:105–140.

Ruby, Bret J.

1997 The Mann Phase: Hopewellian Subsistence and Settlement Adaptations in the Wabash Lowlands of Southwestern Indiana. Unpublished Ph.D. dissertation, Department of Anthropology, Indiana University, Bloomington.

Ruby, Bret J., Christopher Carr, and Douglas K. Charles

2005 Community Organizations in the Scioto, Mann, and Havana Hopewellian Regions: A Comparative Perspective. In *Gathering Hopewell: Society, Ritual, and Ritual Interaction*, edited by Christopher Carr and D. Troy Case, pp. 119–176. Kluwer Academic/Plenum, New York.

Rudolph, Katie Zejdlik

2009 A Taphonomic Analysis of Human Skeletal Material from Aztalan: Cannibalism, Hostility and Mortuary Variability. Unpublished master's thesis, Department of Anthropology, University of Wisconsin, Milwaukee.

Runnings, Anna L., Carl E. Gustafson, and Dave Bentley

1989 Use-Wear on Bone Tools: A Technique for Study under the Scanning Electron Microscope. In *Bone Modification*, edited by Robson Bonnichsen and Marcella H. Sorg, pp. 259–266. Center for the Study of First Americans, University of Maine, Orono.

Sagard-Théodat, Gabriel

1632 *Le Grand Voyage du Pays des Hurons, Situé en l'Amérique vers la Mer Douce, ès Derniers Confins de la Nouvelle France dite Canada*. Denys Moreau, Paris.

1939 *The Long Journey to the Country of the Hurons*. Edited by George M. Wrong. Translated by Hugh H. Langton. Champlain Society, Toronto.

Salzer, Robert J.

1987 Preliminary Report on the Gottschall Site (47Ia80). *Wisconsin Archeologist* 68:419–472.

Salzer, Robert J., and Grace Rajnovich

2000 *The Gottschall Rockshelter: An Archaeological Mystery*. Prairie Smoke, Maplewood, Minnesota.

Sampson, Kelvin W., and Duane Esarey

1993 A Survey of Elaborate Mississippian Copper Artifacts from Illinois. In *High-*

ways to the Past: Essays on Illinois Archaeology in Honor of Charles J. Bareis, edited by Thomas E. Emerson, Andrew C. Fortier, and Dale L. McElrath. Special issue, *Illinois Archaeology* 5:452–480.

Sampson, Kurt A.

2008 Getting to the Point: Typology, Morphology, and Lithic Material Variation in the Milwaukee Public Museum Projectile Point Collection from the Aztalan Site. Unpublished master's thesis, Department of Anthropology, University of Wisconsin, Milwaukee.

Santure, Sharron, Alan D. Harn, and Duane Esarey

1990 *Archaeological Investigations at the Morton Village and Norris Farms 36 Cemetery*. Reports of Investigations No. 45. Illinois State Museum, Springfield.

Savage, Howard

1978 Appendix D. Armstrong: Faunal Analysis. In The Armstrong Site: A Silvernale Phase Oneota Village in Wisconsin by William Hurley, pp. 118–145. *Wisconsin Archeologist* 59(1).

Saxe, Arthur

1970 Social Dimensions of Mortuary Practices. Unpublished Ph.D. dissertation, Department of Anthropology, University of Michigan, Ann Arbor.

Schele, Linda, and David Freidel

1990 *A Forest of Kings: The Untold Story of the Ancient Maya*. HarperCollins, New York.

Schele, Linda, and Mary E. Miller

1986 *The Blood of Kings: Dynasty and Ritual in Maya Art*. Braziller, New York.

Schermer, Shirley J.

1987a *Human Skeletal Remains from 13LO2, the Blood Run National Historic Landmark Site*. Research Papers 12(1). Office of the State Archaeologist, University of Iowa, Iowa City.

1987b *Preliminary Report on the 1986 Limited Survey at the Blood Run National Historic Landmark Site, Lyon County, Iowa*. Contract Completion Report 248. Office of the State Archaeologist, University of Iowa, Iowa City.

2009 Osteological Report for the State Medical Examiner's Office. Manuscript on file, Office of the State Archaeologist, University of Iowa, Iowa City.

Schermer, Shirley J., Linda Forman, Robin M. Lillie, Jill Robinson, and Larry J. Zimmerman

1998 *NAGPRA Inventory and Consultation: Human Remains and Funerary Objects in the Charles R. Keyes Collection*. Research Papers 23(1). Office of the State Archaeologist, University of Iowa, Iowa City.

Schermer, Shirley J., and Robin M. Lillie

2007 Oneota Mortuary Behavior in Iowa. Paper presented at the Midwest Archaeological Conference, South Bend, Indiana. Copy on file, Office of the State Archaeologist, University of Iowa, Iowa City.

Schermer, Shirley J., Robin M. Lillie, and Linda Forman

1995 *Documentation and Consultation under the Native American Graves Protection and*

Repatriation Act for Human Remains and Cultural Items from U.S. Army Corps of Engineers Rock Island District Archaeological Collections at the Office of the State Archaeologist, University of Iowa, Iowa City, Iowa. Contract Completion Report 470. Office of the State Archaeologist, University of Iowa, Iowa City.

Schermer, Shirley J., Robin M. Lillie, Eve A. Hargrave, and Kristin M. Hedman

2008 A Midwestern Perspective on Ritual Use of Human Bone. Poster presented at the Paleopathology Association Meeting, Columbus, Ohio.

Schermer, Shirley J., and Douglas W. Owsley

1989–1990a Osteological Data from 13MC4. Manuscript on file, Office of the State Archaeologist, University of Iowa, Iowa City.

1989–1990b Osteological Data from 13WD8. Manuscript on file, Office of the State Archaeologist, University of Iowa, Iowa City.

Schiffer, Michael B.

1976 *Behavioral Archaeology.* Academic, New York.

1987 *Formation Processes in the Archaeological Record.* University of New Mexico Press, Albuquerque.

Schindelholz, Eric, and Paul S. Storch

2001 A Simple Guide for Archaeological Materials Characterization. Unpublished senior research paper, Department of Anthropology, University of Minnesota, Minneapolis.

Schlesier, Karl H.

1987 *The Wolves of Heaven: Cheyenne Shamanism, Ceremonies, and Prehistoric Origins.* University of Oklahoma Press, Norman.

Schmidt, Christopher, and Criss Helmkamp

1997 Analysis of the Human Dental Remains. In *Hopewell in Mt. Vernon: A Study of the Mt. Vernon Site (12-PO-885)*, edited by General Electric, pp. 67–84. Distributed by Friends of APL, Mt. Vernon, Indiana.

Schmidt, Christopher W., Rachel A. Lockhart Sharkey, Christopher Newman, Anna Serrano, Melissa Zolnierz, Jeffrey A. Plunkett, and Anne Bader

2010 Skeletal Evidence of Cultural Variation: Mutilation Related to Warfare and Mortuary Treatment. In *Human Variation in the Americas: The Integration of Archaeology and Biological Anthropology*, edited by Benjamin M. Auerbach, pp. 215–237. Occasional Paper No. 38. Center for Archaeological Investigations, Carbondale, Illinois.

Schmidt, Edward W.

1909 The Fort Sweney Site. In *The History of Goodhue County*, edited by Franklyn Curtiss-Wedge, pp. 20–22. H. C. Cooper Jr., Chicago.

Schoenbeck, Ethel

1946 Sister Creeks Mound #60 Hopewellian. Original field notes on file, Dickson Mounds Museum, Lewistown, Illinois.

1947 A Seven-Pound Copper Axe among 1946 Hopewell Discoveries. *Illinois Academy of Sciences Transactions* 40:36–42.

Schortman, Edward M.
1989 Interregional Interaction in Prehistory: The Need for a New Perspective. *American Antiquity* 54:52–65.
Schultes, Richard Evans, and Albert Hofmann
1979 *Plants of the Gods: Origins of Hallucinogenic Use.* McGraw-Hill, New York.
Schultz, Jack M.
1992 The Use-Wear Generated by Processing Bison Hides. *Plains Anthropologist* 37(141):333–351.
Schultz, John, Matthew Williamson, Stephen Nawrocki, Anthony Falsetti, and Michael Warren
2003 A Taphonomic Profile to Aid in the Recognition of Human Remains from Historic and/or Cemetery Contexts. *Florida Anthropologist* 56:141–147.
Schutz, Noel William, Jr.
1975 The Study of Shawnee Myth in an Ethnographic and Ethnohistorical Perspective. Unpublished Ph.D. dissertation, Department of Anthropology, Indiana University, Bloomington.
Scott, George Ryley
1996 *Phallic Worship: A History of Sex and Sexual Rites.* Reprinted. Luxor, London. Originally published 1966, Senate, Middlesex, United Kingdom.
Seeman, Mark
1988 Ohio Hopewell Trophy-Skull Artifacts as Evidence for Competition in Middle Woodland Societies circa 50 B.C.–A.D. 350. *American Antiquity* 53: 565–577.
2004 Hopewell Art in Hopewell Places. In *Hero, Hawk, and Open Hand: American Indian Art of the Ancient Midwest and South*, edited by Richard F. Townsend and Robert V. Sharp, pp. 7–72. Yale University Press, New Haven, Connecticut.
2007 Predatory War and Hopewell Trophies. In *The Taking and Displaying of Human Body Parts as Trophies by Amerindians*, edited by Richard J. Chacon and David H. Dye, pp. 167–189. Springer, New York.
Setzler, Frank M.
1930 The Archaeology of the Whitewater Valley. *Indiana History Bulletin* 8(12): 373–418.
Sharapova, Svetlana, and Dmitry Razhev
2011 Skull Deformation during the Iron Age in the Trans-Urals and Western Siberia. In *The Bioarchaeology of the Human Head: Decapitation, Decoration, and Deformation*, edited by Michelle Bonogofsky, pp. 202–227. University Press of Florida, Gainesville.
Shetrone, Henry C.
1922–1925 The Hopewell Group. Field notes on file, Ohio Historical Society, Columbus.
1926 Explorations of the Hopewell Group of Prehistoric Earthworks. *Ohio Archaeological and Historical Quarterly* 35:1–227.

1930 *The Mound-Builders.* Appleton, New York.

Shetrone, Henry C., and Emerson F. Greenman

1931 Explorations of the Seip Group of Prehistoric Earthworks. *Ohio Archaeological and Historical Quarterly* 40:343–509.

Shields, Wayne F.

1978 The Ogden-Fettie Site: An Archaeological Compendium. Manuscript on file, Illinois State Museum, Springfield.

Shipman, Pat

1989 Altered Bones from Olduvai Gorge, Tanzania: Techniques, Problems and Implications of Their Recognition. In *Bone Modification,* edited by Robson Bonnichsen and Marcella H. Sorg, pp. 317–334. Center for the Study of First Americans, University of Maine, Orono.

Simon, James J. K., and Amy F. Steffian

1994 Cannibalism or Complex Mortuary Behavior? An Analysis of Patterned Variability in the Treatment of Human Remains from the Kachemak Tradition of Kodiak Island. In *Reckoning with the Dead: The Larsen Bay Repatriation and the Smithsonian Institution,* edited by Tamara L. Bray and Thomas W. Killion, pp. 75–100. Smithsonian Institution Press, Washington, D.C.

Skinner, Alanson

1913 *Social Life and Ceremonial Bundles of the Menomini Indians.* Anthropological Papers 13, Pt. 1. American Museum of Natural History, New York.

1923 *Observations on the Ethnology of the Sauk Indians.* Bulletin 5. Public Museum of Milwaukee, Milwaukee, Wisconsin.

1924 The Mascoutens or Prairie Potawatomi Indians, Pt. I: Social Life and Ceremonies. *Bulletin* 6(1):1–262. Milwaukee Public Museum, Wisconsin.

1926 Ethnology of the Ioway Indians. *Bulletin* 5(4):181–354. Milwaukee Public Museum, Wisconsin.

Skinner, Henry D.

1916 Maori Necklace and Pendants of Human and Imitation Teeth. *Man* 16: 129–130.

Slattery, Richard G.

1979 Further Testing at the McKinney Oneota Village Site (13LA1). *Journal of the Iowa Archeological Society* 26:81–94.

Slattery, Richard G., George A. Horton, and Michael E. Ruppert

1975 The McKinney Village Site: An Oneota Site in Southeastern Iowa. *Journal of the Iowa Archeological Society* 22:35–57.

Smith, B. Holly

1991 Standards of Human Tooth Formation and Dental Age Assessment. In *Advances in Dental Anthropology,* edited by Marc A. Kelley and Clark S. Larsen, pp. 143–168. Wiley-Liss, New York.

Smith, Fred H.

1974 The Henry County Skull: An Incised Hominid Cranium from Tennessee. *Tennessee Archaeologist* 30:68–79.

Smith, Maria O.

1992 Osteological Indications of Warfare in the Archaic Period of West Tennessee. Paper presented at the 49th Annual Meeting of the Southeastern Archaeological Conference, Little Rock, Arkansas.

1993a A Probable Case of Decapitation at the Late Archaic Robinson Site (40SM4), Smith County, Tennessee. *Tennessee Anthropologist* 18:131–142.

1993b Intergroup Violence among the Prehistoric Hunter-Gatherers from the Kentucky Lake Reservoir. Paper presented at the 62nd Annual Meeting of the American Association of Physical Anthropologists, Toronto, Canada. Abstract in *American Journal of Physical Anthropology, Supplement* 16:183–185.

1995 Scalping in the Archaic: Evidence from the Western Tennessee Valley. *Southeastern Archaeology* 14:60–68.

1997 Intergroup Violence in the Archaic Period of West Tennessee: The Osteological Evidence. In *Troubled Times: Violence and Warfare in the Past*, edited by David W. Frayer and Debra L. Martin, pp. 241–266. Gordon and Breach, New York.

2002 Late Woodland/Early Mississippian Evidence of Intergroup Violence: Emerging Temporal and Spatial Patterning. Abstract. *American Journal of Physical Anthropology* Supplement 34:144.

2003 Beyond Palisades: The Nature and Frequency of Late Prehistoric Deliberate Violent Trauma in the Chickamauga Reservoir of East Tennessee. *American Journal of Physical Anthropology* 121:303–318.

Smith, Marian W.

1937 The War Complex of the Plains Indians. *Proceedings of the American Philosophical Society* 78(3):425–461.

Smith, Teresa S.

1995 *The Island of the Anishnaabeg: Thunderers and Water Monsters in the Traditional Ojibwe Life-World*. University of Idaho Press, Moscow.

Sofaer, Joanna

2006 *The Body as Material Culture: A Theoretical Osteoarchaeology*. Cambridge University Press, Cambridge.

Soffer, Olga, James M. Adovasio, and David C. Hyland

2000 The "Venus" Figurines: Textiles, Basketry, Gender, and Status in the Upper Paleolithic. *Current Anthropology* 41:511–537.

Somers, A. N.

1920 Prehistoric Cannibalism in America. *Wisconsin Archeologist* 19:20–24.

Sorensen, Jorgen Podemann

1986 Three Varieties of Ritual Drama. *Tenemos* 22:79–92.

Speck, Frank G., Leonard Broom, and Will West Long

1993 *Cherokee Dance and Drama*. University of Oklahoma Press, Norman.

Spector, Janet

1993 *What This Awl Means: Feminist Archaeology at a Wahpeton Dakota Village*. Minnesota Historical Society Press, St. Paul.

Spencer, Susan Dale
2007 Cut Marks on Crania at the Late Mississippian Mann Site Cemetery, Posey County, Indiana. Paper presented at the 53rd Annual Meeting of the Midwest Archaeological Conference, South Bend, Indiana.

Spencer, Susan Dale, and Cheryl Ann Munson
2009 Current Research on the Caborn-Welborn Population and Mortuary Practices: Old Bones, New Tricks. Paper presented at the Indiana Archaeological Council Annual Workshop, Strawtown, Indiana.

Spencer, Susan Dale, Cheryl Ann Munson, and Mark Cantin
2007 Mortal Wounds of a Late Mississippian. Paper presented at the 123rd Annual Meeting of the Indiana Academy of Science, Indianapolis.

Spencer, Susan Dale, Cheryl Ann Munson, Jason M. Gresalfi, Kylie Nicole McFarland, Anna-Marie Casserly
2009 A Biocultural Analysis of Late Mississippians from Southwestern Indiana. Paper presented at the 125th Annual Meeting of the Indiana Academy of Science, Kokomo.

Squier, Ephraim G., and Edwin H. Davis
1848 *Ancient Monuments of the Mississippi Valley Comprising the Results of Extensive Original Surveys and Explorations.* Smithsonian Contributions to Knowledge 1. Smithsonian Institution, Washington, D.C.

Standing Bear, Luther
1933 *Land of the Spotted Eagle.* Houghton-Mifflin, Boston.

Starr, Frederick
1891 Dress and Adornment: Religious Dress. *Popular Science* 40(12):194–206.
1895 Summary of the Archaeology of Iowa. *Proceedings of the Davenport Academy of Natural Sciences* 6:53–124.

Steinbring, Jack
1966 The Manufacture and Use of Bone Defleshing Tools. *American Antiquity* 31:575–581.

Steponaitis, Vincas P.
1983 *Ceramics, Chronology, and Community Patterns: An Archaeological Study at Moundville.* Academic, New York.

Steponaitis, Vincas P., and Vernon J. Knight Jr.
2004 Moundville Art in Historical and Social Context. In *Hero, Hawk, and Open Hand: American Indian Art of the Ancient Midwest and South,* edited by Richard F. Townsend and Robert V. Sharp, pp. 166–181. Yale University Press, New Haven, Connecticut.

Sterling, William T.
1920 A Visit to Aztalan in 1838. *Wisconsin Archeologist* 19:18–19.

Stevens, Scott
2007 Cultural Mediations; or, How to Listen to Lewis and Clark's Indian Artifacts. *American Indian Culture and Research Journal* 31(3):181–202.

Stewart, Frank Henderson

2001 Hidatsa. In *Plains*, edited by Raymond J. DeMallie, pp. 329–348. Handbook of North American Indians, Vol. 13, William C. Sturtevant, general editor, Smithsonian Institution, Washington, D.C.

Stipčević, Aleksandar

1977 *The Illyrians: History and Culture*. Translated by Stojana Čulić. Burton Noyes Press, Park Ridge, New Jersey

Straffin, Dean F.

1972a Unraveling the Oneota Mystery. *The College* Spring:3–8.

1972b Archaeological Research in Southeastern Iowa: New Light on the Ancestors to the Ioway Indians. *Iowa Archeological Society Newsletter* 65:4–6.

Stross, Brian

1998 Seven Ingredients in Mesoamerican Ensoulment: Dedication and Termination in Tenejapa. In *The Sowing and Dawning: Termination, Dedication, and Transformation in the Archaeological Record of Mesoamerica*, edited by Shirley B. Mock, pp. 31–40. University of New Mexico Press, Albuquerque.

Struever, Stuart, and Gail L. Houart

1972 An Analysis of the Hopewell Interaction Sphere. In *Social Exchange and Interaction*, edited by Edwin Wilmsen, pp. 47–79. Anthropological Papers No. 46. Museum of Anthropology, University of Michigan, Ann Arbor.

Sublett, Audrey J., and Charles F. Wray

1970 Some Examples of Accidental and Deliberate Human Skeletal Modification in the Northeast. *Journal of the New York State Archaeological Association* 50: 14–26.

Sudarsono, R. M.

1984 *Wong, Wayang: The State Ritual Dance Drama in the Court of Yogyakarta*. Gadjah Mada University Press, Bulaksumur, Yogyakarta, India.

Sullivan, Lynne P., and Robert C. Mainfort Jr.

2010 Mississippian Mortuary Practices and the Quest for Interpretation. In *Mississippian Mortuary Practices: Beyond Hierarchy and Representationist Perspective*, edited by Lynne P. Sullivan and Robert C. Mainfort Jr., pp. 1–13. University Press of Florida, Gainesville.

Sullivan, Lynne P., and Robert C. Mainfort Jr. (editors)

2010 *Mississippian Mortuary Practices: Beyond Hierarchy and the Representationist Perspective*. University Press of Florida, Gainesville.

Sullivan, Norman

1990 The Biological Consequences of the Mississippian Exchange into the Western Great Lakes Region: A Study of Prehistoric Culture Contact. In *Powers of Observation: Alternative Views of Archeology*, edited by Sarah M. Nelson and Alice B. Kehoe, pp. 73–87. Archaeological Papers of the American Anthropological Association No. 2. American Anthropological Association, Washington, D.C.

Swanton, John R.

1928a *Religious Beliefs and Medical Practices of the Creek Indians.* Bureau of American Ethnology Annual Report 42. Smithsonian Institution, Washington, D.C.

1928b *Social Organization and Social Usages of the Indians of the Creek Confederacy.* Bureau of American Ethnology Annual Report 44. Smithsonian Institution, Washington, D.C.

1929 *Myths and Tales of the Southeastern Indians.* Bureau of American Ethnology Bulletin 88. Smithsonian Institution, Washington, D.C.

1946 *The Indians of the Southeastern United States.* Bureau of American Ethnology Bulletin 137. Smithsonian Institution, Washington, D.C.

Tanner, Jeri

1968 The Teeth in Folklore. *Western Folklore* 27:97–105.

Taylor, Colin F.

1994 *The Plains Indians.* Salamander, London.

Taylor, Jay L. B.

1929 Appendix B: Some Researches in the Illinois River Valley near Havana. In *The Cahokia Mounds* by Warren K. Moorehead, Jay L. B. Taylor, Morris M. Leighton, and Frank C. Baker, pp. 155–166. Bulletin Vol. 26, No. 4. University of Illinois, Urbana.

Taylor, Timothy

1996 *The Prehistory of Sex: Four Million Years of Human Sexual Culture.* Bantam, New York.

Thomas, Sidney J.

1941 A Sioux Medicine Bundle. *American Anthropologist*, n.s. 43:605–609.

Thwaites, Reuben (editor)

1959 *The Jesuit Relations and Allied Documents: Travels and Explorations of the Jesuit Missionaries in New France, 1610–1791.* 73 vols. Reprinted. Pageant, New York. Originally published 1896–1901, Burrows Brothers, Cleveland, Ohio.

Tiesler, Vera, and Andrea Cucina (editors)

2007 *New Perspectives on Human Sacrifice and Ritual Body Treatment in Ancient Mayan Society.* Springer, New York.

Tiesler Blos, Vera

2006 *Basos Conceptuales para la Evaluacíon de Restos Humans en Arqueologia.* Ediciones de la Universidad Autónoma de Yucatán, Mérida

Tiffany, A. S.

1876 Mound Explorations in 1875. *Proceedings of the Davenport Academy of Natural Sciences* 1:113–114.

Tiffany, Joseph A.

1979 An Overview of Oneota Sites in Southeastern Iowa: A Perspective from the Ceramic Analysis of the Schmeiser Site, 13DM101, Des Moines County, Iowa. *Proceedings of the Iowa Academy of Science* 86(3):89–101.

1982 Site Catchment Analysis of Southeast Iowa Oneota Sites. In *Oneota Studies,* edited by Guy E. Gibbon, pp. 1–13. Publications in Anthropology No. 1. University of Minnesota, Minneapolis.

1988 Preliminary Report on Excavations at the McKinney Oneota Village Site (13LA1), Louisa County, Iowa. *Wisconsin Archeologist* 69:227–312.

Time-Life Books (editors)

1992 *The European Challenge*. Time-Life, Alexandria, Virginia.

Tomak, Curtis

1994 The Mount Vernon Site: A Remarkable Hopewell Mound in Posey County, Indiana. *Archaeology of Eastern North America* 22:1–46.

Torbenson, Michael, Arthur Aufderheide, and Elden Johnson

1992 Punctured Human Bones of the Laurel Culture from Smith Mound 4, Minnesota. *American Antiquity* 57:506–514.

Townsend, Richard F., and Robert V. Sharp (editors)

2004 *Hero, Hawk, and Open Hand: American Indian Art of the Ancient Midwest and South*. Yale University Press, New Haven, Connecticut.

Trenholm, Virginia Cole

1970 *The Arapahoes, Our People*. University of Oklahoma Press, Norman.

Trigger, Bruce G.

1969 *The Huron: Farmers of the North*. Holt, Rinehart, and Winston, New York.

Tsintjilonis, Dimitri

2000 Death and the Sacrifice of Signs: Measuring the Dead in Tana Toraja. *Oceania* 71:1–17.

Tung, Tiffany A.

2012 *Violence, Ritual, and the Wari Empire: A Social Bioarchaeology of Imperialism in the Ancient Andes*. University Press of Florida, Gainesville.

Turner, Bryan S.

1991 Recent Developments in the Theory of the Body. In *The Body: Social Process and Cultural Theory*, edited by Mike Featherstone, Mike Hepworth, and Bryan S. Turner, pp. 1–36. Sage, London.

Turner, Victor

1957 *Schism and Continuity in an African Society: A Study of Ndembu Village Life*. Manchester University Press, Manchester, United Kingdom.

1967 *The Forest of Symbols: Aspects of Ndembu Ritual*. Cornell University Press, Ithaca, New York.

1968 *Drums of Affliction: A Study of Religious Processes among the Ndembu of Zambia*. Clarendon, Oxford.

1974 *Dramas, Fields, and Metaphors: Symbolic Action in Human Society*. Cornell University Press, Ithaca, New York.

1982 *From Ritual to Theatre: The Human Seriousness of Play*. Performing Arts Journal Publications, New York.

Turpin, Solveig A.

1996 Painting on Bones and Other Unusual Media in the Lower and Trans-Pecos Regions of Texas and Coahuila. *Plains Anthropologist* 41(157):261–272.

Ubelaker, Douglas H.

1978 *Human Skeletal Remains*. Aldine, Chicago.

United States Congress

1865 Congressional Testimony of Mr. John S. Smith and Lt. James D. Cannon. Joint Committee on the Conduct of the War, Massacre of Cheyenne Indians, 39th Cong., 2nd sess., March 14, Washington, D.C. Electronic document, http://www.pbs.org/weta/thewest/resources/archives/four/sandcrk.htm#chivtest, accessed July 27, 2014.

Urcid, Javier

1994 Cannibalism and Curated Skulls: Bone Ritualism on Kodiak Island. In *Reckoning with the Dead: The Larsen Bay Repatriation and the Smithsonian Institution*, edited by Tamara L. Bray and Thomas W. Killion, pp. 101–121. Smithsonian Institution Press, Washington, D.C.

Utley, Robert M.

1963 *The Last Days of the Sioux Nation*. Yale University Press, New Haven, Connecticut.

Valentin, Frederique, and Noemie Rolland

2011 Marquesan Trophy Skulls: Description, Osteological Analyses, and Changing Motivations in the South Pacific. In *The Bioarchaeology of the Human Head: Decapitation, Decoration, and Deformation*, edited by Michelle Bonogofsky, pp. 97–121. University Press of Florida, Gainesville.

Vastokas, Joan

1974–1975 The Shamanic Tree of Life. *ArtsCanada* 30(184–187):125–149.

Vitebsky, Piers

2001 *Shamanism*. University of Oklahoma Press, Norman.

Voegelin, Erminie Wheeler

1944 Mortuary Customs of the Shawnee and Other Eastern Tribes. *Indiana Historical Society, Prehistory Research Series* 2(4):227–444.

von Gernet, Alexander D.

1988 The Transculturation of the Amerindian Pipe/Tobacco/Smoking Complex and Its Impact on the Intellectual Boundaries between "Savagery" and "Civilization," 1535–1935. Unpublished Ph.D. dissertation, Department of Anthropology, McGill University, Montreal.

von Gernet, Alexander D., and Peter Timmins

1987 Pipes and Parakeets: Constructing Meaning in an Early Iroquoian Context. In *Archaeology as Long-Term History*, edited by Ian Hodder, pp. 31–42. Cambridge University Press, Cambridge.

Vradenburg, Joseph

1993 Analysis of Human Skeletal Remains. In *The Tremaine Site Complex: Oneota Occupation in the La Crosse Locality, Wisconsin*, Vol. 1: *The OT Site (47 Lc-262)* by Jodie O'Gorman, pp. 141–156. Archaeology Research Series No. 1. Museum Archaeology Program, State Historical Society of Wisconsin, Madison.

Wade, Nicholas

2010 A Host of Mummies, a Forest of Secrets. *New York Times*. Electronic document, http://www.nytimes.com/2010/3/16/science/16archeo.html?_r=1&emc=&, accessed May 6, 2013.

Walker, James R.

1917 *The Sun Dance of the Oglala*. Anthropological Paper 16, Pt. 2. American Museum of Natural History, New York.

1980 *Lakota Belief and Ritual*. Edited by Raymond J. DeMallie and Elaine A. Jahner. University of Nebraska Press, Lincoln.

Walker, William H.

1998 Where Are the Witches of Prehistory. *Journal of Archaeological Method and Theory* 5:245–308.

Walker, Winslow M.

1952 The Dickison Mound Group, Peoria County, Illinois. In *Hopewellian Communities in Illinois*, edited by Thorne Deuel, pp. 12–41. Scientific Papers Vol. 5. Illinois State Museum, Springfield.

Wallace, Anthony F. C.

1956 Revitalization Movements. *American Antiquity* 58:264–281.

1966 *Religion: An Anthropological View*. Random House, New York.

Wallis, Wilson D.

1947 *The Canadian Dakota*. Anthropological Paper 41, Pt. 1. American Museum of Natural History, New York.

Walthall, John A.

1990 *Prehistoric Indians of the Southeast: Archaeology of Alabama and the Middle South*. University of Alabama Press, Tuscaloosa.

Warwick, Matthew

2002 A Diachronic Study of Animal Exploitation at Aztalan, a Late Prehistoric Village Site in Southeast Wisconsin. Unpublished Master's thesis, Department of Anthropology, University of Wisconsin, Milwaukee.

Webb, William S., and Raymond S. Baby

1957 *The Adena People No. 2*. Ohio Historical Society, Columbus.

Webb, William S., and David L. DeJarnette

1942 *An Archaeological Survey of Pickwick Basin in the Adjacent Portions of the States of Alabama, Mississippi, and Tennessee*. Bureau of American Ethnology Bulletin 129. Smithsonian Institution, Washington, D.C.

Webb, William S., and William G. Haag

1947 The Fisher Site, Fayette County Kentucky. *Reports in Anthropology and Archaeology* 7(2):1–104.

Webb, William S., and Charles E. Snow

1945 *The Adena People*. Reports in Anthropology and Archaeology No. 6. University of Kentucky, Lexington.

Wedel, Mildred M.

2001 Iowa. In *Plains*, edited by Raymond J. DeMallie, pp. 432–446. Handbook of North American Indians, Vol. 13, William C. Sturtevant, general editor, Smithsonian Institution, Washington, D.C.

Wedel, Waldo R.

2001 Plains Village Tradition, Central. In *Plains*, edited by Raymond J. DeMallie, pp. 173–185. Handbook of North American Indians, Vol. 13, William C. Sturtevant, general editor, Smithsonian Institution, Washington, D.C.

Weidenreich, Franz

1951 *Morphology of Solo Man*. Anthropological Papers Vol. 43, Pt. 3. American Museum of Natural History, New York.

Welch, James, and Paul Stekler

1994 *Killing Custer*. Norton, New York.

Welsch, Roger

1981 *Omaha Tribal Myths and Trickster Tales*. Ohio University Press, Athens.

Weltfish, Gene

1965 *The Lost Universe: Pawnee Life and Culture*. University of Nebraska Press, Lincoln.

Wesler, Kit W.

2001 *Excavations at Wickliffe Mounds*. University of Alabama, Tuscaloosa.

Wessells, Hunter, Tom F. Lue, and Jack W. McAninch

1996 Penile Length in the Flaccid and Erect States: Guidelines for Penile Augmentation. *Journal of Urology* 156:995–997.

West, Jolee A., and Julien Louys

2007 Differentiating Bamboo from Stone Tool Cut Marks in the Zooarchaeological Record with a Discussion on the Use of Bamboo Knives. *Journal of Archaeological Science* 34:512–518.

White, Douglas R., George P. Murdock, and Richard Scaglion

1971 Natchez Class and Rank Reconsidered. *Ethnology* 10:369–390.

White, Randall

1993 The Dawn of Adornment. *Natural History* 102(5):60–67.

2007 Systems of Personal Ornamentation in the Early Upper Palaeolithic: Methodological Challenges and New Observations. In *Rethinking the Human Revolution: New Behavioural and Biological Perspectives on the Origin and Dispersal of Modern Humans*, edited by Paul Mellars, Katie Boyle, Ofer Bar-Yosef, and Chris Stringer, pp. 287–302. McDonald Institute Monographs. McDonald Institute for Archaeological Research, Cambridge, United Kingdom.

White, Randall, Dominique Henry-Gambier, and C. Normand

2003 Human-Tooth Ornaments from the French Early Aurignacian: Implications for Early Upper Paleolithic Treatment of the Dead. In *Paleoanthropology Society Abstracts for the 2003 Meetings*. Tempe, Arizona.

White, Tim

1992 *Prehistoric Cannibalism at Mancos 5MTUMR-2346*. Princeton University Press, Princeton, New Jersey.

White, Tim D., and Pieter A. Folkens

2005 *The Human Bone Manual*. Elsevier, Amsterdam.

Wieberg, Danielle A. M., and Daniel J. Wescott
2008 Estimating the Timing of Long Bone Fractures: Correlation between the Postmortem Interval, Bone Moisture Content and Blunt Force Trauma Fracture Characteristics. *Journal of Forensic Sciences* 53:1028–1034.

Wiessner, Polly
1983 Style and Social Information in Kalahari San Projectile Points. *American Antiquity* 49:253–276.

Wilbert, Johannes
1975 Magico-Religious Use of Tobacco among South American Indians. In *Cannabis and Culture*, edited by Vera Rubin, pp. 439–461. Mouton, The Hague.

Wilford, Lloyd A.
1945 Three Village Sites of the Mississippi Pattern in Minnesota. *American Antiquity* 11:32–40.

Willey, Patrick
1990 *Prehistoric Warfare on the Great Plains: Skeletal Analysis of the Crow Creek Massacre Victims*. Garland, New York.

Willey, Patrick, and William M. Bass
1978 A Scalped Skull from Pawnee County. *Kansas Anthropological Association Newsletter* 24(1):1–11.

Williams, Leonard C.
1975 Human Skull Artifacts. *Tennessee Archaeologist* 31:33–36.

Williams, Stephen
1990 The Vacant Quarter and Other Late Events in the Lower Valley. In *Towns and Temples along the Mississippi*, edited by David H. Dye and Cheryl A. Cox, pp. 170–180. University of Alabama Press, Tuscaloosa.

Williamson, Ron
2007 "Otinontsiskiaj Ondaon" ("The House of Cut-Off Heads"): The History and Archaeology of Northern Iroquoian Trophy Taking. In *The Taking and Displaying of Human Body Parts as Trophies by Amerindians*, edited by Richard J. Chacon and David H. Dye, pp. 190–221. Springer, New York.

Willoughby, Charles C.
1932 Notes on the History and Symbolism of the Muskhogeans and the People of Etowah. In *Etowah Papers I: Exploration of the Etowah Site in Georgia*, edited by Warren K. Moorehead, pp. 7–67. Yale University Press, New Haven, Connecticut.

Willoughby, Charles C., and Earnest A. Hooton
1922 *The Turner Group of Earthworks, Hamilton County, Ohio*. Papers of the Peabody Museum of American Archaeology and Ethnology Vol. 8, No. 3. Harvard University, Cambridge, Massachusetts.

Wilson, Lee Anne
1982 Bird and Feline Motifs on Great Lakes Pouches. In *Native North American Art History: Selected Readings*, edited by Zena P. Mathews and Aldona Jonaitis, pp. 429–443. Peek, Palo Alto, California.

Winchell, Newton H. (editor)
1911 *The Aborigines of Minnesota*. Minnesota Historical Society, St. Paul.
Winter, Joseph C. (editor)
2000 *Tobacco Use by Native North Americans: Sacred Smoke and Silent Killer*. University of Oklahoma Press, Norman.
Winters, Howard D.
1974 Some Unusual Grave Goods from a Mississippi Burial Mound. *Indian Notes* 10(2):34–46.
Wissler, Clark
1910 *Material Culture of the Blackfoot Indians*. Anthropological Papers Vol. 5, Pt. 1. American Museum of Natural History, New York.
Witter, Finley M.
1878 Notes on Mounds and Mound-Builders. Paper read before the Muscatine Academy of Science, November 21. *Weekly Tribune*, Muscatine, Iowa.
Woermann, J. W.
1902–1904 *Map of the Illinois and Des Plaines Rivers from Lockport, Illinois to the Mouth of the Illinois River* (Sheet 11). U.S. Army Corps of Engineers, Chicago.
Wood, W. Raymond, and Lee Irwin
2001 Mandan. In *Plains*, edited by Raymond J. DeMallie, pp. 349–364. Handbook of North American Indians, Vol. 13, William C. Sturtevant, general editor, Smithsonian Institution, Washington, D.C.
Woodbury, Nathalie F. S. (editor)
1961 Notes and News. *American Antiquity* 26:580–600.
Wray, Donald E., and Richard S. MacNeish
1961 *The Hopewellian and Weaver Occupations of the Weaver Site, Fulton County, Illinois*. Scientific Papers, Vol. VII, No. 2. Illinois State Museum, Springfield.
Wright, Thomas
2006 [1865] The Worship of the Generative Powers during the Middle Ages of Western Europe. In *Sexual Symbolism: A History of Phallic Worship* by Richard Payne Knight and Thomas Wright, pp. 123–237. Privately printed, London. 2006 facsimile ed. Dover, Mineola, New York.
Young, Gloria A., and Michael P. Hoffman
2001 Quapaw. In *Plains*, edited by Raymond J. DeMallie, pp. 497–514. Handbook of North American Indians, Vol. 13, William C. Sturtevant, general editor, Smithsonian Institution, Washington, D.C.
Young, Marcy A.
1981a Human Remains from the 1979 Excavation of the McKinney Oneota Village Site (13LA1). In *Miscellaneous Reports on Iowa Archaeology*, edited by Robert Burchfield, pp. 10–14. Research Papers 6(1). Office of the State Archaeologist, University of Iowa, Iowa City.
1981b Analysis of Human Skeletal Remains from the 1980 Excavation of the McKinney Site, 13LA1. In *Miscellaneous Reports on Iowa Archaeology*, edited by Robert Burchfield, pp. 308–311. Research Papers 6(4). Office of the State Archaeologist, University of Iowa, Iowa City.

Zedeño, María Nieves
2008 Bundled Worlds: The Roles and Interactions of Complex Objects from the North American Plains. *Journal of Archaeological Method and Theory* 15: 362–378.
Zilhão, João
2007 The Emergence of Ornaments and Art: An Archaeological Perspective on the Origins of "Behavioral Modernity." *Journal of Archaeological Research* 15:1–54.
Zilhão, João, and Francesco d'Errico
1999 Reply, in The Neanderthal Problem Continued. *Current Anthropology* 40: 355–364.

Contributors

Kathleen T. Blue holds a Ph.D. from the University of Chicago and is an associate professor in the Department of Anthropology at Minnesota State University, Mankato. Her areas of interest include juvenile health and growth in past populations, mortuary practices, postmortem bone modification, and forensic taphonomy.

Christopher Carr holds a Ph.D. from the University of Michigan and is a professor at Arizona State University. He is a prehistorian of the Eastern Woodlands of North America with particular interests in the social, political, ritual, and philosophical-religious aspects of the lives of peoples in the midwestern United States during that time. His books include *Gathering Hopewell: Society, Ritual, and Ritual Interaction* (2005) and *The Scioto Hopewell and Their Neighbors* (2008), both coedited with D. Troy Case.

Dawn E. Cobb holds an M.A. from Northern Illinois University and is a physical anthropologist at the Illinois State Museum. She is the former Illinois Human Skeletal Remains Protection coordinator for the Illinois State Historic Preservation Agency, where she oversaw bioarchaeological investigations in the state. Currently working at the Illinois Department of Natural Resources, Cobb conducts workshops across the state on cemetery preservation and has coauthored with Hall Hassan (IDNR) *The Illinois Historic Cemetery Preservation Handbook: A Guide to Basic Preservation (2008).*

Della Collins Cook holds a Ph.D. from the University of Chicago and is a professor of anthropology at Indiana University, Bloomington. Her research interests include the paleopathology of ancient New World populations. She is a contributor to *Tracing Childhood: Bioarchaeological Investigations of Early Lives in Antiquity* (2014), *Bones of the Maya: Studies of Ancient Skeletons (2006)*, and *Bioarchaeology: The Contextual Analysis of Human Remains (2006).*

Paul D. Emanovsky holds an M.S. in human biology from the University of Indianapolis and is currently a Ph.D. candidate at the University of Florida. He works as a forensic anthropologist at the Joint POW/MIA Accounting Command in Hawaii.

Eve A. Hargrave holds an M.A. in anthropology from Pennsylvania State University and is the public engagement coordinator for the Illinois State Archaeological Survey, part of the Prairie Research Institute at the University of Illinois, Urbana-Champaign. Her current research interests include mortuary practices, prehistoric cultural manipulation of human remains, paleopathology, demography, and ancient DNA studies of prehistoric populations in the midwestern United States.

Kristin M. Hedman holds a Ph.D. in physical anthropology from the University of Illinois and is the associate director of the Ancient Technologies and Archaeological Materials Program at the Illinois State Archaeological Survey, part of the Prairie Research Institute at the University of Illinois, Urbana-Champaign. In addition to her interests in paleopathology and the demography of historic and prehistoric populations, her research interests focus on stable isotopic evidence of diet and migration in prehistoric populations.

Cheryl A. Johnston holds a Ph.D. in physical anthropology from the Ohio State University and is a board-certified forensic anthropologist. Johnston is an associate professor of anthropology at Western Carolina University, specializing in the recovery and analysis of human remains from forensic contexts. Her current research is focused on taphonomy and human decomposition.

Anne B. Lee holds an M.A. in anthropology from the Ohio State University. She specializes in the analysis of faunal remains from historic and prehistoric sites of the Ohio valley. Lee is currently a principal investigator for Hardlines Design Company in Columbus, Ohio.

Robin M. Lillie holds an M.A. from Northern Illinois University and is a skeletal biologist for the University of Iowa Office of the State Archaeologist Burials Program. Areas of interest include early historic burials in the Midwest, osteological evidence of trauma, and the cultural manipulation of human skeletal remains.

Cheryl Ann Munson holds an M.A. from the University of Illinois and is an archaeologist and research scientist in the Department of Anthropology, Indiana University, Bloomington. While much of her work has been concentrated on cultural resource management projects, other research has focused on the late prehistoric cultures of southern Indiana and the Ohio valley. She has directed or codirected investigations at numerous Mississippian sites. This work led to the definition of the Mississippian Caborn-Welborn phase, dating A.D. 1400–1650.

Stephen P. Nawrocki holds a Ph.D. in anthropology from SUNY, Binghamton, and has taught anatomy and human biology at the University of Indianapolis since 1991. He is a board-certified forensic anthropologist and serves as the primary forensic consultant for the state of Indiana.

Anna Novotny is a Ph.D. candidate in bioarchaeology at Arizona State University. Her focus is on the prehistory and ethnology of the Maya people, especially their religion, mortuary practices, and ancestor veneration. Her field excavation and laboratory studies in Mesoamerica have been at the sites of Chan, Teotihuacan, Holmul, Cancuen, Palmarejo, and El Coyote.

Mary Lucas Powell holds a Ph.D. from Northwestern University and is the former editor of the *Paleopathology Newsletter*. She has spent more than a quarter century conducting bioarchaeological investigations of health and disease in ancient Native American populations in the U.S. Midwest and Southeast. With Della Collins Cook, she edited *The Myth of Syphilis: The Natural History of Treponematosis in North America (2005).*

Shirley J. Schermer holds an M.A. from the University of Iowa and is the retired director of the Burials Program for the University of Iowa Office of the State Archaeologist. With over 30 years of experience in archaeology and human osteology in the Midwest and Plains, her research interests include bioarchaeology, mortuary practices, cultural ideology related to death, and paleopathology.

Maria Ostendorf Smith holds a Ph.D. from the University of Tennessee, Knoxville, and is a professor of anthropology at Illinois State University. She is a bioarchaeologist and paleopathologist who specializes in the precolumbian peoples of the upper and west-central Tennessee River valley. Her research includes the pattern and antiquity of intergroup violence and investigating community health parameters within and between sociopolitical and subsistence strategy changes in the Tennessee osteoarchaeological samples.

Linea Sundstrom holds a Ph.D. from the University of Kansas and is an adjunct professor of anthropology at the University of Wisconsin, Milwaukee. Her research interests focus on the archaeology and ethnohistory of the northern Great Plains. She is the author of *Indian Rock Art of the Black Hills Country*, *Enduring Motives: The Archaeology of Tradition and Religion in Native America* and numerous articles on Plains Indian religion, sacred sites, and symbolism.

Katie J. Zejdlik holds an M.A. from the University of Wisconsin, Milwaukee, and is a Ph.D. candidate in anthropology at Indiana University, Bloomington. Her research interests include dental anthropology, biological distance, population movement and interaction, skeletal indicators of violence and their social correlates, mortuary practices, and women's roles in indigenous American history.

Index